Textbook of
Obstetric
Anesthesia

Editors

Amit Padvi
MBBS, MD, Fellowship in Pediatric Anesthesiology
Consultant Anesthesiologist
Kokilaben Dhirubhai Ambani Hospital, Mumbai
Formerly worked as Assistant Professor
Department of Anesthesia
Faculty Member of Department of Pediatric Anesthesia
Seth GS Medical College and KEM Hospital
Mumbai

Namita Padvi
MBBS, MD, DNB, Fellowship in Pediatric Anesthesiology
Assistant Professor, Department of Anesthesia
Topiwala National Medical College and BYL Nair Charitable Hospital
Mumbai

Sushila Baldwa
MBBS, MD, DGO
Currently Consulting Obstetrician and Gynecologist
Apollo Clinic, Mumbai and Nakoda Foundation, Mumbai
Formerly Served as Faculty at BJ Medical College, Pune and
Sassoon General Hospital, Pune

Mahesh Baldwa
MBBS, MD (Pediatrics), DCH, LLB, LLM, PhD (Law) MBA FIAP
Consultant Pediatrician, Baldwa Hospital, Mumbai
Ex-Assistant Professor of Pediatrics, TN Medical College and Nair Hospital, Mumbai
Ex-Assistant Professor, JJ Hospital, Grant Medical College, Mumbai
Ex-Visiting Professor, Paper Setter and Examiner
Department of Law, University of Mumbai

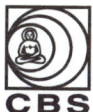

CBS Publishers & Distributors Pvt Ltd
New Delhi • Bengaluru • Chennai • Kochi • Kolkata • Mumbai
Hyderabad • Nagpur • Patna • Pune • Vijayawada

Disclaimer

Science and technology are constantly changing fields. New research and experience broaden the scope of information and knowledge. The editors have tried their best in giving information available to them while preparing the material for this book. Although all efforts have been made to ensure optimum accuracy of the material, yet it is quite possible some errors might have been left uncorrected. The publisher, the printer and the editors will not be held responsible for any inadvertent errors, omissions or inaccuracies.

Textbook of
**Obstetric
Anesthesia**

ISBN: 978-93-85915-23-9

Copyright © Editors and Publisher

First Edition 2016

All rights reserved. No part of this book may be reproduced or transmitted in any form or by any means, electronic or mechanical, including photocopying, recording, or any information storage and retrieval system without permission, in writing, from the editors and the publisher.

Published by Satish Kumar Jain and produced by Varun Jain for
CBS Publishers & Distributors Pvt Ltd
4819/XI Prahlad Street, 24 Ansari Road, Daryaganj, New Delhi 110 002, India.
Ph: 23289259, 23266861, 23266867   Fax: 011-23243014   Website: www.cbspd.com
e-mail: delhi@cbspd.com; cbspubs@airtelmail.in.

Corporate Office: 204 FIE, Industrial Area, Patparganj, Delhi 110 092
Ph: 4934 4934   Fax: 4934 4935   e-mail: publishing@cbspd.com; publicity@cbspd.com

Branches

• **Bengaluru:** Seema House 2975, 17th Cross, K.R. Road, Banasankari 2nd Stage, Bengaluru 560 070, Karnataka
   Ph: +91-80-26771678/79   Fax: +91-80-26771680   e-mail: bangalore@cbspd.com
• **Chennai:** 7, Subbaraya Street, Shenoy Nagar, Chennai 600 030, Tamil Nadu
   Ph: +91-44-26680620, 26681266   Fax: +91-44-42032115   e-mail: chennai@cbspd.com
• **Kochi:** Ashana House, 39/1904, AM Thomas Road, Valanjambalam,
   Eranakulam 682 018, Kochi, Kerala
   Ph: +91-484-4059061-62-64-65   Fax: +91-484-4059065   e-mail: kochi@cbspd.com
• **Kolkata:** 6/B, Ground Floor, Rameswar Shaw Road, Kolkata 700 014, West Bengal
   Ph: +91-33-2289-1126, 1127, 1128,   e-mail: Kolkata@cbspd.com
• **Mumbai:** 83-C, Dr E Moses Road, Worli, Mumbai-400018, Maharashtra
   Ph: +91-22-24902340/41   Fax: +91-22-24902342   e-mail: mumbai@cbspd.com

Representatives

• **Hyderabad**   0-9885175004   • **Nagpur**   0-9021734563   • **Patna**   0-9334159340
• **Pune**   0-9623451994   • **Vijayawada**   0-9000660880

Printed at : Goyal Offset Printers

to

our cherished possession
Baby Parneeka
and
Baby Diya

Textbook of
Obstetric
Anesthesia

Disclaimer

Medical field is always in a dynamic state, with continuous influx of new knowledge and practices. Everyday results of new researches broaden our understanding of the subject, improve our medical practices and change the research methods.

Clinicians and researchers should use their own clinical acumen, experience, skill and knowledge in evaluating and using any information, drugs, techniques, procedures, equipment or experiments described herein. In clinically applying such knowledge or methods, they should be careful of their own safety as well as that of others, including parties for whom they have a professional liability.

When using any drug described herewith, readers are advised to check the most current information provided by the manufacturer. They should verify the recommended dose or formula, the method, route and duration of administration, side effects and contraindications. Clinician should assess each patient individually and use their own knowledge, skill and experience to make diagnosis and determine the best perioperative or procedural anesthetic regime for each patient.

Contributors are individually responsible for their respective opinions, views, information and figures assimilated in their respective chapters and are hereof individually responsible for the source of such information.

To the fullest extent of the law, neither the publisher, nor the authors, contributors or editors assume any liability for any injury and/or damage to persons or property as a matter of product liability, negligence or otherwise, or from any use or operation of any methods, products, instructions, or ideas contained in the material herein.

Foreword

Obstetric anaesthesia is unique in that the anaesthesiologist has to care for two lives at the same time with safety and quality as the prime objectives. To effectively achieve this, the anaesthesiologists still have to be equipped with an evidence-based, specific and extensive knowledge. This is what a textbook should aim to provide.

The *Textbook of Obstetric Anesthesia* has been successful in achieving the above said objective, with excellence. It has been authored by a team of young and knowledgeable anesthesia professionals, with excellent clinical and academic commitment. They have taken pains to study the exhaustive literature that is available to condense and organize the contents into a very useful, user-friendly and authentic textbook.

The book has adopted a refreshing approach to the speciality of obstetric anesthesia by covering all aspects of the speciality ranging from history to the most recent developments. Addition of chapters on medicolegal aspects of obstetric anesthetic practice, record keeping, 'grey areas' and controversies and cardiopulmonary resuscitation has enhanced the value of the book significantly.

I am sure, this book will prove to be a worthy companion to the residents and trainees and a reliable source of reference to both obstetric anaesthesiologists and for anaesthesiologists who anaesthetize obstetric patients frequently.

Dr. Raveendra US MD, DNB
Professor
Department Anaesthesiology
KS Hedge Medical Academy
Mangalore

Editor
Nitte University Journal of Health Science
Mangalore

Contributors

Babita Gupta MBBS, MD
Additional Professor
Department of Anaesthesiology
Pain Medicine and Critical Care
All India Institute of Medical Sciences, New Delhi

Antara Gokhale MBBS, MD, EDIC
Senior Consultant
Royal Hospital, Muscat

Charulata Deshpande MBBS, MD
Professor
Department of Anaesthesia
Topiwala National Medical College and
BYL Nair Charitable Hospital, Mumbai

Rita Wahal MD, DA(UK), FFARCS, FICA
Professor
King George's Medical University, Lucknow

Sarita Fernandes MBBS, MD
Additional Professor
Department of Anaesthesia
Topiwala National Medical College and
BYL Nair Charitable Hospital, Mumbai

Namita Padvi MBBS, MD (University topper) DNB Fellowship in
Pediatric Anesthesiology
Assistant Professor
Department of Anaesthesia
Topiwala National Medical College and
BYL Nair Charitable Hospital, Mumbai

Varsha Gupta MBBS, MD
Bhagwati General Hospital, Mumbai

Mahesh Baldwa MBBS, MD (Pediatrics), DCH, FIAP, LLM,
PhD (Law), MBA
Consultant Pediatrician
Baldwa Hospital, Mumbai

Ex-Assistant Professor of Pediatrics
Topiwala National Medical College and
BYL Nair Charitable Hospital, Mumbai

Amit Padvi MBBS, MD, Fellowship in Paediatric Anaesthesiology
Consultant in Department of Anesthesia
Kokilaben Dhirubhai Ambani Hospital, Mumbai

Chinmayi Patkar MBBS, MD, DNB
Assistant Professor
Department of Anaesthesia
Topiwala National Medical College and
BYL Nair Charitable Hospital, Mumbai

Ashish Mali MBBS, MD
Assistant Professor
Department of Anaesthesia
Topiwala National Medical College and
BYL Nair Charitable Hospital, Mumbai

Sushila Baldwa MBBS, MD
Senior Consultant Obstetrician and Gynecologist
Apollo Clinic, Mumbai

Anjana Sahu MBBS, MD
Senior Assistant Professor
Department of Anaesthesia
Topiwala National Medical College and
BYL Nair Charitable Hospital, Mumbai

Sushama Tandale MBBS, MD, Fellowship in Paediatric
Anaesthesiology
Assistant Professor
Department of Anaesthesia
Rajeev Gandhi Medical College and
Chatrapati Shivaji Maharaj Hospital, Mumbai

Minal Harde MBBS, MD, DNB
Associate Professor
Department of Anaesthesia
Topiwala National Medical College and
BYL Nair Charitable Hospital, Mumbai

Namrata Padvi MBBS, MD
Formerly Assistant Professor
Government Medical College, Dhule, Maharashtra

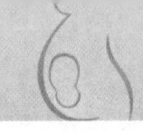

Dinesh Kumar Sahu MBBS, MD (Anaesthesiology), Fellowship in Pain Management (ISSP)
Consultant
Jagjivanram Railway Hospital, Mumbai

Rakesh Garg MBBS, MD, DNB, PGCCHM, MNAMS, FCCS, CCEPC
Assistant Professor, Department of Anaesthesiology
Intensive Care, Pain and Palliative Care Dr BRAIRCH
All India Institute of Medical Sciences, New Delhi

Anju Gupta MBBS, MD
Assistant Professor, Department of Anesthesiology
Chacha Nehru Bal Chikitsalaya, New Delhi

Ekta Rai MBBS, MD, MRCA
Professor
Department of Anaesthesia
Christian Medical College, Vellore, Tamil Nadu

Anity Singh MBBS, DA, MD, DNB
Assistant Professor
Department of Anaesthesia,
Christian Medical College, Vellore, Tamil Nadu

Sandeep Sahu MBBS, MD, PDCC, MNAMS, FICCM, FACEE, ICMR-International Fellow
Associate Professor
Department of Anaesthesiology
Sanjay Gandhi Postgraduate Institute of
Medical Sciences, Lucknow

Sanjay Agarwal MBBS, MD, PDCC
Consultant Anaesthesiologist
Department of Anaesthesiology
Fortis Hospital, Noida

Chetna Shamshery MBBS, MD, PDCC
Senior Resident
Department of Anaesthesiology
Sanjay Gandhi Postgraduate Institute of
Medical Sciences, Lucknow

Indu Lata MBBS, MD, MNAMS, MICOG, FICMCH, FICOG
Associate Professor
Department of Maternal and Reproductive Health
Sanjay Gandhi Postgraduate Institute of
Medical Sciences, Lucknow

Gayathri Bhat MBBS, MD
Professor
Department of Anaesthesiology and Critical Care
KS Hegde Medical Academy, Mangalore

Kausalya Chakravarthy MBBS, MD (Anaesthesia), DGO, Fellowship in Obstetric Anaesthesia
Assistant Professor Anesthesia
Niloufer Hospital for Women and Children
Osmania Medical College, Hyderabad

Indrani Hemantkumar MBBS, MD, DA, DNB
Professor and HOD
Department of Anaesthesia
Seth GS Medical College and
KEM Hospital, Mumbai

Sona Dave MBBS, MD, DNB
Professor
Department of Anaesthesia
Topiwala National Medical College and
BYL Nair Charitable Hospital, Mumbai

Anita Malik MBBS, MD, FICA
Professor
Department of Anaesthesiology and Critical Care
King George's Medical University, Lucknow

Namisha Malik MBBS, DA, DNB
Resident
Vivekananda Polyclinic and Institute of
Medical Sciences, Lucknow

Roopali V Telang MBBS, MD, Fellowship in Paediatric Anaesthesiology
Associate Consultant
Department of Anaesthesiology
PD Hinduja National Hospital, Mumbai

Pradnya Bhalerao MBBS, MD
Associate Professor
Department of Anaesthesiology and Critical Care
BJ Government Medical College and
Sassoon General Hospitals, Pune

Preface

If you can dream it, you can do it.

—*Walt Disney*

Textbook of Obstetric Anesthesia is immediate sequel to successful writing of *Textbook of Paediatric Anaesthesia*. We will never forget the intellectual challenges, joys which we had during our interactions with various enlightened and accomplished contributors of the various chapters and once again we thank one and all from bottom of heart and place them on the pedestal they deserve.

All the contributors have filled copyright forms and have tried their best to give due credit to the source of variety of information. This is with the sole aim that intellectual's right of property must be respected. For all copyrighted author works, books, information sources which are not acknowledged anywhere in this book hence, we seek their forgiveness and overtly apologize for not doing so. We assure them of doing so in the next edition of this book.

Obstetric anesthesia is fast getting recognition as a separate specialty on its own. At present it is not a superspecialty branch of medicine in India. Anesthesiologists in several institutes are assigned obstetric specialty anesthesia work by rotation.

This book is aimed to take the knowledge and skills of obstetric anesthesiology to newer heights.

How will the new topics help the reader?

It will provide new insight for postgraduate students pursuing anesthesia and practitioners practising obstetric anesthesia. The topics related to anatomy, physiology, and topical, regional and general anesthesia with respect to specialty or special situations along with medicolegal and ethical aspects are discussed in detail. They shall help the readers in improving their skills, knowledge and provide practical insight about obstetric anesthesia.

What is special about the style of presentation in the proposed book?

It has usual textbook style covering each topic with each chapter being made reader friendly by adding "clinical pearls". Summary is given at the end of each topic for better understanding and providing a bird's eye view of the topic.

The book delivers the knowledge essential to the safe practice of obstetric anesthesia. It covers history of obstetric anesthesia, general obstetric physiology and pharmacology, preoperative, intraoperative, and postoperative care; anesthesia for a full range of specific surgical procedures. Geared primarily for learners of obstetric anesthesia, these tightly focused, user-friendly chapters make it ideal for both general anesthesiologist as well as postgraduate students, and as a reference for everyday clinical practice.

Obstetric anethesiologists in the West have been quicker to respond to the need for obstetric anesthesiology knowledge. There is ample literature generated from the West which analyses the issues related to obstetric anesthesiology thoroughly. There is scanty literature on this subject in India where the volume of patients surpasses many times bigger than most of the western countries. We should have our own literature, written in simple English suited to our milieu. With the phenomenal increase in the patient volume in India, the need for indigenous literature related to obstetric anesthesiology is going to be even greater in the future.

The editors sincerely hope that this book will serve to fill the void effectively for practising anesthesiologists. This book looks beyond the problems and moves on to solutions. It comprehensively provides solutions to obstetric anesthesiologists in almost all vulnerable areas of this subspecialty. They can extrapolate and integrate the obstetric anesthesiology wisdom in broad specialty of anesthesiology on many divergent occasions in practical ways. Whereas extrapolating wisdom in broad specialty of anesthesiology to obstetric anesthesiology may turn out risky. It will be better to accept changes in broad specialty of anesthesiology, giving its own space to obstetric anesthesiology as a separate subspecialty branch.

Amit Padvi
Namita Padvi
Sushila Baldwa
Mahesh Baldwa

Acknowledgements

The editors wish to acknowledge the hard work of all those who have made this edition of the book possible, especially the contributors, without whose expertise this book would not exist.

We would also like to acknowledge all of those who have taught and mentored us throughout our lives.

We acknowledge editorial help of Dr (Mrs) Varsha Gupta and Ankit Gupta.

We also acknowledge the role of our parents, friends, colleagues, students, critics and God almighty for shaping our thinking and motivating us to bring this book.

Finally, we are grateful to the outstanding staff of CBS Publishers & Distributors Pvt Ltd, especially Mr SK Jain (Chairman), Mr Ramesh Krishnamachari, Mrs Ritu Chawla (AGM– Production) and Mr Surendra Jha.

We invite appreciations, suggestions and criticism by email on *2015toa@gmail.com.*

It is a well known fact that ignorance breeds and feeds uncertainty; uncertainty breeds and feeds unfounded fears; and this leads to inaction. Let us learn and drive away ignorance. Happy reading.

Amit Padvi
Namita Padvi
Sushila Baldwa
Mahesh Baldwa

Contents

Section 4
Medicolegal and Ethical Principels in Obstetric Anesthesia

General Topics

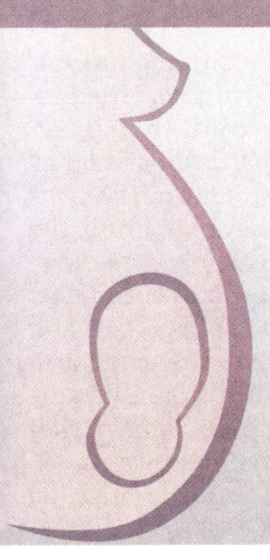

History of Obstetric Anesthesia

Namita Padvi, Sushila Baldwa, Mahesh Baldwa, Varsha Gupta

The quality of obstetric care in a society can be considered a criterion for the level of civilization it has achieved. Modern obstetric anesthesia has evolved from the crude practices of older ages to todays balanced anesthesia techniques. History of obstetric anesthesiology cannot be dissected from general historic development in anesthesiology, non-invasive obstetrics, general surgery, obstetric surgery, pharmacology and medical science as a whole.[1]

HISTORY

History in General

Many surgeons had strong notions that average men and women should tolerate pain caused by labor pain and surgery and thus kept patients away from administering anesthesia during the same. Humans have inhabited the earth for 200,000 years, yet the public demonstration of surgical general anesthesia happened only in 1846.[1]

History in Specific to Obstetric Anesthesia

Women have been bearing the pain of labor since generations and multiple attempts have been made to relieve the same since ages. The Chinese administered opium and alcohol to parturients, while the Egyptians in Pharaonic times burnt turpentine near a woman in labor, or concocted a vinegar and marble dust mixture to rub on her abdomen. The Babylonians and Greeks before Christ practiced goddess-worship and placation with sacrifices. Hippocrates noted that a primipara woman suffers the most in labor. Many ancient methods were non-pharmacological and sometimes barbaric. Witchcraft anesthesia was practiced in medieval times. In 1591, Eufame McCulzean was burnt to death as a witch in Edinburgh attempted to cast labor pains onto a dog. In the 18th century, Mesmer induced a trance-like state in his patients, which was the beginning of present-day hypnotism.

Anesthesia during childbirth has been constantly evolving and changing ever since ether anesthesia was introduced to medical/dental practice from 1847. The agents and methods used for analgesia and anesthesia are of many types.[2]

GENERAL ANESTHESIA IN OBSTETRICS

Unique pain of childbirth has been recognized since time immemorial. People at large believed that calamities—disease, drought, poverty, and pain—signified divine retribution inflicted as punishment for sin. According to Scripture, childbirth pain originated when God punished Eve and her descendants for Eve's disobedience in the Garden of Eden. They believed that it was wrong to avoid the pain of divine punishment. James Young Simpson, a successful obstetrician and chair of midwifery in Edinburgh, was the first to use general anesthesia in obstetrics. On 19th January 1847, he used ether for the relief of labor pains. He used diethyl ether to anesthetize a woman with a deformed pelvis for childbirth. This was closely on the heels of WTG Morton's first open demonstration of ether anesthesia on 16th October 1846. He continued to use ether during 1847, but was not satisfied with it and began searching for an alternative. On 4th November 1847, Simpson experimented with chloroform on self and close friends making them unconscious. Within six days of experiment, he reported to the Edinburgh Medico-Chirurgical Society, the use of chloroform in 30 painless deliveries. In next two weeks, his success with chloroform was published in The Lancet.[3] Quoting from the Bible "In sorrow thou shalt bring forth children."— Genesis 3:16. The clergymen discredited Simpson as an agent of evil. They argued that relief of labor pain is against God's Will. Simpson, who was also a student of the Bible, presented God as the first anesthetist by quoting Genesis 2:21, "And the Lord God caused a deep sleep to fall upon Adam, and he put to sleep; and He then took one of his diseased rib out, and closed up the flesh instead thereof". He argued, "What god did himself, could not be sinful". He stated that pain during labor/childbirth was not due to any religious curse but is the result of anatomic, physiologic reasons supported by scientific explanations. Simpson prophesied the role of public opinion in the acceptance of obstetric anesthesia, a fact not lost on his adversaries. Arguments also arose regarding the safety of anesthesia on mother and fetus as well as the altering of the birthing process. Early in the controversy he wrote, "Medical men may oppose for a time the super-induction of anesthesia in parturition but they will oppose it in vain; for certainly our patients themselves will force use of it upon the profession. The whole question is, even now, one merely of time."[4] Simpson as such failed to change the perception of obstetricians and physicians about pain relief during childbirth and labor.[3] By 1860, Simpson's prophecy came true; anesthesia for childbirth became part of medical practice by public acclaim.

Simpson's Method

Although Simpson strongly advocated the use of anesthesia for parturients, he ignored the safety issues related thereof. He anesthetized the obstetric patients during first stage of labor and kept them unconscious until after the delivery of placenta. Simpson failed to recognize the adverse effects of anesthesia on uterine contractions and on the newborn, which led to widespread criticism by the fellow physicians.[5] The whole controversy centered around Meigs from USA and Simpson from UK. There was a difference in their interpretation of the nature of labor and the

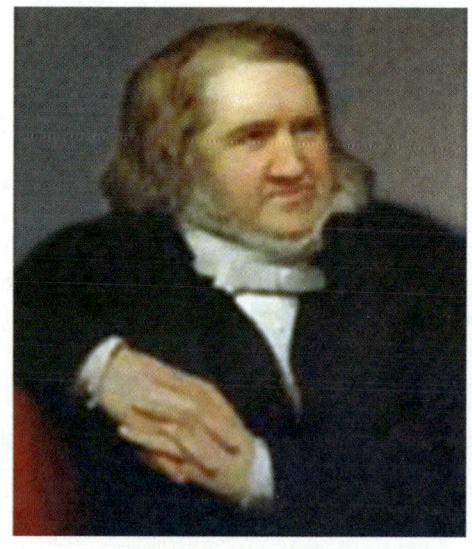

James Young Simpson

significance of labor pain. Simpson maintained that all pain, labor pain included, is without physiologic value. He said that pain only degrades and destroys those who experience it. In contrast, Meigs argued that labor pain has purpose, that uterine pain is inseparable from contractions, and that any drug that abolishes pain will alter contractions. Meigs also believed that pregnancy and labor are normal processes that usually end quite well. He said that physicians should, therefore, not intervene with powerful, potentially disruptive drugs.[7]

John Snow

John Snow (1813–1858) was an excellent physician, and epidemiologist who became famous as an obstetric anesthetist by administering labor analgesia to Queen Victoria for her last of the two deliveries. Snow held deep insight and knowledge of anesthetic physiology and pharmacology and performed experiments to demonstrate the effects of anesthesia on the body. Snow anesthetized 77 obstetric patients with chloroform. He initiated anesthesia

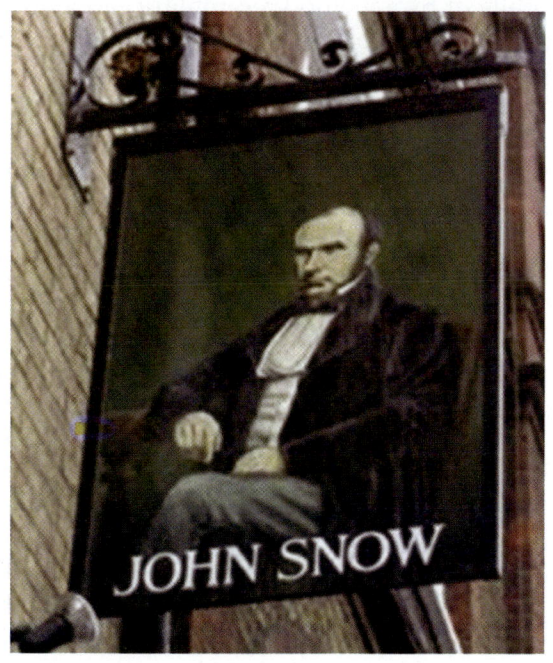

John Snow

during second stage of labor only and titrated the dose of chloroform to maintain a semi-conscious state. Light anesthetic had minimal effect on labor or the neonate but provided adequate analgesia and many women were able to obey commands during childbirth.[5] Queen Victoria had analgesia by open drop technique—giving analgesic doses of chloroform on a folded handkerchief, named and termed as "chloroform a la reine". The method had been used for the birth of Victoria's eighth child in 1853 by John Snow. This replaced the term 'narcose au chloroforme' (first coined by James Young Simpson). Pleased with the pain relief, in 1853 she wrote in her journal, "Dr. Snow gave that blessed chloroform and the effect was soothing, quieting, and delightful beyond measure."[3] According to private records, John Snow anesthetized the Queen for the delivery of Prince Leopold at the request of her personal physicians. Although no one made a formal announcement of that end, rumors surfaced and provoked strong public criticism. Thomas Wakley, the founding editor of *The Lancet*, remarked that he could not imagine that anyone had incurred the awful responsibility of advising the administration of chloroform to her Majesty during a perfectly natural labor with a seventh child. (It was her eighth child, but Wakley had apparently lost count.) Court physicians did not defend their decision to use ether. Perhaps not wanting a public confrontation, they simply denied that the Queen had received any anesthetic. In fact, they first acknowledged use of a royal anesthetic 4 years later when the Queen delivered her ninth and last child, Princess Beatrice. Queen Victoria undaunted by the clergy chose to use an anesthetic during labor and the clergy's position crumpled like the great wall of 'Berlin'. Queen's endorsement to use of obstetric anesthesia herself ended religious opposition. By that time, however, the issue was no longer controversial in public as well as amongst physicians.[12]

But Snow discouraged the open drop technique and introduced inhalers to anesthetize with varied concentrations of anesthetic agents. John Snow's meticulous clinical skills changed the fellow obstetricians' and physicians' point of view about labor analgesia and earned him the title of the Queen's "anesthetist". So it was John Snow who succeeded in lifting the taboo on labor analgesia and guiding the light further. Chloroform anesthesia/analgesia became one of the most prized and important possessions in medical practice. In the next three decades, it became popular throughout the world.

OBSTETRIC ANESTHESIA IN EUROPE AND USA

The first use of modern anesthetic for childbirth happened just 3 months after Morton's historic demonstration of the anesthetic properties of ether at the Massachusetts General Hospital in Boston, Massachusetts. Adam Hammer was the first person in Germany to use ether for pain relief during labor on February 18th 1847.[7] It was Nathan Cooley Keep, who administered the first obstetric anesthetic in the United States on 7th April 1847. The lady who received it was Fanny Appleton Longfellow, wife of the famous poet and scholar Henry Wadsworth Longfellow. She wrote

"….Henry's faith gave me courage and I had heard such a thing had succeeded in abroad where the surgeons extend this great blessing more boldly and universally than our timid doctors…. This is certainly the greatest blessing of this age."[8]

Klikowitsh of Russia used nitrous oxide and oxygen inhalational anesthesia for labor analgesia in 1880. He observed that three or four inhalations would make uterine contractions painless without clouding of consciousness. From then on, it achieved widespread popularity till Eastman showed that incorrect administration could cause asphyxia neonatorum. In 1933, Minnit developed a self-administered nitrous oxide and air apparatus, which was in use till 1970. Its successor Entonox (50% nitrous oxide and 50% oxygen premixed in one cylinder) was introduced in 1961. Trichloroethylene was also used for the same for about 40 years, until its withdrawal in 1984.

OPIOIDS IN OBSTETRIC ANESTHESIA

The next major innovation in obstetric anesthesia came in 1906. *Dämmerschlaf*, which means "twilight sleep," was a technique developed by von Steinbüchel[13] of Graz and popularized by Gauss[9] of Freiburg. It was a combination of opioids with scopolamine to make women amnestic and somewhat comfortable during labor. Until that time, opioids had hardly been used for obstetric practice. Although opium had been part of medical practice since the Roman Empire, it was not used extensively, because of the difficulty of obtaining consistent results with the crude extracts available at that time. In 1809, Sertürner, a German pharmacologist, isolated codeine and morphine from a crude extract of the poppy seed. However, the methods for administering the drugs remained unsophisticated. Physicians gave morphine orally or by a method resembling vaccination, in which they placed a drop of solution on the skin and then made multiple small puncture holes with a sharp instrument to facilitate absorption. Approximately 50 years later, the technical advancement of needle and syringe simplified the administration of opioids and facilitated the development of twilight sleep.[10] Twilight sleep" or "Dammerschlaf' was the term used to describe a "state of clouded consciousness" induced by the use of morphine and scopolamine. In 1903, von Steinbuchel of Austria first used twilight sleep for obstetrics. It was popularized by Carl Gauss of Freiburg through public lectures and publications. Gauss recommended only 10 mg of morphine for entire labor but gave scopolamine as necessary, depending on the patient's response to a "memory test". On the contrary, the obstetricians felt that twilight sleep could not provide adequate analgesia and believed it could suppress uterine contractions and cause neonatal respiratory depression. Despite their skepticism, twilight sleep became the trend for pain relief in labor. It soon came to light that twilight sleep failed to provide adequate pain relief; hence physicians started combining it with barbiturates. In 1934, Irving et al published their research on popular labor analgesia methods prevalent during that time. They concluded that the incidence of neonatal apnea was 35 to 67% in the analgesic group compared to 2% in the non-analgesic group. Nembutal (pentobarbitone sodium) with scopolamine was found to be the most effective method for labor analgesia.

EFFECTS OF ANESTHESIA ON NEWBORN

Slowly but steadily various physicians raised their voice on the adverse effects of anesthesia on the newborn. Paul Zweifel advocated that drugs administered to the mother can cross the placental barrier and affect the fetus. Physicians started considering that anesthetic drugs can cause neonatal asphyxia. In 1953, Apgar described a simple, reliable system for evaluating newborns immediately after birth. She showed that it was sufficiently sensitive to detect differences in the condition of the neonates whose mothers had been anesthetized. for cesarean section by different techniques.[11] Infants born to women, who were given spinal anesthesia, had higher scores than those delivered with general anesthesia. Apgar score changed the quality of newborn's assessment and care. First, it replaced simple observation of neonates with a reproducible measurement—that is, it substituted a numerical score for the ambiguities of words such as *oligopnea* and *asphyxia*. Thus it established the possibility of the documentation and systematic comparison of different treatments. Second, it provided objective criteria for the initiation of neonatal resuscitation. Third, and most important, it helped change the focus of obstetric care. Until

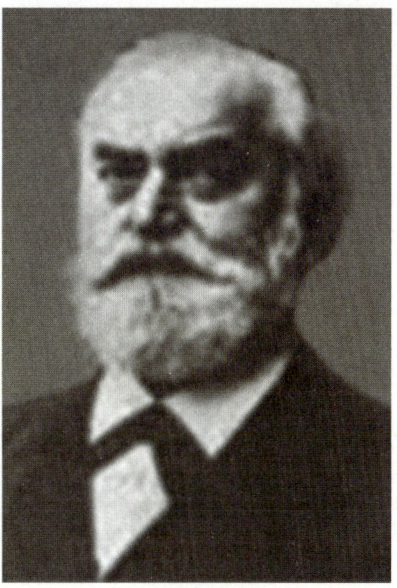

Paul Zweifel

that time, the primary criterion for success or failure had been the survival and well-being of the mother, a natural goal considering the maternal risks of childbirth until that time. After 1900, as maternal risks diminished, the well-being of the mother no longer served as a sensitive measure of outcome. The Apgar score called attention to the child and made its condition the new standard for evaluating obstetric management.

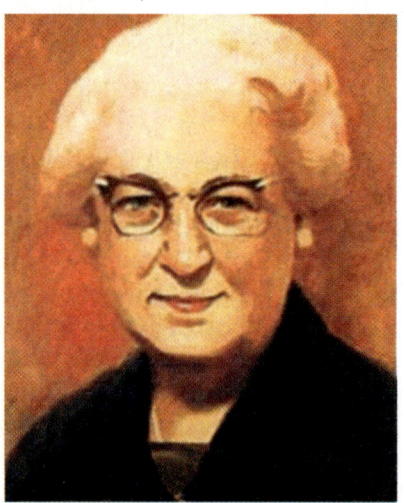

Virginia Apgar

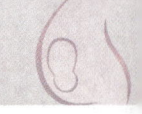

REGIONAL ANESTHESIA FOR CONTROL OF PAIN

In 1901, Oskar Kreis of Germany used spinal anesthesia for labor analgesia in 6 pregnant women. 5 out of 6 parturients suffered nausea, vomiting and severe postpartum headache. In 1909, Walter Stoeckel of Germany injected cocaine solution in the epidural space, through sacral hiatus. Stoeckel described a series of 141 cases of obstetric epidural analgesia in an article entitled 'Uber Sakrale Anasthesie'. In 1928, George Pitkin was the first person to use hyperbaric spinal anaesthesia for delivery, which he called 'controllable spinal anesthesia' in obstetrics.' In 1933, regional anesthesia in obstetrics had a major breakthrough when John GP Cleland described the pathway of uterine pain. He used paravertebral block and low caudal analgesia to control the pain during first and second stage of labor respectively. In 1938, Graffagnino of New Orleans used epidural anesthesia in obstetrics, through modification of the original technique of Pages of Spain and Dogliotti of Italy. In August 1942, Edwards (obstetrician-gynecologist) and Hingson (anesthesiologist) used continuous (intermittent) caudal anesthesia (CCA) for obstetric analgesia. They used a malleable needle as had Lemon and Paschal for continuous spinal anesthesia and highlighted the principal advantages of CCA: "The babies were just as alert and wide awake at birth as those of the mothers who had no form of sedation or anesthesia, and the parturients remained "relaxed," "at ease," "alert," and "usually cheerful". In 1949, Curbelo applied continuous thoracic epidural block for surgical procedures using the technique described by Tuohy for continuous spinal anesthesia. In 1949, Flowers et al described continuous epidural block for labor, delivery, and cesarean section inserting plastic tubing via the lumbar interspaces using a similar technique. They stated, "The site of election (for inserting the needle) is the second lumbar interspace as this is the largest peridural space in the lumbar area". Despite this, it took two decades for lumbar epidural anesthesia to replace continuous caudal anesthesia because of lack of availability of sterile single use plastic tubing. The availability of sterile single use plastic tubing in containers started the era of epidural analgesia in labor. As the years passed by, epidural anesthesia underwent major changes in three spheres.

Drugs: Local anesthetics, which had negligible effect on newborn and with less motor block were preferred. Opioids were added to provide walking epidurals.

Dose: Dilute local anesthetics with less volumes were used.

Method of administration: With the invention of infusion pumps in the 1980s, it became possible to address changing patterns of pain during the course of labor; epidural blocks became more consistent and predictable.

Factors that Influenced the Evolution of Obstetric Anesthesia

Effects of Anesthesia on Labor and Newborn

From the beginning, physicians were worried about the adverse effects of anesthesia on uterine contractions and fetus. As early as the 1900s, Oskar Kreis found that spinal anesthesia had no effect on uterine contractions. Hence the success of regional anesthesia in obstetrics, which had minimal influence on the mother and baby. But high incidence of nausea and vomiting, fluctuations in blood pressure, shorter duration made spinal anesthesia unpopular. Epidural, pudendal and paracervical blocks were the only regional techniques to survive into the second half of the twentieth century.

Improvements in Pharmacology

Local anesthetics with longer duration of action, fewer side effects, and that would preferentially block sensory nerves, were searched. Small amounts of opioids were used to effectively block the first stage of labor.

Economic Factors

With time, labor analgesia became costly and there was a shortage of anesthetists as well. To overcome this problem, midwives were trained to give anesthesia and new equipment for self-administration of anesthetic gases was devised. Obstetricians were able to provide pain relief to more than one patient at a time when the intravenous drugs and regional anesthesia came into practice.

Obstetric Practice

This also shaped the use of anesthesia. When the practice changed from extensive use of forceps, dense blocks were replaced by mobile epidurals. With the rise in cesarean section, rate and the appreciation of risk of general anesthesia, epidurals were instituted early in labor.

Patient's Expectation

This was the most important factor, which influenced obstetric anesthesia. Public support for the inhalation anesthesia and later on for pain free deliveries, forced the physicians to use them on laboring women in spite of their drawbacks. With the increasing public awareness about the safety of anesthesia drugs on the fetus, women preferred the technique of natural, painless, gentle birth. The public interest in labor analgesia was renewed with the introduction and development of epidural anesthesia, which was relatively safe and provided effective pain relief.

History is important in proportion to the lessons it teaches. With respect to obstetric anesthesia, three lessons stand out. First, every new drug and technique comes with its inherent risks. Physicians who first used obstetric anesthesia seemed reluctant to accept this fact, perhaps because of their inexperience with potent drugs (pharmacology was in its infancy) or because they gave in too quickly to patients who wanted relief from pain and who had little understanding of the technical issues confronting physicians. This age of denial lasted almost half a century, until 1900. In another half a century, obstetricians learned to modify their practice to limit the effects of anesthetics on the child.

During the nineteenth century, physicians learned to apply principles of anatomy, physiology, and chemistry to the study and treatment of disease. The same applied to obstetric anesthesia. Studies on placenta revealed the pathway for the transmission of drugs and their potential effects on the fetus. Similarly, studies of the physiology and anatomy of the uterus helped elucidate potential effects of anesthesia on labor. Thus, lessons from basic sciences helped improve patient care.

OBSTETRIC ANESTHESIA—PAST AND PRESENT

Today is the era of patient-controlled epidural analgesia (PCEA) for labor analgesia. This has the advantage of giving the patient more control over her analgesia and comfort. With the use of neuraxial opioids, which produce selective analgesia with minimum sensory and motor changes, the face of obstetric anesthesia is continually evolving.

Evolution of Aspiration Prophylaxis

The paper that bought to light a major cause of mortality during anesthesia in laboring women was published in 1946. Its credit goes to Curtis Lester Mendelson, an obstetrician at the New York Lying–In Hospital. He reviewed the records of 44016 pregnancies from 1932 to 1945 and found 66 cases of aspiration of gastric contents during general anesthesia. A crucial investigation was undertaken by the Association of Anesthetists into the cases of regurgitation that proved fatal during anesthesia. It was published by Morton and Wylie (Anæsthetic deaths due to regurgitation or vomiting. Anaesthesia Volume 6, Issue 4, pp 190–201, Oct. 1951, UK):

1. Emptying of stomach with a gastric tube before induction of anesthesia

2. Use of cuffed endotracheal tube

3. Inhalational induction in supine position

4. Intravenous induction in reverse Trendelenburg position

The solutions put forward:

1. **Protect the airway**

2. **Cricoid pressure:** The biggest advance came in 1961 in the form of a simple maneuver, which is still being used. Brian Arthur Sellick was a consultant Anesthetist at the Middlesex Hospital in London. His communication to The Lancet in 1961 advocated the use of cricoid pressure for all full stomachs, particularly for operative obstetrics and emergency general surgery. He was aware that this technique should not be relied on totally and there were drawbacks in its use. He described preoxygenation, an open vein and implied the importance of ready suction and a tipping trolley.

3. **Reduction of gastric acidity—articulate alkalosis:** The next big step was to neutralize the acid in the stomach. Mendelson (1964) and Dinmick (1957) had suggested the use of particulate alkalosis in laboring women. Taylor and Pryse-Davies (1966) showed that antacids in laboring women increase gastric pH. In 1974, Roberts and Shirley suggested that low pH was more dangerous than volume. They arbitrarily defined that a patient with at least 25 mL of gastric juice of pH less than 2.5 in the stomach at delivery is risky.

4. **Empty the stomach:** Preoperative dietary restriction was practiced from late 1940s to reduce the stomach contents during labor. Howard and Sharp in 1973 investigated the effect of metoclopramide on gastric emptying during labor. Holdsworth et al in 1974 published a comparison between two methods of emptying the stomach before general anesthesia: aspiration by a stomach tube and apomorphine-induced vomiting.

5. **Delayed gastric emptying proved:** It was well known that labor delayed gastric emptying and this was usually due to the administration of narcotic analgesics. This was shown conclusively by Nimmo et al in 1975. They found that metoclopramide did not counteract the effect of diamorphine and pethidine on gastric emptying.

6. **Second look at reduction of gastric acidity—clear alkalosis:** Gibbs et al in 1982 showed a rapid increase in rapid pH with sodium citrate (30 mL dose of 0.3 M). H_2 blockers: Dundee's team in 1981 used cimetidine intravenously in preoperative parturients. Thompson et al in 1984 advocated the use of oral ranitidine 150 mg and saline antacids for aspiration prophylaxis. Tordoff and Sweeney in 1990 confirmed routine use of ranitidine and sodium citrate for acid aspiration prophylaxis by a survey of 288 UK obstetric anesthesia departments.

SUMMARY

In this fascinating story, ranging over 150 years, we have come a long way, still in India, women approach labor with trepidation. Over the ages, with the change in public attitude in favor of obstetric anesthesia, anesthetics were used increasingly for labor pain. The absence of pain, at least in part led to drop in maternal and infant mortality and morbidity by permitting the midwife, or obstetrician to work unhindered in difficult labors. The Old Testament curse of womankind has been finally repudiated in the New Testament prophecy "She shall be saved in childbearing if they continue in faith and charity and holiness with sobriety" and it is due to the hard work and dedication from several researchers, physicians, obstetricians, anesthesiologists, pharmaceutical organizations,

Key Notes Milestones in obstetric anesthesia to remember

1. Introduction of inhalational agents in 1847, the expanded use of opioids in the early decades of the twentieth century, and the refinement of regional anesthesia starting in the mid-twentieth century.
2. Physicians have debated the safety of obstetric anesthesia since 1847, when James Young Simpson first administered anesthesia for delivery.
3. Despite controversy, physicians quickly incorporated general anesthesia into clinical practice, largely because of their patients' desire to avoid childbirth pain.
4. Mainly two issues have dominated the debate, firstly, the effects of general anesthesia on labor and secondly, the effects of anesthesia on the newborn.
5. Outstanding conceptual developments included:
   (a) Zweifel's idea that drugs given to the mother cross the placenta and affect the fetus, and
   (b) Apgar's idea that the condition of the newborn can be assessed objectively after general or neuraxial anesthetic care of the mother.
6. Neuraxial blocks have become more popular for cesarean section displacing general anesthesia.
7. Patient controlled epidural analgesia (PCEA) for painless normal delivery.
8. Preventing Mendelson syndrome.

and professional societies in the last century. They have made obstetric anesthesia safe for pregnant women seeking pain-free childbirth, making their birthing experience a pleasurable memory to be cherished for a long time.

REFERENCES

1. Padvi N, Padvi A, Gupta V, Baldwa M. Textbook of Paediatric Anaesthesia, CBS Publishers & Distributors Pvt Ltd, Delhi, 2015, pp.3–16.
2. Lull CB, Hingson RA. Control of pain in childbirth (3rd ed.). Philadelphia: Lippincott Co., 1948, pp. 139–152. 2. Toski JA, Bacon DR, Calverley RK. The History of Anesthesiology. In: Barash PG, Cullen BF, Stoelting RK. Clinical Anesthesia. Philadelphia: Lippincott Williams & Wilkins, 2006; pp 5–6. 3. Caton D. John Snow's Practice of Obstetric Anesthesia [Special Article]. Anesthesiology 2000;92:247–52. 4. Goerig M, Streckfuss W. Adam Hammer (1818–1878)—remarks on a forgotten pioneer of ether anaesthesia in obstetrics. Anasthesiol Intensivmed Noffallmed Schmerzther 2004;39(5):265–75. 5. Clark RB. Fanny Longfellow and Nathan Keep. A SA News Letter Sept. 1997 Vol 61.
3. Caton D. "In the Present State of Our Knowledge": Early Use of Opioids in Obstetrics. Anesthesiology 1995;82:779–84. 7. Caton D. Review of "John Snow: Anaesthetist to Queen and Epidemiologist to a Nation. A Biography". Anesthesia and Analgesia 1995;82:223. (8) Kreis O. Ober medullar-narkose bei gebarenden. Centralblatt fur Gynakologie 1900;28:724–9. 9. Moore DC. Memories of the early years of regional anesthesia for childbirth. Regional Anesthesia and Pain Medicine 2003;28:466–69. 10. Doughty A. Walter Stoeckel (1871–1961) A pioneer of regional analgesia in obstetrics. Anaesthesia, 1990;45:468–71. 11. Cleland JGP. Paravertebral anesthesia in obstetrics: experimental and clinical basis. Surg, Gynecol Obstet 1933;57:51–62. 12. Hingson RA, Edwards WB. Continuous caudal analgesia. An analysis of the first ten thousand confinements thus managed with a report of the authors' first thousand cases. Journal of the American Medical Association 1943;123:538–46. 13. Caton D, Frolich MA, Euliano TY. Anesthesia for Childbirth: Controversy and change [The Nature and Management of Labour Pain: Peer-Reviewed Papers from an Evidence-Based Symposium]. American Journal of Obstetrics and Gynecology 2002;186(Suppl.)S25–30.
4. In: Simpson WG (Ed.) The Works of Sir JY Simpson, Vol II: Anesthesia, Edinburgh: Adam and Charles Black; 1871:177.
5. Regarding anaesthesia for women in labour, the statement "Simpson disregarded the adverse effects on uterine contractions or on the newborn" deserves a counter-balance. In an article in the Edin Monthly I of Med Science in March 1847 Simpson wrote: "it will be necessary to ascertain anaesthesia's precise effects, both upon the action of the uterus and on the assistant abdominal muscles, its influence, if any, upon the child;

whether it has a tendency to haemorrhage or other complications."

6. Caton D. Obstetric anesthesia: The first ten years. Anesthesiology 1970;33:102–9.

7. The extent to which clergymen discredited Simpson has been much debated. See papers by Adams and Maltby in The History of Anae,sthcsia Society Proceedings 2001;29:42–57.

8. Did John Snow become famous as an obstetric anaesthetist by chloroforming Queen Victoria for labour analgesia? As Connor and Connor (Anaesthesia 1996;51:955–7) have pointed out, it was not until 1859 that a major newspaper, when commenting on the obituary of John Snow, informed of the Queen's use of chloroform in 1853 and 1857.

9. Gauss CJ. Die Anwendung des Skopolamin-Morphium-Dämmerschlafes in der Geburtshilfe. Medizinische Klinik 1906;2:136–8.

10. Macht DI: History of opium and some of its preparations and alkaloids. JAMA 1915;6:477–81.

11. Apgar V. A proposal for a new method of evaluation of the newborn infant. Curr Res Anesth Analg 1953;32:260–7.

12. Sykes WS: Anesthesiology, I. Essays on the First Hundred Years of Anaesthesia, Park Ridge, Ill: Wood Library Museum of Anesthesiology; 1982

13. Von Steinbüchel R. Vorläufige Mittheilung über die Anwendung von Skopolamin-Morphium-Injektionen in der Geburtshilfe. Centralblatt Gyn 1902;30:1304–6.

General Physiological Principles in Obstetric Anesthesia

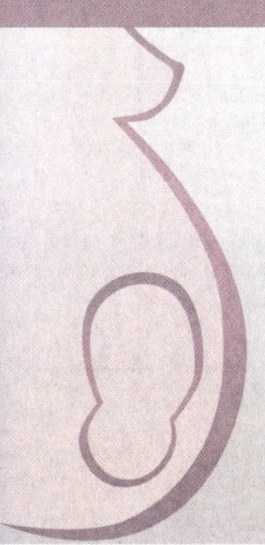

Essentials of Physiological Changes of Pregnancy in Respiratory System and Metabolism

Roopali V Telang

Pregnancy is a state of altered body physiology. The surge in estrogen-progesterone, progressive enlargement of the gravid uterus, increased metabolic demands during pregnancy cause many physiological and anatomical changes in the respiratory system.[1,2] Proper understanding of these changes is of great importance for the obstetric anesthesiologists. These changes affect anesthetic physiology, pharmacology and management techniques during pregnancy and are even more important in patients with comorbidities. It has been found in literature that failure to intubate trachea is 7–10 times more common in pregnant than in nonpregnant women. Therefore, to accurately diagnose and treat any abnormality in the respiratory system, it is important to understand the altered physiology of respiratory system and effects of it on pharmacokinetics of drugs.

ANATOMIC CHANGES

Upper Airway

Increase in estrogen during pregnancy leads to increased vascularity and edema of upper respiratory mucosa involving oropharynx, nasopharynx, glottis and arytenoids. In addition, there is edema because of fluid overload associated with pregnancy which is exaggerated in pregnancy-induced hypertension (PIH). It can give rise to nasal stuffiness and epistaxis in pregnant women. Some women develop a benign nasal growth, mostly unilateral called as nasal granuloma gravidarum or telangiectatic polyp or pregnancy tumor. They present with nasal blockage and epistaxis.[3] In most cases, this growth usually

Increased tissue friability and edema of mucosal lining increases risk of bleeding while manipulating upper airway, difficult ventilation and intubation of trachea. Careful handling of upper airway is a must. Nasal instrumentation should best be avoided. Laryngoscopy should be done gently. Due to edema, tracheal intubation should be done with small size endotracheal tube, e.g. 6, 6.5 no. There should be minimum attempts for intubation. There can be exaggerated airway edema in patient with upper respiratory tract infection, fluid overload and pre-eclampsia. Laryngoscopy may be difficult because of gain in weight, especially in obese and short stature and due to enlarged breast tissue. Difficult airway cart, best intubating position must be ensured before attempting intubation. Due to airway handling, there is risk of airway obstruction post-extubation.

resolves post-delivery. If epistaxis and nasal blockage is significant, the polyp can be excised under local anesthesia.

Chest, Lungs and Diaphragm

Changes in thorax and abdomen start as early as first trimester. In pregnancy, chest becomes barrel-shaped.

This is because of following changes:

1. The diaphragm is gradually moved upward by the gravid uterus which causes 4 cm elevation of diaphragm.[4]
2. Despite the upward displacement, the movement of diaphragm during respiration increases by up to 2 cm in the pregnant females compared to the nonpregnant.[5]
3. Ligaments loosening and rib flaring leads to increase in the anteroposterior and transverse diameters of the chest by 2 cm.[4]
4. Increase in subcostal angle from 68° to sometimes up to 103°.[6,7]

Hence, during gestation, diaphragmatic breathing pattern is more than thoracic. Overall, in pregnancy, chest wall compliance decreases and compliance of lung does not change (Table 2.1).

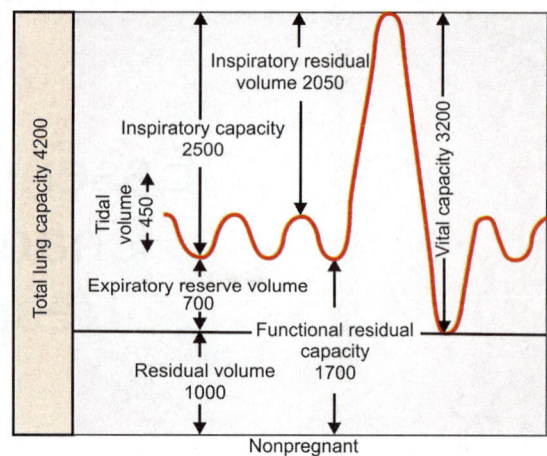

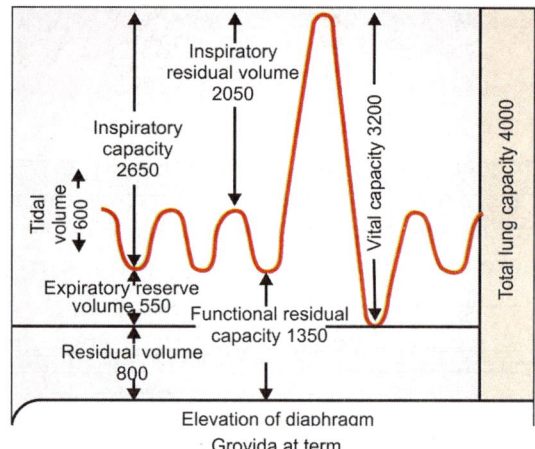

Fig. 2.1. Changes in lung capacity in pregnancy

Table 2.1: Anatomical changes in respiratory system in pregnancy	
Component of respiratory	Change
Upper airway	Edema
Chest wall compliance	Decreased
Thoracic AP and transverse diameter	Increased
Diaphragm	Elevated
Lung compliance	Unchanged

PHYSIOLOGICAL CHANGES

Lung Volumes and Capacities, Ventilation, Oxygen Consumption

In pregnancy, there is overall increase in lung capacity. As stated, because of better movement of diaphragm and compensatory increase in AP and transverse diameter of chest, tidal volume is increased than in nonpregnant state (Fig. 2.1). Thus in pregnancy, minute ventilation increases from 30% at seventh week to 50% at term (Table 2.2, Fig. 2.2). Respiratory rate is not changed much. As a result of increased area of apposition between diaphragm and chest wall, the expiratory reserve volume (ERV) decreases by 25%.[8,9] Gravid uterus increases abdominal pressure and thus chest wall compliance is reduced by 35–40%.[10] Due to reduced chest wall compliance, functional residual capacity (FRC) decreases. Decreases in FRC and ERV are the consistent changes throughout pregnancy starting at 12 weeks of gestation.

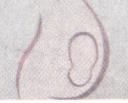

Table 2.2: Approximate percentage change in lung parameters

Lung parameter	Change in pregnancy
1. Tidal volume (TV)	+45%
2. Functional residual capacity (FRC)	−20%
3. End residual volume (ERV)	−25%
4. Dead space	+45%
5. Respiratory rate	No change
6. Minute ventilation	+45%
7. Alveolar ventilation	+45%

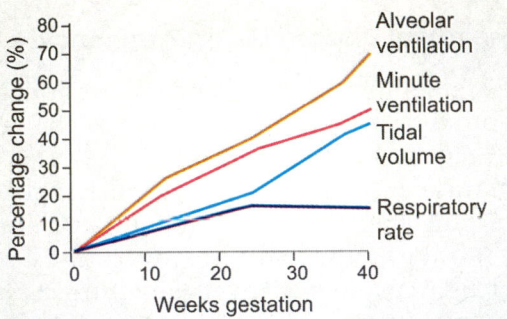

Fig. 2.2. Percentage change in lung parameters over period of gestation

Supine and lithotomy position exaggerates this reduction in residual volume and FRC.

Throughout pregnancy, there is no change in vital capacity (VC) in upright position. Thus during pregnancy, a significant change in VC may indicate cardiorespiratory dysfunction.

During pregnancy, there is almost no change in FEV_1 and FEV_1/FVC ratio, and peak expiratory flow rate (PEFR).[11–14] The pulmonary function test (PFT) values of non-pregnant females can be used for interpretation in pregnant. The flow volume loop, and absolute flow rate at low lung volumes are normal in pregnant females.[15,16] Large airway conductance is either increased or normal.[12,17] Closing volume which is a measure of small airway function is normal.[18,19] Due to decrease in FRC in supine position, during tidal breathing, small airways can close while lying down.

In one-third to one-half of supine pregnant women, FRC is less than closing capacity causing hypoxemia and impaired organ perfusion. General anesthesia induction should always be preceded by pre-oxygenation to decrease risk of hypoxemia. Also decrease in FRC accompanied with increase in minute ventilation results in faster induction and recovery from inhalational anesthetic agents.

Blood Gases and Acid-Base Status

In pregnancy, there is 20% increase in oxygen consumption. This results from increased metabolic demands of maternal organs, fetoplacental unit.[20] However, minute ventilation is increased which increases partial pressure of oxygen in arterial blood and alveoli (PaO_2 and PO_2). During pregnancy, PaO_2 is around 100–110 mm Hg (Table 2.3).[22–24]

Table 2.3: Changes in blood gas parameters in pregnancy

1. pH	Normal to slightly alkalotic (7.4 to 7.45)
2. $PaCO_2$	Decreased to 30 mm Hg
3. PaO_2	Increased up to 105 mm Hg
4. Bicarbonate	Decreased up to 15 mEq/L
5. $\Delta PaCO_2$- $EtCO_2$	0

Level of progesterone rises gradually from 6 weeks (25 ng/mL) to term (150 ng/mL).[21] Raised progesterone level causes hyperpnea. Progesterone is considered as respiratory stimulant as it increases chemoreceptor sensitivity. Increase in minute ventilation due to increase in tidal volume reduces arterial CO_2 ($PaCO_2$) from 40 mm Hg (pre-pregnant) to 30–32 mm Hg in pregnancy.[22,23] Kidney compensates for this respiratory alkalosis by increasing bicarbonate excretion and bicarbonate level is 15–20 mEq/L in pregnancy. This metabolic compensation by bicarbonates leads to mild alkalotic pH in pregnancy.[25] Thus during pregnancy, blood gas picture is of chronic respiratory alkalosis. Chronic alkalosis and anemia of pregnancy stimulates 2,3-diphophoglycerate synthesis which causes

Nausea and vomiting is common during first trimester. In severe form known as hyperemesis gravidarum, the associated intractable vomiting can cause fluid and electrolyte disturbances. Patient may develop metabolic alkalosis and ketosis, if oral intake is poor. Ketosis can occur more rapidly in pregnant than in non-pregnant women with fasting. In later months of pregnancy, pregnant females are prone to ketosis in less than 16 hours of fasting in comparison to more than 24 hours of fasting in non-pregnant women. Mild ketosis of fasting does not have any adverse effects on mother and fetus. Ketoacidosis due to maternal diabetes is more serious and can have adverse effects on fetus. If pregnant female is on diuretic treatment due to other medical condition, diuretic use is associated with metabolic alkalosis. The resulting picture is mixed alkalosis due to hyperventilation-induced low PCO_2.

rightward shifting of oxygen dissociation curve. This helps in transfer of oxygen across placenta by helping unloading of oxygen. Hypoxic ventilatory response doubles in pregnancy.

Metabolism and Respiration during Labor

During labor, due to pain, the parturient hyperventilates which causes respiratory alkalosis and this shifts oxyhemoglobin curve to left. This causes decreased release of oxygen from maternal Hb across placenta, causing fetal hypoxemia. Minute ventilation increases by 70 to 140% in first stage and 120 to 200% in the second stage of labor as compared to prepregnant level.[26] Hypocarbia due to hyperventilation in mother causes uterine artery vasoconstriction. These changes are aggravated by supine and lithotomy position. Consumption of oxygen is increased by 40% and 75% in first and second stages of labor respectively in comparison to pre-labor consumption.[26,27] There is also elevated lactate level due to anaerobic metabolism in view of increased demand of oxygen.[27,28] Effective epidural analgesia can markedly diminish maternal hyperventilation and oxygen consumption.[27,28]

Metabolism and Respiration during the Puerperium

Oxygen consumption, tidal volume, and minute ventilation remain elevated 6 to 8 weeks post-delivery, although minute ventilation decreases halfway towards pre-pregnant value by 72 hours. Alveolar and mixed venous PCO_2 increases slowly, by 6 to 8 weeks postpartum the values are slightly lower than non-pregnant state. FRC increases after delivery but is less than pre-pregnant values for 1 to 2 weeks.[29]

Respiratory Disease during Pregnancy

Most women with mild to moderate respiratory insufficiency are able to continue pregnancy. Women with severe respiratory insufficiency may have adverse maternal and fetal outcome.[30] VO_2 max is 34 mL/kg/min to 38 mL/kg/min, increases by 20% due to increased requirement by maternal organs and growing fetus. Increased minute ventilation during pregnancy is often perceived as shortness of breath. As much as 75% females have exertional dyspnea by 30 weeks of pregnancy.[31–34] Physiological dyspnea is dyspnea at rest or with mild exertion is common during pregnancy. It is due to increased minute ventilation and effect of enlarging uterus that increases work of breathing. Other contributing factors are increased pulmonary blood flow, anemia, and nasal congestion.

It is challenging to differentiate physiologic dyspnea from pathologic. Following points are important for diagnosis:

• History
• Duration of symptoms
• Onset—sudden onset or paroxysmal dyspnea
• Respiratory rate >20/minute
• PCO_2 <30 and >35 mm Hg
• Hypoxemia
• Abnormal spirometry or ECHO

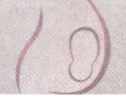

Asthma

Asthma is currently affecting ~300 million people globally. At a given time approximately 8% pregnant women are suffering from asthma. Though incidence of asthma is increasing worldwide its morbidity and mortality is decreasing due to better medical care. Asthma is a disease of variable intensity with symptoms of airway obstruction, inflammation and hyper-responsiveness.

Risk factors implicated in etiology of asthma are given in Table 2.4.

Diagnosis: In pregnant patients, history, signs and symptoms of asthma (wheezing, dyspnea, shortness of breath, chest tightness) are similar to non-pregnant.

The diagnosis of asthma is confirmed by objective lung function test

- **Pulmonary function test:** Pregnancy does not affect FEV_1, FEV_1/FVC and PEFR.[11–14] Hence values during non-pregnant state can be used for comparison. Spirometry test shows airflow limitation with reduced FEV_1, FEV_1/FVC ratio and PEFR. Reversibility 15 minutes after inhaled beta agonist or in some patients, after 2 to 3 weeks of oral glucocorticoids is demonstrated as >12% or 200 mL increase in FEV_1. Diurnal variation in symptoms can be confirmed by measuring PEFR twice daily.

- **Airway responsiveness:** Measured by methacholine or histamine challenge, not so useful in clinical practice.

- **Hematological test:** Total serum IgE and specific IgE to inhaled allergens.
- **Imaging:** High resolution computerized tomography (HRCT) can show bronchial wall thickening or bronchiectatic picture, but are not diagnostic of asthma.
- **Skin test:** This is reactive in allergic asthma. It tests sensitivity to common allergens.

Effects of pregnancy on asthma: During pregnancy, asthma in one-third patients improves, one-third deteriorates and one-third remains stable. This improvement is thought to be due to bronchodilator effect of progesterone. Following are the patterns of asthma during pregnancy:

- If there is deterioration, symptoms aggravates between 29 and 36 weeks of gestation.
- Asthma severity is less during ninth month of pregnancy.
- No worsening of asthma with labor and delivery.
- If there is improvement, it is gradual throughout gestation period.
- Asthma severity follows similar patterns in subsequent pregnancy.

Pregnancy-induced hypertension (PIH), if present in asthmatic patients, should be treated cautiously. Low dose aspirin is used in these patients. Aspirin can cause spasm in patient sensitive to it.[35] β-blockers are usually used in non-pregnant non-asthmatic patients. In pre-eclampsia, labetalol is commonly used. β-blockers, particularly non-β1 selective, can

Table 2.4: Risk factors implicated in etiology of asthma

Exogenous/environmental factor	Endogenous factor	Triggers
Allergen—indoor, outdoor	Genetic predisposition	Allergens
Occupational sensitizers	Atopy	Exercise and hyperventilation
Passive smoking	Airway hyper-responsiveness	Upper respiratory tract viral infections
Respiratory infections	Gender	Cold air
		Drugs (beta-blockers, aspirin)
		Stress
		Irritants (e.g. perfumes)

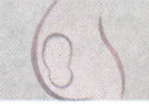

bring on bronchospasm, therefore, should not be used. Vasodilators, e.g. calcium channel blocker, nitroglycerine, hydralazine, and nitropruside, can be used in pre-eclampsia. These agents interfere with hypoxic pulmonary vasoconstriction. This can cause ventilation perfusion mismatch. Thus can cause additive hypoxia in asthmatics

Effects of asthma on pregnancy: Asthma exacerbation can lead to fetal hypoxia. It has been found that women with asthma have higher risk of pre-eclamsia, preterm labor, IUGR, perinatal mortality, postpartum hemorrhage, and congenital malformation of fetus.[36]

There is increased risk of postpartum hemorrhage in asthmatic parturient. The probable causes are use of β-agonist, abnormalities of smooth muscle and neural regulation of contraction.[37] Prostaglandin F2α (prostodin) should be used with caution to treat postpartum hemorrhage (PPH). Oxytocin should be used in PPH as it does not precipitate bronchospasm and can be given in incremental doses, taking care of hypotension. Methergine too can cause bronchospasm. Ergot alkaloid (methergine) or prostodin should be used with preparedness to treat bronchospasm.

Medical management:
- Avoid known allergen
- Drug therapy is divided into two parts:
  1. Control of acute symptoms, e.g. bronchodilators
  2. Control of inflammation (disease controller)

Bronchodilators: As given in Table 2.5.

Corticosteroids:
- Inhaled corticosteroids (ICSs): Most effective anti-inflammatory
- Reduce the number of inflammatory cells and their activation in airway.
- Dose twice daily
- Improve symptoms of asthma rapidly and lung functions improve over several weeks
- Minimal systemic side effects.

Systemic corticosteroids: To treat acute exacerbations (IV hydrocortisone, methylprednisolone).

Several studies have proved oral steroids prednisone or prednisolone in dose of 30 to 45

Table 2.5: Types of bronchodilators

	Mechanism of action	Duration dosing	Other actions	
β2 agonist	Activate β2 receptor ↑Adenylyl cyclase Airway smooth muscle relaxation Inflammatory cell inhibition	Short-acting (SABA) DOA—3 to 4 hours Rapid symptom release Long-acting (LABA) DOA >12 hours Used with corticosteroids	Functional antagonists Inhibit all known bronchoconstrictors Inhibit mast cell mediator release Prevent plasma exudation Inhibit sensory nerve activation	SABA—Albuterol Terbutaline LABA—Salmeterol
Anti-cholinergic	Muscarinic receptor antagonist Inhibit cholinergic nerve-induced bronchoconstriction mucus secretion		None	Ipratropium Bromide Used as add on drug
Theophylline	Phosphodiesterase inhibitor	Sustained release tablet OD or BD		

mg OD for 5–10 days can be used to treat acute exacerbation. No tapering is needed. Around 1% patients need maintenance dose, lowest possible dose should be determined. Steroid use may cause hypertension in these patients.

Management of asthma exacerbation:

During pregnancy, about 5.8% women are hospitalized for exacerbation.[38] Management of these patients requires multidisciplinary approach involving obstetrician, intensivist, pulmonologist, pediatrician and anesthesiologist.

ABG analysis should be done keeping in mind respiratory alkalosis of pregnancy. Arterial blood gas shows marked respiratory alkalosis. Marked alkalosis due to exacerbation affects oxygen delivery to fetus due to decreased placental blood flow.[39] Acute respiratory acidosis on the other hand indicates maternal exhaustion. If maternal venous PCO_2 is increased, it may affect offloading of fetal PCO_2.[40]

Aims of treatment:
- To correct maternal hypoxemia
- To correct maternal hypercarbia.
- Reversal of bronchospasm by inhaled β2 agonist and systemic steroids

Treatment:
- Supplemental oxygen—to maintain oxygen SpO_2 >95%.
- Inhaled salbutamol every 20 minutes maximum 3 doses in first hour.
- In severe cases, ipratropium bromide is administered simultaneously.
- Systemic steroids—oral or intravenous.

Patient is monitored closely for any sign of maternal exhaustion like increasing $PaCO_2$ which mandates initiation of mechanical ventilation to avoid hypercarbia, fetal acidosis. Depending on period of gestation, electronic and biophysical monitoring of fetus is done.

Obstetric management: Induction of labor should be done cautiously as prostaglandin

F2α causes bronchoconstriction *in vivo* and *in vitro*. Prostaglandin E2 causes bronchoconstriction when taken as aerosol *in vivo* but dilates airway *in vitro*. Bronchoconstriction is probably due to irritant effect. Nevertheless vaginal use of prostaglandin E2 should be done cautiously.

Management during labor and delivery: Aim of labor analgesia is:
- To provide adequate pain relief
- Stress relief
- Avoid maternal hyperventilation.
- Technique used should cause minimal sedation, minimal respiratory muscle paralysis, should have minimal effect on fetus.

Following are the different methods:

- *Opioids:* Systemic opioids are useful to avoid stress and hyperventilation especially during first stage. Non-histamine releasing opioids, e.g. fentanyl, remifentanyl, are better choice than morphine. Opioids can be administered by intrathecal or epidural route without causing motor block. They should be administered judiciously in patients with active wheezing to avoid respiratory depression in parturient and fetus.

- *Continuous lumbar epidural:* It provides good pain relief avoiding maternal stress, hyperventilation and respiratory depression. Level of analgesia is maintained at T10 thoracic level to avoid respiratory muscle paralysis (using low dose local anesthetic with opioid). Besides, lumbar epidural can be used for anesthesia in cesarean section is an added advantage.

- *Paracervical and pudendal nerve blocks:* Paracervical and pudendal nerve blocks can be administered by obstetrician during first and second stages of labor respectively provide pain relief without sedation and to provide respiratory compromise.

- *Lumbar sympathetic block:* It can be used in first stage with same benefits of paracervical and pudendal nerve blocks.

Anesthesia for cesarean delivery: The choice of anesthesia depends on underlying respiratory status. Neuraxial anesthesia is better than general anesthesia due to avoidance of airway manipulation. Neuraxial anesthesia is associated with lower incidence of bronchospasm than general anesthesia. Patient with stable respiratory status can be given spinal or epidural anesthesia. However, neuraxial anesthesia is hazardous in unstable patient with labored respiration as it can compromise respiratory function further.

If general anesthesia is planned, induction is rapid sequence to avoid risk of aspiration. Either propofol or ketamine can be used. Ketamine relaxes smooth muscles of airway and inhibits neural reflexes. Propofol is also better than thiopentone with respect to airway. Inhalation induction with sevoflurane in patient with status asthmaticus has also been reported in literature.[41] After baby delivery, for maintenance, high concentration of volatile agents is used. This affects airway smooth muscle, and inhibits airway reflexes. This may give rise to hemorrhage following cesarean section due to uterine relaxation. Oxytocin should be first line of drug to control PPH.

Cigarette Smoking

Over last few decades, smoking rates have fallen in males and increased amongst females. The Journal of American Medical Association (JAMA) has conducted a study in 187 countries between 1980 and 2012 to know the prevalence of smoking and cigarette consumption. Data from India showed that rate of cigarette smoking among Indian men has fallen from 33.8% in 1980 to 23% in 2012, whereas it has risen from 3 to 3.2% in Indian women over the same period.[42] In India, the number of female smokers has increased from about 5.3 million to 12.2 million over similar duration. Approximately, 50% females quit smoking in pregnancy, of which 50 to 60% return back to smoking 6 months postpartum.

Pharmacology: Tobacco contains more than 4000 chemicals like nicotine, carbon monoxide, cyanides, etc. Carbon monoxide (CO) has 200 times more affinity for hemoglobin as compared to oxygen. Endogenous production of CO (from hemoglobin metabolism) and atmospheric pollution account for carboxyhemoglobin (COHb) concentration of about 2.5% in non-smokers. In smokers, the level ranges from 3 to 15%. COHb causes absolute decrease in oxygen content by decreasing hemoglobin available to bind oxygen and shifts oxygen dissociation curve to left producing increased affinity of hemoglobin for oxygen. This results in decreased oxygen supply at tissue level. Chronic hypoxia at tissue level is compensated by increase in red blood cell count which leads to increased blood viscosity. Increased blood viscosity may affect cardiovascular performance. CO also exerts negative inotropic effect.

Nicotine acts on sympathoadrenal system by release of catecholamines.

Effects of cigarette smoking: Clinical manifestations of smoking are due to its acute pharmacologic effects and comorbid conditions as a result of chronic smoking. Nicotine increases maternal heart rate, blood pressure, causes peripheral vasoconstriction. Chronic smoking is associated with atherosclerosis, and poor wound healing. Smoking leads to airway hyperactivity, increased mucus secretion, thick mucus, small airway narrowing, altered lung volumes, bronchitis and COPD. Smoking causes feeling of increased alertness, euphoria, and dependence.

Smoking cessation is associated with withdrawal symptoms like headache, irritable mood, poor concentration, drowsiness, easy fatigability, nausea, sleep disturbance, and anxiety. Smoking cessation can be dealt with counseling, hypnosis, acupuncture and pharmacologic therapy. Nicotine replacement therapy has not undergone much evaluation in pregnant patients hence its use is reserved when all other measures fail. The benefits of smoking cessation evolve over several weeks to months.

Effects on pregnancy: Smoking can affect oxygen delivery to fetus due to COHb and decreased uteroplacental circulation. Nicotine crosses placenta due to its low molecular rate. There is increased incidence of placenta previa, placental abruption and spontaneous abortion. Smoking adversely affects fetal growth. Low birth weight, IUGR, and sudden infant death syndrome are known. Smoking may have long-term effects on babies like asthma, attention deficit disorder, and cognitive dysfunction.

COHb levels come to non-smoker level in 48 hours and there is rise in oxygen content and availability. Pregnant women have demonstrated 8% increase in available oxygen with cessation of 48 hours. As mentioned, smoking leads to airway hyperactivity, increased mucus production and decreased mucociliary action. Airway manipulation can cause bronchospasm. Approximately six weeks are needed for improvement in airway parameters. For labor and delivery, intravenous and regional anesthesia is preferred. If general anesthesia is needed, one should be ready to tackle problem associated with airway manipulations.

Cystic Fibrosis

Cystic fibrosis, also known as mucoviscidosis, is an autosomal recessive disorder. It affects mostly lungs but also pancreas, liver, kidneys and intestine. It is caused by mutation in the gene which is needed for cystic fibrosis transmembrane conductance regulator (CFTR) protein synthesis. The product of this gene is a chloride channel involved in production of sweat, digestive juices and mucus. It affects exocrine gland function. In cystic fibrosis, all these secretions become thick.

Patients have following symptoms:

- Difficulty in breathing, repeated chest infection due to impaired mucociliary clearance.
- Sinus infection, poor growth, fatty stool, clubbing, and infertility in males.
- Patients develop bacterial pneumonia, allergic bronchopulmonary aspergilosis, and infection due to *Mycobacterium avium complex.*
- In long term, patient develops bronchiectasis due to repeated lung infection and lung damage. Chronic hypoxemia can cause pulmonary hypertension, corpulmonale and respiratory failure. Other symptoms include pancreatitis, and malabsorption.

Diagnosis of cystic fibrosis: On the basis of clinical and laboratory, diagnosis of cystic fibrosis is given in Table 2.6.

Effects of pregnancy on cystic fibrosis: Pregnancy may affect cystic fibrosis by increasing:

1. Work of breathing
2. Airway responsiveness

Table 2.6: Diagnosis of cystic fibrosis based on clinical and laboratory findings	
Clinical criteria	**Laboratory findings**
• Family history	• Sweat chloride concentration >60 mEq/L
• Chronic obstructive pulmonary diseases and colonization with *Pseudomonas aeruginosa* before age of 20 years	• CFTR genotype with two known cystic fibrosis mutations
	• CFTR dysfunction detection by nasal potential difference test
	• Other findings
• Exocrine pancreatic insufficiency	• X-ray chest—hyperinflation of lung
	• ABG—hypoxemia
	• PFT—restrictive or obstructive pattern PFT ↑residual volume, ↓ FEV_1 severity of disease

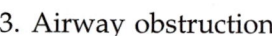

3. Airway obstruction
4. Blood volume.

Congestive cardiac failure and pulmonary hypertension can happen due to increased blood volume. However, pregnancy does not affect long-term outcome of cystic fibrosis.

Effects of cystic fibrosis on pregnancy: In cystic fibrosis, chronic hypoxemia and poor maternal nutrition (due to repeated infections) lead to LBW and preterm labor. With better antenatal care, pregnancy outcome can be improved. Fetal outcome depends on preconception maternal status. Prepregnancy low BMI and FEV_1 suggest poor fetal outcome.

Medical management: Respiratory system management is symptomatic. Inhalation of hypertonic saline to clear mucus and recombinant deribonuclease I to decrease viscosity can be tried.[43] Mechanical airway clearance can be done in patients producing copious mucus. Bronchodilators may be useful in patients with airway obstruction which is reversible. For chronic hypoxemia, cor pulmonale oxygen therapy is used. Long-term antibiotic therapy is required for repeated chest infections and exacerbation of symptoms. Use of long-term azithromycin reduces exacerbations of cystic fibrosis is reported.[44] Teratogenic effects on

---

Management During Labor and Delivery

Due to underlying lung condition, monitor for hypoxemia. Continuous SpO_2 monitoring to be done and appropriate oxygen therapy should be started as required. Labor analgesia avoids maternal hyperventilation by giving pain relief. Labor analgesia should be administered judiciously to avoid high level thoracic block and respiratory depression to protect effective cough. Administration of intravenous opioid may cause respiratory depression and hypoxemia. Intrathecal opioid is an alternative with close patient monitoring. For labor and cesarean section, epidural analgesia is a better option. Low dose bupivacaine with or without opioids provides good analgesia during labor with minimal respiratory depression and high thoracic blockade. General anesthesia may be needed in patients with severe respiratory function compromise.

---

fetus due to antibiotic use for long duration are not known. Gene therapy and lung transplantation are other treatment modalities.

Obstetric management: Decision for continuation of pregnancy depends on prepregnant condition of patient. Patient should be counseled for hereditary transmission of the disease. Multidisciplinary approach is needed involving obstetrician, chest physician, pediatrician, specialist of fetal medicine and dietician. Diet planning with addition of extra 300 kcal/day to daily caloric requirement and pancreatic enzyme supplement.[45]

Respiratory Failure

Respiratory failure is relatively rare during pregnancy. It is associated with significant maternal and fetal morbidity and mortality.

Causes: Causes of respiratory failure during pregnancy are given in Table 2.7.

Effects of respiratory failure on pregnancy: Respiratory failure increases morbidity and mortality in pregnant patients. In respiratory failure, fetal oxygen delivery is decreased. This is due to maternal arterial hypoxemia and hypotension. Hypotension is due to predisposing disease condition and raised airway pressures due to mechanical ventilation. First trimester abortion is the most common reason for pregnancy loss. Outcomes during second and third trimesters are IUFD, preterm delivery, and stillbirth.

Effects of pregnancy on respiratory failure: Course and outcome of respiratory failure is not affected by pregnancy.

Medical management: Medical management is same as in non-pregnant patients. Goal is to maintain oxygenation, perfusion of mother and treat the underlying cause. All arrangements of vaginal delivery, neonatal resuscitation, and cesarean section to be kept ready in ICU.

Table 2.7: Causes of respiratory failure during pregnancy

Pregnancy specific:	Causes of adult respiratory distress syndrome (ARDS)
• Pre-eclampsia, pulmonary edema	• Infection
• Amniotic fluid embolism	• Bacterial or viral pneumonia
• Tocolytics	• Pyelonephritis
Aggravated by pregnancy:	• Sepsis
• Gastric acid aspiration	• Endometritis
• Sepsis, ARDS	• Hemorrhage
• Venous thromboembolism	• Multiple blood transfusion
• Cardiac failure	• DIC
Others:	• Drugs
• Pneumonia	• Salicylates, opioids
• Asthma	• Gastric acid aspiration
• Neuromuscular disease	• Embolism
• Cystic fibrosis	

ARDS is an acute onset diffuse injury of lungs leading to arterial hypoxemia, pulmonary infiltrates on chest X-ray and decreased lung compliance in the presence of predisposing cause. Overall mortality is 50–60%.[46–48]

Non-invasive ventilation (NIV) may be used to prevent upper airway handling and sedation. NIV is associated with risk of aspiration. Indications for tracheal intubation with mechanical ventilation in pregnant patients are not different from non-pregnant. Hyperventilation should be avoided to prevent respiratory alkalosis-induced decrease in uterine blood flow. To avoid aortocaval compression, left uterine displacement should be maintained. In few patients where conventional methods fail, alternative forms of treatment like extracorporeal membrane oxygenation (ECMO), inhaled nitric oxide and high frequency oscillatory ventilation are tried. Safety of these methods during pregnancy is not known.

Obstetric management: It is unproven whether delivery improves outcome in respiratory failure. There is limited data to prove whether normal delivery or cesarean section improves the outcome. Normal delivery is reported in mechanically ventilated

Management during Labor and Delivery

Intravenous opioid can be used for labor analgesia in a mechanically ventilated patients who are already receiving opioids for sedation. Lumbar epidural analgesia can be given, if underlying condition and treatment permits. Patient's intravascular volume, coagulation profile, presence of sepsis are all to be looked for before epidural. In mechanically ventilated patients, general anesthesia can be given for cesarean section. Apart from medical management, the anesthetic management is same as in patients without respiratory failure.

patients.[49,50] Normal delivery can also avoid problems associated with intra-abdominal surgery in a critically ill patient.

CONCLUSION

Pregnancy induces multiple changes in body physiology. Basic understanding of this physiology helps one to differentiate and diagnose disease and its management. Managing respiratory diseases needs a team approach for maternal and fetal wellbeing.

Key Points

1. Increase in estrogen during pregnancy leads to increased vascularity and edema of upper respiratory mucosa involving oropharynx, nasopharynx, glottis and arytenoids in pregnancy.
2. Increased tissue friability and edema of mucosal lining increases risk of bleeding while manipulating upper airway, difficult ventilation and intubation of trachea.
3. During gestation, diaphragmatic breathing pattern is more than thoracic. Overall, in pregnancy, chest wall compliance decreases and compliance of lung does not change.
4. In pregnancy, there is overall increase in lung capacity.
5. In pregnancy, there is 20% increase in oxygen consumption.
6. During labor, due to pain, the parturient hyperventilates, which causes respiratory alkalosis and this shifts oxyhemoglobin curve to left. This causes decreased release of oxygen from maternal Hb across placenta, causing fetal hypoxemia.
7. Asthmatic pregnants are approximately 8% in incidence at any given point of time and need special anesthetic attention.
8. In pregnancy with cystic fibrosis, chronic hypoxemia and poor maternal nutrition (due to repeated infections) leads to LBW and preterm labor.

REFERENCES

1. Cheek TG, Gutsche BB. Maternal physiologic alterations. In: Hughes SC, Levinson G, Rosen MA (Eds). Shnider and Levinson Anesthesia for Obstetrics, 4th ed. Philadelphia: Lippincot Williams & Wilkins, 2002, p.3.
2. Gaiser R. Physiologic changes of pregnancy. In: Chestnut DH, Polley LS, Tsen LC, et al (Eds). Chestnut's Obstetric Anesthesia: Principles and Practice, 4th ed. Philadelphia: Elsevier, 2009, p15.
3. Ellegard EK. Pregnancy rhinitis. Immunol Allergy Clinic North America 2006;26:119.
4. Weinberger SE, Weiss ST, Cohen WR, et al. Pregnancy and the lung. American Review Respiratory Disease 1980;121:559.
5. Gilroy RJ, Mangura BT, Lavietes MH. Rib cage and abdominal volume displacements during breathing in pregnancy. Am Rev Respir Dis 1988;137:668–72.
6. Turner AF. The chest radiograph in pregnancy. Clinical Obstet Gynecol 1975;18:65.
7. Thomson K, Cohen M. Studies on the circulation in normal pregnancy: II, Vital capacity observations in normal pregnant women. Surg Gynecol Obstet 1938:66:591.
8. Bonica J. Principles and Practice of obstetric analgesia and anesthesia. Philadelphia: FA Davis CO, 1962.
9. BonicaJJ. Maternal respiratory changes during pregnancy and parturition. Clin Anesth 1974;10: 1–19.
10. Mark GF, Murthy PK, Orlin LR. Static compliance before and after vaginal delivery. Br J Anesth 1970;42:1100–4.
11. Milne JA. The respiratory response to pregnancy. Postgrad Med J 1979;55:318–24.
12. Milne JA, Mills RJ, Howie AD, Pack AI. Large airway function during normal pregnancy. Br J Obstet Gynecol 1977;84:448–51.
13. Mokkpatti R, Prasad EC, Venkatraman, Fatima K. Ventilatory functions in pregnancy. Indian J Physiol Pharmacol 1991;35:237–40.
14. Brancazio LR, Laifer SA, Schwartz T. Peal expiratory flow rate in normal pregnancy. Obstet Gynecol 1997;89:383–6.
15. Baldwin GR, Moorthi DS, Whelton JA, Mac Donnell KF. New lung functions and pregnancy. Am J Obstet Gynecol 1977;127:235–9.
16. Norregaard O, Schultz P, Ostergaard A, Dahl R. Lung function and postural changes in pregnancy. Respir Med 1989;83:467–70.
17. Gee JB, Packer BS, Millen JE, Robin ED. Pulmonary mechanics during pregnancy. J Clin Invest 1967;46:945–52.
18. Bevan DR, Holdcroft A, Loh L, MacGregor WG, O'Sullivan JC, Sykes MK. Closing volume and pregnancy. Br Med J 1974;1:13–5.
19. Russell IF, Chambers WA. Closing volume in normal pregnancy. Br J Anaest 1981;53:1043–7.
20. Powse CM, Gaensler EA. Respiratory and acid base changes during pregnancy. Anesthesiology 1965;26:381–92.

21. Yannone ME, McCurdy JR, Goldfien A. Plasma progesterone levels in normal pregnancy, labor, and the puerperium. II. Clinical data. Am J Obstet Gynecol 1968;101:1058.

22. Liberatore SM, Pistelli R, Patalano F, et al. Respiratory function during pregnancy. Respiration 1984;46:145–50.

23. Pernoll ML, Metcalfe J, Kovach PA, Watchtel R, Dunham MJ. Ventilation during rest and exercise in pregnancy and postpartum. Respir Physiol 1975;25:295–310.

24. Artol R, Wiswell R, Romen Y, Dorey F. Pulmonary responses to exercise in pregnancy. Am J Obstet Gynecol 1986;154:378–83.

25. Lim VS, Katz AI, Lindhelmer MD. Acid base regulation in pregnancy. Am J Physiol 1976;231:1764.

26. Hagedral M, Morgan CW, Summer AE, Gutsche BB. Minute ventilation and oxygen consumption during labor with epidural analgesia. Anesthesiology 1983;59:425–7.

27. Pearson JF, Davies P. The effect of continuous lumbar epidural analgesia on maternal acid base balance and arterial lactate concentration during second stage of labor. J Obstet Gynaecol Br Common 1973;80:225–9.

28. Pearson JF, Davies P. The effect of continuous lumbar epidural analgesia on acid base status of maternal blood during first stage of labor. J Obstet Gynaecol Br Common 1973;80:218–24.

29. Robert Gaiser. Physiological changes of pregnacy. In: Davis H Chestnut, Cythiawong, Lawrence C Tsen, et al (Eds). Chestnut's Obstetric Anesthesia: Principles and Practice, 5th ed. Philadelphia: Elsevier, 2014.

30. Graves, CR. Acute pulmonary complications in pregnancy. In: Fink, MP, Abraham, E, Vincent, J, Kochanek, PM (Eds). Textbook of Critical Care. Philadelphia: Elsevier, 2005, p.1551.

31. Gilbert R, Auchincloss JH Jr. Dyspnea of pregnancy. Clinical and physiological observations. Am J Med Sci 1966;252:270–6.

32. Milne JA, Howie AD, Pack AI. Dyspnoea during normal pregnancy. Br J Obstet Gynaecol 1978;85:260–3.

33. Tenholder MF, South-Paul JE. Dyspnea in pregnancy. Chest 1989;96:381–8.

34. Zeldis SM. Dyspnea during pregnancy. Distinguishing cardiac from pulmonary causes. Clin Chest Med 1992;13:567–85.

35. Stevenson DD, Szczeklik A. Clinical and pathologic perspectives on aspirin sensitivity and asthma. J Allergy Clin Immunol 2006;118(4): 773–86.

36. Arif M Seyal. The pregnant patient with asthma. In: Meric Gershwin, Timothy E. Albertson (Eds). Bronchial Asthma: A Guide for Practical Understanding and Treatment, 5th ed, p. 207.

37. Carlisle AS. Perioperative management of the pregnant patient with asthma. In: Hughes SC (Ed). Shnider and Levinson's Anesthesia for Obstetrics. Philadelphia, Lippincott Williams & Wilkins; 2001, p.487.

38. Murphy VE, Gibson P, Talbot PI, et al. Severe asthma exacerbations during pregnancy. Obstet Gynecol 2005;106(5 pt 1):1046–54.

39. Stenius-Aarniala BS, Hedman J, Teramo KA. Acute asthma during pregnancy. Thorax 1996;51: 411–4.

40. Hanania NA, Belfort MA. Acute asthma in pregnancy. Crit Care Med 2005;33:5319–24.

41. Que JC, Lusaya VO. Sevoflurane induction for emergency cesarean section in a parturient in status asthmaticus. Anesthesiology 1999;90: 1475–76.

42. Ng M, Freeman MK, Fleming TD, et al. Smoking Prevalence and Cigarette Consumption in 187 Countries, 1980–2012. JAMA 2014;311(2):183–92.

43. Saeed Z, Wojewodka G, Marion D, Guilbault C, Radzioch D. Novel pharmaceutical approaches for treating patients with cystic fibrosis. Curr Pharm Des 2007;13(31):3252–63.

44. McArdle JR, Talwalkar JS. Macrolides in cystic fibrosis. Clin Chest Med 2007;28(2):347–60.

45. Rush D, Johnstone FD, King JC. Nutrition ang Pregnancy. In: Burrow GN, Ferris TF (Eds). Medical Complications in Pregnancy, 3rd ed. Philadelphia: Saunders,1988, pp.117–35.

46. Mabie WC, Barton JR, Sibai BM. Adult respiratory distress syndrome in pregnancy. Am J Obstet Gynecol 1992;167:950–7.

47. Fowler AA, Hamman RF, Zerbe GO, et al. Adult respiratory distress syndrome: prognosis after onset. Am Rev Respir Dis 1985;132:472–8.

48. Montgomery AB, Stager MA, Carrico CJ, et al. Causes of mortality in patient with adult respiratory distress syndrome. Am Rev Respir Dis 1985;132:485–9.

49. Jenkins TM, Troiano NH, Graves CR, et al. Mechanical ventilation in an obstetric population: Characteristics and delivery rates. Am J Obstet Gynecol 2003;188:549–52.

50. Pacheco LD, Gei AF, VanHook JW, et al. Burns in pregnancy. Obstet Gynecol 2005;106:1210–2.

CHAPTER 3

Essentials of Physiological Changes of Pregnancy in Cardiovascular System

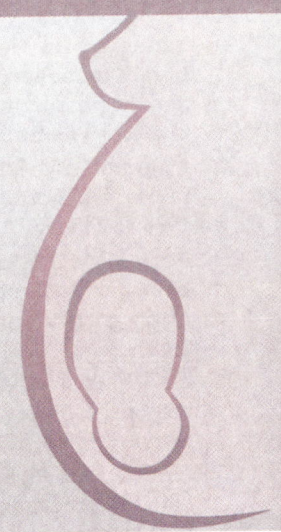

Charulata Deshpande, Ashish Mali

Physiological changes occur in almost each and every organ system of the body during pregnancy. The changes in cardiovascular system during pregnancy and labor are significant and while majority of women tolerate them well, a previously undiagnosed pregnant patient may decompensate and managing such patient can be a nightmare for the attending anesthesiologist.

INTRODUCTION

The physiological changes in cardiovascular system in pregnancy occur in response to and to adapt to the increasing metabolic demands of the mother and the fetus.

The enlarging uterus, the growing fetus and placenta, changes in peripheral tissues such as the growing breasts, new fat and protein deposition increase the metabolic needs of the mother.

Increased hormonal secretion from the ovaries and placenta (estrogen, progesterone, relaxin) and endorphins directly or indirectly contribute towards the physiological changes in the cardiovascular system.

The act of labor further increases the cardiac work load and demands on the cardiovascular system.

During early to mid-pregnancy, the changes in cardiovascular system are more of physiological in nature whereas during mid and late pregnancy, the mechanical pressure from the enlarging uterus also leads to anatomical changes by affecting the heart position.

CLINICAL EXAMINATION OF CARDIOVASCULAR SYSTEM

Characteristic changes are noticed during the clinical examination and investigations of the cardiovascular system during pregnancy. Some of them mimic the signs and symptoms of a cardiac disease.

History

- History of dyspnea on exertion (DOE)
- History of easy fatiguability
- History of palpitations
- History of edema feet

Examination[1]

- Tachycardia
- Sharp full bounding/collapsing pulse
- Normal systolic blood pressure with slightly lower diastolic blood pressure
- Apex impulse and apex beat shifts cephalad to 4th left intercostal space and leftwards
- Accentuation of first heart sound (S1)
- Accentuated splitting of mitral and tricuspid components of S1
- Third heart sound (S3) may be heard in third trimester
- Fourth heart sound (S4) is heard in 16% pregnant women in third trimester and is not of clinical significance.
- Grade I or II ejection systolic murmur over tricuspid area is common. This is a benign flow murmur due to dilatation of tricuspid annulus resulting in tricuspid regurgitation. Dilatation of tricuspid annulus results from increased right ventricular chamber size due to increased preload.
- Continuous murmur from venous hum or mammary souffle.

XRC Findings

Heart appears enlarged on X-ray chest PA view as heart is pushed upwards, leftward and anteriorly.

In X-ray chest lateral view, the most common finding is slight prominence of pulmonary conus and slight left atrial enlargement.

ECG Findings[2–4]

- Sinus tachycardia
- Small right axis deviation in first trimester followed by small left axis deviation in third trimester
- Shortened PR interval and shortened uncorrected QT interval
- Transient depressed ST segment
- Inversion or flattening of T wave in standard lead III and isoelectric low voltage T waves in left-sided limb leads and precordial leads
- Atrial premature contractions and ventricular premature contractions
- Less frequently, atrial arrhythmias may be present due to atrial enlargement.

Clinical Application

Pregnant women with 'long QT syndrome' have reduced risk of adverse cardiac events during pregnancy (risk ratio of 0.38) while the risk increases in postpartum period (risk ratio of 2.7) suggesting that postpartum period is associated with prolonged QT interval.[2] The incidence of adverse cardiac events such as syncope or sudden death can occur following delivery in 9th month.

Beta-blockers reduce the incidence of cardiac events during the high-risk postpartum period.[2]

Echocardiography Findings[5–7]

- Left ventricular hypertrophy
- Increased left ventricular wall thickness
- Increased left ventricular end diastolic volume
- Normal left ventricular end systolic volume
- Increased left ventricular ejection fraction
- Dilatation of tricuspid, pulmonary and mitral valve annulus with no change in aortic annulus
- Tricuspid and pulmonary regurgitation is observed in 94% pregnant women while mitral regurgitation is seen in 27% pregnant women.
- Mild pericardial effusion may be seen.

The cardiovascular changes in pregnancy often mimic heart disease on clinical examination, and it is important for the anesthesiologist to differentiate between the pathological findings of a heart disease from the physiological changes of pregnancy.

Hallmarks of a Cardiac Disease

- DOE of >grade II
- Systolic murmur of higher grade (grade III and IV)
- Presence of a diastolic murmur is always pathognomonic of heart disease
- Severe dysrhythmias
- Cardiac enlargement which is unequivocal in nature on X-ray chest and 2D echo-cardiography.
- Increase in central venous pressure, pulmonary artery diastolic pressure and pulmonary capillary wedge pressure.

> *Points to remember*
> The incidence of adverse cardiac events, such as syncope or sudden death, can occur following delivery in 9th month in patients with long QT interval.

PHYSIOLOGICAL CHANGES IN CARDIO-VASCULAR SYSTEM (Table 3.1, Figs 3.1 and 3.2)

The physiological changes in the cardio-vascular system ensure that adequate amount of oxygenated and nutrient-rich blood is delivered to the growing fetus, uterus and other peripheral organs. These physiological changes occur in all components of the cardiovascular system: the preload (the circulating blood volume), the heart (myocardial contractility and function), the afterload (systemic vascular resistance), heart rate and less frequently heart rhythm and the neuro-hormonal system.

Circulating Blood Volume: Hypervolemia of Pregnancy[8–11]

The circulating blood volume begins to increase from the 6th gestational week. The blood volume increases progressively throughout the first and second trimester. There is some debate over the increase in blood volume during third trimester with some studies indicating that the increase in blood volume plateaus in third trimester while others indicate a continuous progressive increase.

The circulating blood volume reaches approximately 50% more than the prepregnant value by 32–34 weeks of gestation. The increase in blood volume is significantly more in twin or multiple pregnancies.

The red blood cell mass increases by 20–30% and the plasma volume increases by 40–50%. This disproportionate increase in plasma volume results in hemodilution or physiological anemia of pregnancy.

This increase in blood volume is responsible for 1–2 kg weight gain in the mother and the enlarged capacity of the uteroplacental, breast, renal, striated muscle and cutaneous vascular systems accommodates it.

The preload to the heart is increased as a larger blood volume is delivered to the ventricle. Echocardiography in normal

Table 3.1: Physiological changes in CVS during pregnancy

Parameter	Pregnancy	Labor	Postpartum	Peak % change during pregnancy	Peak time frame during pregnancy
Heart rate	↑	↑	↓	Increases by 15–25%	32 weeks
Systolic blood pressure	↓	↑	↑	Minimal	28 weeks
Diastolic blood pressure	↓	↑	↑	Decreases by 5–20%	28 weeks
Cardiac output	↑	↑	↓	Increases by 40–50%	28 weeks
Stroke volume	↑	↑	↓	Increases by 30–35%	32 weeks
Systemic vascular resistance	↓	↑	↑	Decreases by 15–20%	32 weeks
Blood volume	↑	↑	↓	Increases by 40–50%	32–34 weeks

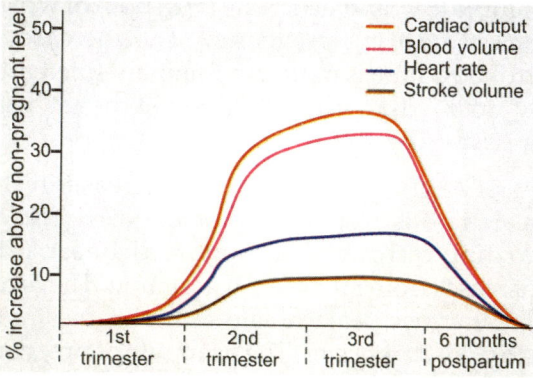

Fig. 3.1. Physiological changes in cardiovascular parameters in pregnancy

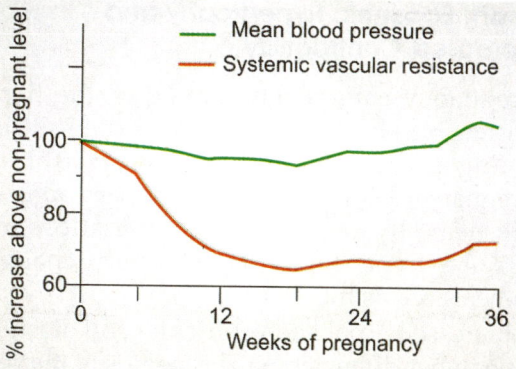

Fig. 3.2. Physiological changes depicting mean blood pressure and systemic vascular resistance with reference to pregnant and non-pregnant state

pregnancy shows an increase in the left ventricular end-diastolic volume as early as 10th week of gestation and peak values during third trimester. Increase in the diastolic dimensions of left atrium, right atrium and right ventricle is also seen.

The increased blood volume facilitates the transfer of respiratory gases, nutrients and products of metabolism between maternal and fetal circulation. It also compensates for the maternal blood loss during delivery which can be approximately 500 mL during vaginal delivery and 1000 mL during cesarean section by autotransfusion of blood during uterine contraction.

The various mechanisms postulated to be responsible for bringing about the increase in blood volume are:

• Increased estrogen levels leading to increased plasma renin levels which in turn leads to sodium and water retention.

• Increased total body water resulting from fluid retention: Increased circulating levels of various pregnancy hormones (prolactin, placental lactogen) as well as growth hormone and prostaglandins are responsible for fluid retention.

• Alterations in the metabolism of vasopressin

• Decreased osmotic threshold for thirst

• Increased erythropoietin levels which increase circulating red blood cell volume.

The circulating blood volume decreases by 10% within the first 3 days following delivery and continues to decrease over the next few weeks to reach pre-pregnant value by 6–9 weeks after delivery.

Clinical pearl

In a normal pregnant woman, cardiac filling pressures (central venous pressure and pulmonary artery wedge pressure) do not increase in spite of distention of cardiac chambers from the increased circulating blood volume. This is due to the fact that the normal heart is capable of adapting to the chronic volume overload of pregnancy.

However, in pregnant women with stenotic valvular lesions (mitral or aortic stenosis), dilated cardiomyopathy or pulmonary hypertension, the heart is not capable of handling volume overload and these women can decompensate any time during pregnancy usually at around 32–34 weeks of pregnancy when the circulating blood volume levels peak.

In pregnant women with hypertrophic obstructive cardiomyopathy, increased preload and cardiac chamber distention may reduce the left ventricular outflow tract obstruction and improve cardiac output and hemodynamic status of the patient.

Heart: Eccentric Hypertrophy and Increased Contractility[12–14]

Pregnancy causes remodeling of the heart which has been compared to the similar changes seen in the heart of an athlete. Pregnancy leads to eccentric hypertrophy of the heart by both chamber dilatation and chamber hypertrophy. The structural changes in heart are as follows:

- Increased atrial and ventricular end diastolic chamber dimensions: This begins in the first trimester and continues till the end of third trimester.
- Increased left ventricular muscle mass: It increases by 23% by third trimester and 50% by term.
- Increased left ventricular wall thickness.
- Increased left ventricular end-diastolic volume and normal end-systolic volume.
- Increased myocardial contractility resulting in greater left ventricular ejection fraction.
- Increased annulus diameters of mitral, tricuspid and pulmonary valves.

The eccentric cardiac hypertrophy results from both increased stretch on the ventricular wall by the increased circulating blood volume and by hypertrophy of cardiac myosites due to pregnancy hormones.

By mid-pregnancy, the enlarging uterus causes upward displacement of diaphragm due to which heart shifts upwards, anteriorly and towards left. This shift in the anatomical position of heart along with eccentric hypertrophy leads to various changes in clinical findings of assessment of heart as discussed earlier.

The structural changes in the heart are reversible and the heart rapidly returns to prepregnant status within 3–6 months postpartum.

Cardiac Output[15,16]

Cardiac output is the simplest and most commonly measured parameter of systolic myocardial function or contractility of the heart. Cardiac output is a product of stroke volume (SV) and heart rate (HR) both of which increase during pregnancy. The increase in stroke volume is more predominant (increases by 35%) than the increase in heart rate (increases by 15%).

Heart rate and rhythm: The increase in the heart rate is responsible for the early rise in cardiac output. The maternal heart rate increases from 5th week of gestation. The heart rate increase peaks at late second trimester to early third trimester. The heart rate of pregnant woman at term is 10–12 beats higher than baseline heart rate.

Although most pregnant women maintain sinus rhythm, premature atrial and ventricular beats are frequently seen.

The heart rate decreases soon after delivery and returns to pre-pregnancy value by two weeks.

> **Clinical pearl**
> Pregnancy may increase the incidence of supra-ventricular and ventricular arrhythmias in women with a previous history of the same and these women are at increased risk of adverse cardiac events during pregnancy.

Stroke volume: The stroke volume increases progressively from 5th–8th week of pregnancy and is responsible for the sustained increase in cardiac output.

The increase in stroke volume is the result of decreased afterload (systemic vascular resistance), increased left ventricular muscle mass and contractility in addition to the increased left ventricular end diastolic volume.

Cardiac output: During pregnancy, cardiac output increases by about 40–50%. First increase in the cardiac output is noted at the 5th gestational week. Cardiac output in pregnant woman increases by 30–40% by the end of first trimester. The increase in cardiac output continues throughout the first and second trimester till it reaches 50% by the end of second trimester and maximum prelabor cardiac output level is reached at around 28 weeks of pregnancy.

Cardiac output increases over and above the prelabor value during labor and delivery. Cardiac output increases above the prelabor value by 15% during first or latent stage, by 30% during the second or active stage and by 45% during the expulsive stage of labor. Cardiac output increases by an additional 10–25% with each uterine contraction. The labor and immediate postpartum period is associated with further increase in cardiac output due to:

- Increased sympathetic stimulation due to anxiety and pain but more importantly due to
- Autotransfusion of 300–500 mL of blood into the central circulation with each uterine contraction.

Cardiac output increases by as much as 60–80% above prelabor value immediately after delivery of fetus due to:

- Relief of aortocaval compression
- Autotransfusion of blood via contracting uterus.

Cardiac output returns to prelabor value within one hour and below prelabor value within 24 hours. Cardiac output returns to prepregnancy value after as long as 12 weeks postpartum.

Pregnant women with stenotic valvular lesions, such as mitral stenosis or aortic stenosis, are at higher risk of decompensation at any time during pregnancy and most commonly at around 28 weeks of gestation when the prelabor cardiac output reaches peak. Increased sympathetic stimulation and autotransfusion of large volume of blood from the contracting uterus during labor and

---

Clinical pearl

Increased cardiac output increases the cardiac workload. Most healthy pregnant patients with good cardiac reserve can tolerate this increase in cardiac output without any adverse events. However, pregnant women with fixed cardiac output conditions or who require elevated filling pressures to increase cardiac output may decompensate from right-sided or left-sided heart failure.

---

immediately postpartum may precipitate cardiac decompensation in a pregnant woman who has tolerated the increased cardiac output till 28 weeks of pregnancy. Inability to increase the cardiac output to the required level in these pregnant women may also lead to adverse fetal events such as IUGR.

The increase in cardiac output along with reduced colloid osmotic pressure seen in pregnancy makes these patients susceptible to pulmonary edema at delivery or in the postpartum period. If associated with pre-eclampsia, the risk of pulmonary edema is even greater from increased pulmonary capillary permeability. Therefore, intravenous fluids should be administered extremely judiciously in these patients.

These patients benefit from labor analgesia as the pain and anxiety-induced sympathetic system stimulation is attenuated.

Increased cardiac workload with resultant increased myocardial oxygen requirement may induce myocardial ischemia in pregnant woman with coronary artery disease.

There is increased risk of aortic dissection from increased blood volume, cardiac output and pregnancy induced hormonal changes in pregnant woman with Marfan syndrome.

Afterload: Increased Systemic Vascular Compliance and Decreased Systemic Vascular Resistance

Fall in the systemic vascular resistance (SVR) is the very first physiological change noticed in the cardiovascular system of a pregnant patient beginning at the 5 weeks of gestation. SVR decreases by 20% during pregnancy and is at its lowest between 20 and 32 weeks of gestation. Studies have shown that the SVR decreases from 1,530 dyn s/cm^5 to 1,210 dyn s/cm^5 during pregnancy. After 32 weeks, SVR slowly increases till term. SVR increases by 30% within 2 weeks postpartum.

The decreased SVR is the result of:

- Increased production of potent vaso-dilator—prostacyclin

- Progesterone-mediated vascular smooth muscle relaxation
- Low resistance uteroplacental circulation (systemic circulation is in parallel with uteroplacental circulation. By law of resistance the total resistance will be lower than the individual resistance.)
- Physiological anemia of pregnancy: decreased viscosity of blood

The pulmonary vascular resistance decreases by 30% during pregnancy by the same mechanisms.

Blood Pressure[17]

The systemic ventricular afterload can be approximated by measuring arterial systolic pressure in a normal pregnant patient.

The blood pressure in a pregnant patient is affected by maternal age, gestational age, parity and positioning. Blood pressure increases with maternal age. Nulliparous woman has higher blood pressure than parous woman of the same age. The systolic, mean and diastolic blood pressure in a normal pregnant woman decreases from first trimester to mid-pregnancy corresponding to decrease in SVR. The fall in diastolic pressure is more than the fall in systolic pressure. The diastolic pressure falls by 20% at mid-pregnancy. The syncopal episodes during the first trimester are usually attributed to the fall in blood pressure. Blood pressure is highest in supine position and lowest in lateral position when measured in brachial artery.

Blood pressure increases during labor above the prelabor value and there is further increase with each uterine contraction due to increased cardiac output.

The systolic and diastolic blood pressure remains at late pregnancy value till 12 weeks postpartum after which it increases to prepregnancy value.

The decrease in SVR along with increase in cardiac output increases blood flow in multiple vascular beds. Uterine blood flow increases from a baseline of 50 mL/min to more than 500 mL/min at term. This ensures adequate perfusion in the intervillous spaces of placenta. Renal blood flow increases by 60–80% by the third trimester with 50% increase in the glomerular filtration rate. Blood flow to the extremities increases with a three to four times increase in the cutaneous blood flow. This results in warm and erythematous hands and feet. Increased blood flow to nasal mucosa leads to nasal congestion and occasional nose bleeds. Blood flow to mucosa of airway is increased and leads to increased susceptibility to airway edema. Increased mammary blood flow leads to engorged breasts, dilatation of superficial veins and presence of continuous murmur over breasts called as mammary soufflé.

Increased peripheral vascular compliance leads to sluggish peripheral venous blood flow, this along with hypercoagulable state of pregnancy increases the risk of deep venous thrombosis. The absorption of intramuscular or subcutaneously administered drugs is also delayed.

> **Clinical pearl**
> In pregnant patients with regurgitant valve lesions, the decrease in afterload helps to reduce the severity of regurgitation.

However, in pregnant women with right to left shunt such as cyanotic heart disease or Eisenmenger syndrome, the fall in SVR causes the right to left shunt to increase during pregnancy leading to increased cyanosis, packed cell volume and hypoxemia. Fetal perfusion suffers with increased risk of fetal adverse effects including fetal loss.

AORTOCAVAL COMPRESSION IN PREGNANCY[18–22] (Fig. 3.3)

During pregnancy, as the size of the gravid uterus increases, there is anatomical compression of the inferior vena cava (IVC) and abdominal aorta. The degree of compression of the inferior vena cava and aorta is proportional to the gestational week of pregnancy and position of the pregnant woman.

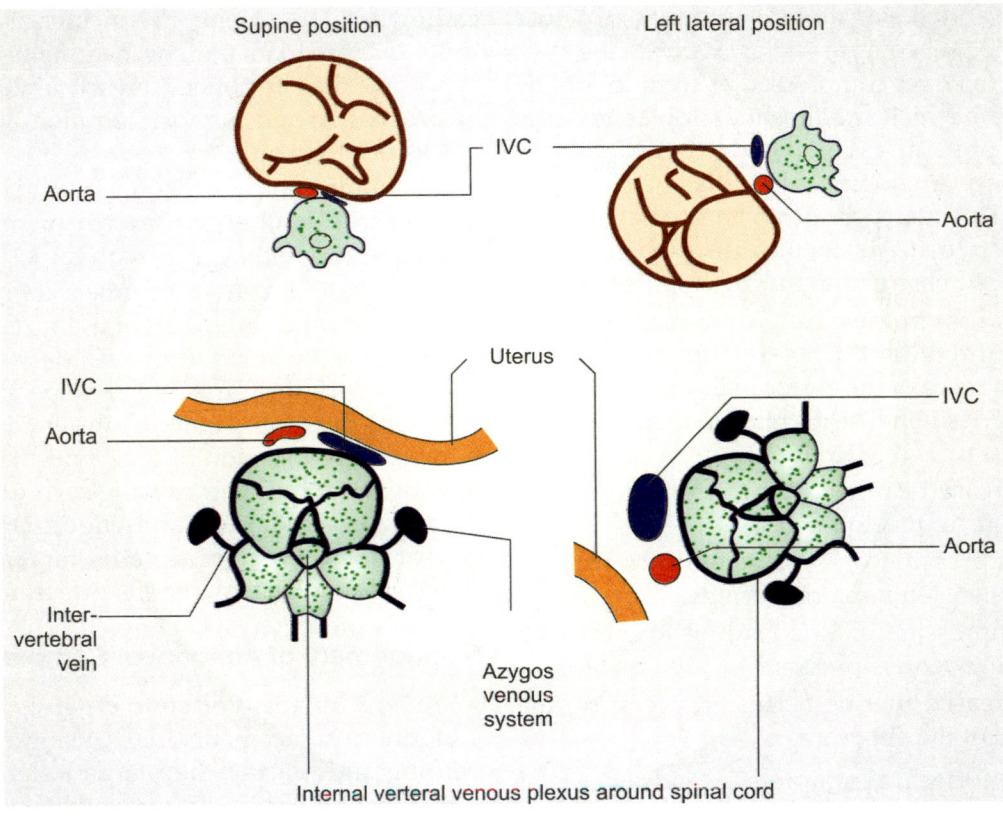

Fig. 3.3. Aortocaval compression in pregnancy

The compression of inferior vena cava begins as early as 13 to 16 weeks of pregnancy. It has been shown that at 13–16 weeks of pregnancy, the femoral venous pressure decreases by 50% in supine. As the size of the gravid uterus increases, the compression of the IVC increases. At term, near total compression of IVC takes place in supine position and partial compression in lateral position as seen by imaging studies. There is 2.5 times increased pressure in femoral vein and lower inferior vana cava in pregnant woman in supine position than in non-pregnant woman at term while in lateral position, the value is 75% above the non-pregnant value.

The decreased venous return to the heart results in lower right atrial filling pressures. This leads to a 10–24% decrease in stroke volume and cardiac output, 20% decrease in blood supply to uterus, and 50% decrease in blood supply to lower limbs in supine position at term.

During caval compression, the venous blood from lower extremity passes to the heart through the alternative venous pathways formed by intraosseous vertebral veins, paravertebral veins and epidural veins draining into azygos vein. This collateral circulation is not as efficient as circulation through IVC leading to lower right atrial pressure in supine position. However, the collateral circulation maintains the right ventricular filling pressure which is relatively unaltered in lateral position. In most unanesthetized women, there is compensatory increased sympathetic tone which leads to increased SVR and heart rate on assuming supine position. This compensatory mechanism gets attenuated or abolished under anesthesia leading to precipitous hypotension.

The aorta being a more muscular structure does not get compressed as easily as the IVC. Aorta may get compressed at term in supine position which manifests as lower femoral artery pressure as compared to brachial artery pressure. Angiographic studies have shown partial obstruction of aorta at the level of lumbar lordosis in supine position and enhanced obstruction during hypotension.

Fetal hypoxia from decreased utero-placental blood flow is the deleterious consequence of the aortocaval compression in supine position. The decrease in uteroplacental blood flow is due to:

- Decreased cardiac output from decreased venous return to the heart
- Compression of aorta leading to arterial hypotension in uterine arteries
- Compression of IVC leading to increased uterine venous pressure
- Decreased uterine perfusion pressure due to all of the above

The aortocaval compression ends once fetal head gets fixed.

Supine Hypotension Syndrome

The group of symptoms such as sweating, pallor, nausea, vomiting, bradycardia, hypotension and mental changes seen in a pregnant patient on assuming supine position is termed as supine hypotension syndrome. This is due to aortocaval compression in supine position leading to exaggerated fall in venous return which cannot be compensated by the

Clinical pearl

Suspicion, prevention, recognition and management of aortocaval compression are critical for safe fetal and maternal management. Anesthesia drugs and techniques which reduce SVR cause decrease in venous return to the heart over and above the decreased venous return due to IVC compression. Central neuraxial block abolishes the vasoconstriction in response to the reduced venous return. Both these can lead to precipitous hypotension in a pregnant woman in supine position.

cardiovascular system. The incidence is seen in 10–15% pregnant patients nearing term. The syndrome may be noticed as early as 20 weeks of pregnancy and is most common at 36–38 weeks of pregnancy.

The syndrome is more common and marked in pregnant women with twin or multiple pregnancy as well as polyhydramnios.

The collateral venous channels comprising of paravertebral, intervertebral and epidural veins divert the blood from IVC to the azygos vein which drains directly into superior vena cava and thus into right atrium. Inadvertent intravascular injection of local anesthetic can directly reach the heart causing severe cardiac depression. Dilatation and engorgement of epidural, paravertebral veins increase the chance of inadvertent venous puncture.

Management of Aortocaval Compression

- Prevent aortocaval compression by left uterine displacement (LUD) using manual lifting and placing the uterus to left or by 15° table tilt or by a 15 cm wedge under the right hip. It has been noted that the placental intervillous perfusion is better with LUD than right uterine displacement.
- Rapid treatment of hypotension by adminis-tration of intravenous fluids and vaso-pressors like phenylephrine and ephedrine to avoid fetal hypoxia.
- Oxygen supplementation

Ankle edema, varicose veins and hemor-rhoids are side effects of IVC compression in pregnancy.

NEUROHORMONAL SYSTEM

Vascular tone in a pregnant patient is more dependent on and sensitive to sympathetic nervous system regulation than in a non-pregnant woman. There is down regulation of alpha and beta receptors in pregnancy. Pregnant women are more dependent on sympathetic nervous system for stable hemodynamics and this dependence increases as the pregnancy progresses and peaks at term.

There is also parasympathetic deactivation near term which results in increased heart rate and cardiac output at rest. Depression of baroreceptor reflexes due to complex hormonal interaction makes pregnant patients more hypotension prone. The result is that conditions causing sympathetic blockade such as central neuraxial block result in more marked and rapid fall in blood pressure.

Fall in peripheral vascular resistance during pregnancy activate the baroreceptors in pregnant woman. Activated baroreceptors in turn stimulate rennin-angiotensin-aldosterone system, sympathetic nervous system and natriuretic peptide system in pregnancy. The circulating levels of angiotensin II is also increased.

Hemodynamic changes of pregnancy return slowly to baseline value and this may take 6 months after delivery.

SUMMARY

The physiological changes are well tolerated by women without heart disease but in women with heart disease these changes can lead to heart failure, arrhythmias and high risk of death from cardiac decompensation. A previously unrecognized heart disease may become evident first time during pregnancy. It is extremely important for the anesthesiologist to know and understand these physiological changes of pregnancy and labor so that appropriate analgesia and anesthesia is provided for a safe mother and fetal outcome.

REFERENCES

1. Cutforth R, MacDonald C. Heart sound and murmurs in pregnancy. American Heart journal 1966;71:741–7.
2. Shotan A, Ostrzega E, Mehra A. Incidences of arrhythmias in normal pregnancy and relation to palpitation, dizziness, and syncope. American Journal Cardiology 1997;79:1061–4.
3. Seth R, Moss A, McNitt S, et al. Long QT syndrome and pregnancy. Journal of American Coll Cardiol 2007;49:1009–18.
4. Carruth JE, Mivis SB, Brogan DR, Wenger NK. The electrocardiogram in normal pregnancy. Am Heart J 1981;102:1075–8.
5. Campos O, Andrade JL, Bocanera J, et al. Physiologic multivalvular regurgitation during pregnancy: a longitudinal Doppler echocardiographic study. Int Cardiol 1993;40:265–72.
6. Rubler S, Damani PM, Pinto ER. Cardiac size and performance during pregnancy estimated with echocardiography. Am J Cardiol 1977;40:534–40.
7. Fox WY, Chan LY, Wong JT, et al. Left ventricular diastolic function during pregnancy: Assesment by spectral tissue doppler imaging. Ultrasound Obstet Gynecol 2006;28:789–93.
8. Pritchard J. Changes in blood volume during pregnancy and delivery. Anaesthesiology 1965;26:393–9.
9. Popas A, Shroff S. Korkarz C. Serial assessment of the cardiovascular system in normal pregnancy. Role of arterial compliance and pulsatile arterial load. Circulation 1997;95(10):2407–2415.
10. Rovinsky JJ, Jaffin H. Cardiovascular haemodynamics in pregnancy. I. Blood and plasma volumes in multiple pregnancy. Am J Obstet Gynecol 1965;93:1–15.
11. Lund CJ, Donavan JC. Blood volume during pregnancy. Significance of plasma and red cell volumes. Am J Obstet Gynecol 1967;98:394–403.
12. Capeless EL, Clapp JF. Cardiovascular changes in early phases of pregnancy. Am J Obstet Gynecol 1989;16:1449–53.
13. Eghbali M, Wang Y, Toro L, Stefani E. Heart hypertrophy during pregnancy: A better functioning heart? Trends Cardiovasc Med 2006;16:285–91.
14. Shannwell CM, Schneppenhein M, Zimmerman T, et al. Left ventricular hypertrophy and diastolic dysfunction in healthy pregnant women. Cardiology 2002;97:73–8.
15. Robson SC, Hunter S, Boys RJ, Dunlop W. Serial study of factors influencing changes in cardiac output during human pregnancy. Am J Physiol 1989;256:H1060–5.
16. Robson SC, Dunlop W, Boys RJ, Hunter S. Cardiac output during Labour. British Med J 1987;295:1169–72.
17. Iwaski R, Ohkuch A, Furuta I, et al. Relationship between blood pressure level in early pregnancy and subsequent changes in blood pressure during pregnancy. Acta Obstet Gynecol Scand 2002;81:918–25.

18. Bieniarz I, Crottogini J, Curachet E. Aortocaval compression by the uterus in late human pregnancy. Am J Obstet Gynecol 1968;100:203–17.

19. Ueland K, Hansen J. Maternal cardiovascular dynamics. II. Posture and uterine contractions. Am J Obstet Gynaecol 1969;103:1–7.

20. Howard B, Goodson J, Mengert W. Supine hypotension syndrome in late pregnancy. Obstet Gynaecol 1953;1:371–7.

21. Kim Y, Chandra P, Marx G. Succesful management of severe aortocaval compression in twin pregnancy. Obstet Gynecol 1975;46:362–4.

22. Kinsella SM, Lohmann G. Supine hypotension syndrome. Obste Gynecol 1994;83:774–88.

23. Shnider and Levinson. Anesthesia for Obstetrics, 5th ed. Wolters Kluwer, Lippincott Williams and Wilkins. 2013, pp. 1–6.

24. David H Chestnut, Linda S Polley, Lawrence C Tsen, Cynthia A Wong. Chestnut Anesthesia Principles and Practice, 4th ed. Mosby Elsevier Publisher. 2009, pp. 16–19.

25. Celia Oakley, Carole A Warnes. Heart Disease in Pregnancy, 2nd ed. Blackwell Publishing. 2007.

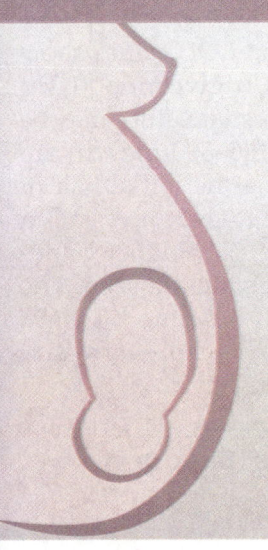

Essentials of Physiological Changes of Pregnancy in Hepatic, Renal, Gastrointestinal and Endocrine Systems

Sarita Fernandes, Chinmayi Patkar

PREGNANCY AND LIVER FUNCTION

The anesthesiologist has to bear in mind certain physiological and biochemical changes that occur in the hepatobiliary system; these have an impact on the course of anesthesia management.

Anatomic Changes

The gravid uterus tends to shift the liver upwards and posteriorly but the liver size and morphology remains almost the same as in the non-pregnant state. The cardiac output increases by 40% during pregnancy but the blood flow to the liver does not change significantly.[1] A slight increase in the diameter of the portal vein and its blood flow is noted.

Biochemical Changes

Serum alanine and aspartate aminotransferase levels remain within the normal limits fixed for non-pregnant women. Therefore, the measurement of serum aminotransferase levels is preferred for the routine diagnosis of liver diseases during pregnancy. Placental production of alkaline phosphatase (ALP) can cause maternal serum ALP levels to rise by 200 to 400%. Raised ALP can also occur in HELLP syndrome, liver or bone disease, intrahepatic cholestasis,[2] etc. Certain liver enzymes, such as lactate dehydrogenase (LDH), glucose-6-phosphatase dehydrogenase (G-6-PD) and amino levulinic acid synthetase, show enhanced activities usually after the fifth month of gestation. Serum 5' nucleotidase activity increases slightly in the second and third trimesters. There is an increase in liver ribonucleic acid content whereas gamma glutamyl transpeptidase (GGT) levels either fall slightly or remain the same. The total bile acid concentrations during pregnancy are not different from non-pregnant women. Serum bilirubin values are lower as compared to non-pregnant women during all three trimesters. Albumin is the significant transport protein for bilirubin and hemodilution during pregnancy may explain the lowered bilirubin levels.[1]

A 25–30% drop in plasma cholinesterase activity is observed from the tenth week of pregnancy up to sixth week postpartum.[3] Enzyme levels may be reduced to 33% of the non-pregnant state on the third postpartum day. Hemodilution and reduced hepatic synthesis are contributory factors. This may be a cause for concern in patients with HELLP syndrome as more than 60% have below normal pseudocholinesterase activity. There is usually no need to adjust the succinylcholine dosage in fit parturients as sensitivity to succinylcholine is not seen until enzyme function reduces by 50%.

Plasma Proteins

The serum albumin to globulin ratio changes during pregnancy. Consequent to the expansion in plasma volume, albumin levels drop by 20–30% and remain low until six to seven weeks postpartum while serum globulin values marginally increase. The decrease in plasma protein concentration leads to a drop in colloid oncotic pressure. Alpha 2-macroglobulin, alpha 1-antitrypsin, and ceruloplasmin levels increase. Pregnancy is a thrombogenic state as evidenced by increased levels of coagulation factors (II, VIII, IX and XII) and fibrinogen. Also protein S levels decrease and fibrinolysis is inhibited.[1] These adaptations help limit the bleeding during childbirth but predispose to thromboembolism during pregnancy and the postpartum period.

Clinical pearl

Decreased serum albumin levels can result in elevated free blood levels of highly protein bound drugs, hence appropriate dose reduction of highly protein bound drugs is warranted during pregnancy. Prothrombin time can be used as a diagnostic and prognostic indicator of liver disease as it does not undergo any variation in the pregnant state.

Lipid Profile

The hyperlipidemic state associated with pregnancy is beneficial as it enables efficient glucose delivery to the fetus.[1] The altered lipid profile is not associated with increased risk of atherosclerosis in normal parturients. In women with pre-existing hyperlipidemia, there is a possibility of temporary deterioration of their lipid profiles as they have to stop the HMG CoA reductase inhibitors during pregnancy.[4]

The total cholesterol and LDL values show a 50–60% rise. Increased triglyceride (TGL) levels up to 2–3 times the usual values may be seen and term levels of 200–300 mg/dL are considered normal. During the initial half of gestation, HDL levels are higher, they fall in the second half and by term 15% higher values than in the non-pregnant state are seen. The TGL levels come back to baseline by eight weeks after delivery but the cholesterol and LDL levels remain elevated.

Clinical Evaluation of Liver Disease in Pregnancy

Symptoms, like nausea, vomiting and pruritus, are common to pregnancy and hepatic disorders. Clinical signs of liver disease, such as spider nevi and palmar erythema, may occur during normal pregnancy thereby masking the diagnosis of liver disease. The full term gravid uterus makes palpation of the liver difficult. When nausea or vomiting persists beyond the first trimester, pathologic conditions should be ruled out and specific investigations like serum aminotransferases performed. It should be borne in mind that jaundice and generalized pruritus are never considered as normal features in pregnancy.

Clinical pearl

Any elevations of serum transaminases, bilirubin, and prothrombin time (PT) indicate a pathologic state during pregnancy and deserve further detailed evaluation.

Biliary Changes

Pregnant women, especially during the second and third trimesters, display an increased frequency of gallstones. Decreased gallbladder evacuation, increased cholesterol levels, impaired transport of bile acids, decrease in the contractile response to cholecystokinin, inhibition of cholecystokinin release from the intestinal mucosa by progesterone are all contributory factors.

Laboratory Values of Liver Function Tests in Non-pregnant and Pregnant		
Hepatic parameter	**Non-pregnant**	**Pregnant**
Total bilirubin (mg/dL)	≤1.0	Unchanged
Serum cholesterol (mg/dL)	120–200	Increase
Serum alkaline phosphatase (U/L)	30–120	Increase
SGPT/SGOT (U/L)	20–40	Unchanged
Serum proteins (g/dL)		
• Total	6.4–8.3	5.5–7.5
• Albumin	3.5–5.0	Slight increase
• Globulin	2.3–3.4	3.0–4.0
Prothrombin time (seconds)	11–14	Unchanged

PREGNANCY AND KIDNEY FUNCTION

The expanding gravid uterus, the metabolic demands of the growing fetus and hormonal influences affect the renal function in many ways.

Anatomic Changes

The kidneys increase in size by about 1 to 1.5 cm and revert back to normal by six months after delivery. Increase in volume by up to 30% is due to dilatation of the pelvicalyceal system and renal vasculature.[5] Compression of the ureters by the growing uterus and hormonal influences of progesterone cause the pelvicalyceal system to dilate.[6] Hydronephrosis and hydroureter may be found in 80% of the pregnant females; the right ureter being more commonly affected due to dextrorotation of the gravid uterus.[6] Progesterone diminishes the tone, peristalsis and force of contraction of the ureter.[7] The expanding uterus decreases the bladder capacity and the trigone is elevated leading to urinary incontinence, frequency and urgency of micturition. Microhematuria although rare can occur due to increase in tortuosity of the bladder vessels.

Clinical pearl

All the aforementioned factors make the pregnant female prone to urinary stasis, asymptomatic bacteriuria and pyelonephritis.

Changes in RBF and GFR

As gestation progresses, maternal cardiac output increases and so does the renal plasma flow (approximately 50%). Consequently, there occurs an increase in the glomerular filtration rate (GFR) by 40 to 65% beginning immediately post-conception and attains a peak value at the end of the first trimester. The GFR stays elevated until the middle of the third trimester when renal blood flow begins to decline toward prepregnancy levels.[8]

In response to the elevated GFR, serum creatinine falls by an average of 0.4 mg/dL (range of 0.4 to 0.8 mg/dL is considered normal during pregnancy).[9] The average normal level of creatinine clearance in pregnancy rises to 150–200 mL/min (normal value being 120 mL/min in the non-pregnant state) by 5 to 7 weeks of gestation and stays elevated until the third trimester. Hence, a serum creatinine value of 1.0 mg/dL which would otherwise be considered normal in a non-pregnant individual reflects renal impairment in a pregnant woman. The blood urea nitrogen (BUN) also shows a parallel decline from about 13 mg/dL in the non-pregnant state to about 8 to 10 mg/dL during gestation. The GFR and BUN concentrations slowly return back to the pre-pregnant values by the sixth postpartum week.[10]

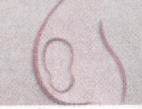

> **Clinical pearl**
>
> GFR and creatinine clearance values are best estimated by 24-hour urine collection technique. Serum creatinine and urea levels at the upper end of normal range indicate decreased renal function in pregnancy.

Changes in the Renin-Angiotensin-Aldosterone System

The fluctuating hormonal milieu in pregnancy plays a key role in activation of the renin-angiotension-aldosterone system leading to salt and water retention. By 8 weeks of gestation, aldosterone levels begin to rise and reach 3- to 6-fold the upper limit of normal (80–100 ng/dL) in the third trimester. The pregnant women retains about 1.1 to 1.6 litres and blood volume increases by 30 to 50%.[7] There also occurs a retention of about 950 mmol of sodium; hence a certain amount of clinical edema occurs in most pregnant women.[11]

Changes in Tubular Function

There is a compensatory increase in tubular reabsorption of solutes and this appears to balance the increased GFR. There is a fall in serum uric acid levels due to increased excretion and decreased proximal tubular reabsorption. The enhanced clearance helps to excrete the additional burden from the fetoplacental unit. Serum uric acid levels drop to about 2 to 3.0 mg/dL by 22 to 24 weeks, followed by gradual rise to normal by term,[7] which can be ascribed to increased renal tubular absorption of water.[12]

Increase in the glomerular basement membrane permeability coupled with the rise in GFR causes proteinuria even in normal pregnancy, especially after 20 weeks of gestation. As such, the upper limits of normal 24-hour urine protein are considered to be 300 mg/day in the pregnant women which is twice the normal value of 150 mg/day in non-pregnant individuals.

The glucose which gets filtered at the glomerulus is mostly reabsorbed by the proximal tubule and the remaining amount in the collecting tubule. Glucosuria is a common occurrence during pregnancy when the tubular reabsorptive capacity is exceeded and it cannot keep up with the increased GFR. Hence, the higher limit of glucosuria has been fixed at 10 gram per 24-hour urine collection in pregnant women.

> **Clinical pearl**
>
> Proteinuria and glucosuria in the pregnant women need to be interpreted correctly after taking into consideration the normal values established during pregnancy. Significant proteinuria is defined as > 300 mg/day and significant glucosuria is considered as >10 gm/day during pregnancy.

Changes in Renal Water and Electrolyte Handling

During pregnancy, the osmotic threshold is reset as it falls by 8–10 mOsmol/kg and reaches a new setpoint of 270 mOsmol/kg. The renal ability to excrete a water load is normally maintained, albeit at a lower osmotic set point.

It has been observed that the osmotic threshold at which arginine vasopressin or antidiuretic hormone is released is lowered. Since the osmotic threshold for thirst also declines; the pregnant woman tends to drink more water to maintain the lower osmolality.

Renin activity which increases during gestation returns to normal by 2 to 7 days after delivery.[13] The serum sodium concentration typically decreases by 4–5 mmol/L below nonpregnant levels even as 500–950 mmol of sodium are retained. Another unexpected finding at term is the net gain of 320 mmol of potassium despite sodium retention by aldosterone. This is attributed to the antikaliuretic effects of progesterone. Under the influence of increased levels of calcitriol, intestinal calcium reabsorption is enhanced but urinary calcium excretion increases. Bicarbonate reabsorption remains normal as renal acidifying mechanisms are unchanged.

Laboratory Values of Renal Function Tests in Non-pregnant and Pregnant		
Renal parameter	Non-pregnant	Pregnant
Bladder capacity (mL)	1300	1500
Renal plasma flow (RPF) (mL/min)	500–700	↑ by 25–30%
Glomerular filtration rate (GFR) (mL/min)	88–128	↑ by 30–50%
Blood urea nitrogen (BUN) (mg/dL)	10–20	Decreases
Serum creatinine (mg/dL)	0.5–1.1	Decreases
Serum uric acid (mg/dL)	2.7–7.3	Decreases
Intravenous pyelogram (IVP)	Normal	Slight to moderate hydronephrosis and hydroureter, right kidney > left kidney

Diabetes Insipidus (DI) of Pregnancy

Vasopressinase, an enzyme secreted by the placenta, hydrolyzes arginine vasopressin. Rarely a transient state of DI may occur during the second trimester and disappears after delivery.[14] It is a consequence of raised vasopressinase levels and can occur in normal pregnancy; the cause of this phenomenon is not exactly known.

PREGNANCY AND GASTROINTESTINAL SYSTEM

Gastrointestinal Motility and Secretions

As the uterus expands, the axis of the stomach is rotated approximately 45° to the right and it is pushed upwards to the left of the diaphragm. Consequently, the intra-abdominal segment of the esophagus is displaced into the thorax in most pregnant women. These women are susceptible to reflux of gastric contents due to reduced tone of the lower esophageal high pressure zone. The increase in lower esophageal tone that normally accompanies the rise in intragastric pressure is also prevented.[15] Lower esophageal sphincter (LES) tone remains relatively unchanged till around 16 weeks after which it gradually weakens reaching a nadir at 36 weeks. Pressure difference between the stomach and esophagus in non-pregnant is 7 mm Hg while it reduces in pregnancy to 4 mm Hg.

Most women experience nausea with or without vomiting due to elevated levels of hCG. It usually begins at 4 to 6 weeks gestation and subsides by the end of first trimester. As the metabolic demand rises by the second trimester, appetite is stimulated. Raised levels of estrogen may cause gums to become congested and bleed easily.

Gastrin increases the volume and decreases the pH of gastric contents, strengthens LES tone and inhibits the pyloric sphincter. During pregnancy, gastrin is also secreted by the fetus and placenta. Although there is no change in serum concentration during the first trimester, levels of gastrin progressively rise during second and third trimesters as well as during labor. The volume of acid secreted by the stomach, pancreas and small intestine also increases. Estrogen has a protective effect on peptic ulcer formation or exacerbation by decreasing the hydrochloric acid formation.

Progesterone decreases the smooth muscle tone and motility causing reverse peristalsis, thereby slowing gastric emptying time and causing esophageal regurgitation. Small and large intestine transit time is prolonged. Constipation is a common complaint during pregnancy. Usual causes are iron supplements, low dietary fiber intake, lack of exercise, etc. Increased progesterone may also contribute to constipation by decreasing water absorption from the colon. The pregnant uterus gradually displaces the appendix upwards away from the McBurney's point, making the diagnosis of acute appendicitis difficult.

Gastric Function during Labor

Contrary to the common belief, gastric emptying is not delayed in the non-laboring term parturient. However, it is decreased with the onset of labor, pain, anxiety or administration of opioids via any route systemic, epidural or subarachnoid.[16] The surge in sympathetic drive at the onset of labor further delays gastric emptying. Increased volume of gastric contents above 25 mL or decreased pH of less than 2.5 can further increase the risk for aspiration. The gastric emptying time for solids is delayed further than that for liquids. Acid aspiration prophylaxis in the form of non-particulate antacid and an H_2-receptor blocker is a must for all women at risk of intervention during labor.

Clinical pearl

It is recommended that the oral intake of solid foods be restricted while allowing modest amounts of clear liquids in uncomplicated laboring patients.

Effects of Analgesia on Gastric Function during Labor

Epidural analgesia using local anesthetics alone does not further delay gastric emptying. In contrast, epidural boluses of fentanyl do delay gastric emptying, which may not be reversed by metoclopramide.[17] Epidural fentanyl administered in a bolus dose of 100 µg, significantly delays gastric emptying during labor and after cesarean section although a 50 µg bolus may be without effect. An epidural fentanyl infusion (2.5 µg/mL with 0.0625% bupivacaine) without a preceding fentanyl bolus does not alter gastric emptying during labor.

Gastric Function during Puerperium

Gastric emptying is delayed during the early postpartum period, but beyond 18 hours postpartum it is comparable to that of non-pregnant women. Plasma progesterone concentrations return to non-pregnant levels within 24 hours of delivery and GE reflux is decreased within 48 hours. Period of risk of aspiration thus extends to a poorly defined time after delivery and appropriate general anesthesia management is somewhat controversial. A rapid-sequence induction of anesthesia, application of cricoid pressure, and intubation with a cuffed endotracheal tube are recommended for pregnant women receiving general anesthesia from the 12th week of gestation to the early postpartum period.[18]

PREGNANCY AND ENDOCRINE SYSTEM

The maternal endocrine system undergoes physiologic changes that support the embryo in growth and development.

Pituitary and Placental Hormones

Increase in size of the anterior pituitary gland occurs mainly due to enhanced size and number of lactotrophs. It manifests as an increase in height and convexity of the pituitary on MRI.[19] This enlargement makes the parturient prone to Sheehan syndrome as massive blood loss can alter the blood supply to the pituitary making it susceptible to postpartum infarction.

There is a feedback suppression of the anterior pituitary hormones, i.e. follicle stimulating hormone (FSH) and luteinizing hormone (LH) caused by elevated levels of estrogen and progesterone. Hence maturation of the follicle and ovulation do not occur. In preparation for childbirth, there is relaxation of pelvic ligaments and joints under the influence of estrogen. Progesterone is needed for sustaining pregnancy; it induces uterine smooth muscle relaxation and prevents miscarriage.

Maternal pituitary growth hormone (GH) production is suppressed due to the action of placental GH variant on the hypothalamus and pituitary; the serum levels of GH may increase as a result of synthesis of GH from the placenta.[20] There is an increase in number of oxytocin receptors in the uterus as pregnancy progresses as well as enhanced affinity to these receptors.[21] Oxytocin levels increase from 10 pg/mL in the first trimester to 30 pg/mL in the third trimester and peak at about 75 pg/mL during labor.

Another anterior pituitary hormone is prolactin whose levels begin to rise at 5–8 weeks gestation and peak at term. In non-lactating women, prolactin levels return to normal by three months postpartum. Melanocyte-stimulating hormone (MSH), produced by the placenta increases skin pigmentation late in pregnancy. Human chorionic somatomamotropin or human placental lactogen (HPL) functions as a growth hormone and is responsible for breast development. The placenta also produces the β subunit of human chorionic gonadotropin (β-hCG), a trophic hormone that, like FSH and LH, maintains the corpus luteum and thereby prevents ovulation.

Thyroid Function

In the presence of optimum iodine intake, the thyroid does not show much variation in size or marginally increases. Iodine requirements during pregnancy are higher due to increased renal loss and transfer to the fetus. Since the fetus is unable to synthesize thyroid hormones until after 12 weeks gestation, it relies on maternal transfer and deficiency hampers its neurological development. Iodine deficiency may cause increase in thyroid size up to 25% and appearance of goitre in 10% women. This is histologically reflected by an increase in vascularity with follicular hyperplasia.[22] Thyroxin-binding globulin (TBG) increases due to the stimulation of hepatocytes by estrogen. The concentration of total T4 increases in parallel with the increase in TBG from a normal range of 5–12 mg/dL in non-pregnant women to 9–16 mg/dL during pregnancy. However, the free T4 and free T3 levels are not affected, hence these assays are relied upon. TSH levels temporarily decrease during the first trimester but return to pre-pregnant levels by the end of this trimester and then remain stable for the remainder of gestation.

Due to the similarity between the alpha subunits of beta-human chorionic gonado-tropin (β-hCG) and TSH, it is found that hCG has weak thyroid stimulating activity. This could lead to a state of gestational transient thyrotoxicosis in some women. During pregnancy, the incidence of hypothyroidism (2–3%) appears to be higher than that of hyper-thyroidism (0.1–0.4%). In women affected before pregnancy, it is recommended to adjust the dose in order to have a pre-pregnancy TSH lower than 2.5 mIU/L and to maintain the same TSH level during the first trimester and not to exceed 3.0 mIU/L during the second and third trimesters.[23]

Clinical pearl

Free T4, free T3 and TSH levels are used to diagnose and follow thyroid disorders in pregnancy.

Physiologic Changes in Pregnancy that Influence Thyroid Function Tests	
Physiologic change	Thyroid function test change
↑ Thyroid-binding globulin (TBG)	↑ Serum total T4 and T3 concentration
First trimester hCG elevation	↑ Free T4 and ↓ TSH
↑ Plasma volume	↑ T4 and T3 pool size
Thyroid enlargement	↓ Serum thyroglobulin
↑ Iodine clearance	↓ Hormone production in iodine deficient areas

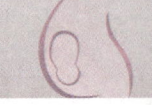

Parathyroid Function

It was initially thought that there exists a state of relative hyperparathyroidism during gestation in order to meet the enhanced fetal demand for skeletal growth and development. Newer PTH assays have now demonstrated that maternal PTH levels remain in the low normal range throughout gestation. The levels of 25-hydroxy vitamin D usually do not change in pregnancy. However, the levels of 1,25-dihydroxy vitamin D is increased due to production by maternal kidneys and the fetoplacental unit and is independent of PTH control. Calcitonin levels also rise by 20% and may help protect the maternal skeleton from excess bone loss.[24]

Adrenal Cortical Function

Pregnancy is associated with a state of physiologic hypercortisolism with increased serum levels of aldosterone, deoxycorticosterone, corticosteroid-binding globulin, cortisol and ACTH.[25] Estrogen stimulates the liver production of corticosteroid-binding globulin (CBG) and their levels almost double during pregnancy. The elevated CBG results in a 100% increase in the plasma cortisol concentration at the end of the first trimester and a 200% increase at term.[26] The increased production is accompanied by a decreased clearance resulting in increase in free cortisol.

As compared to the non-pregnant state, the maternal ACTH or corticotropin levels are about four times higher between 7 and 10 weeks of gestation. It continues to increase due to placental production of corticotropin-releasing hormone (CRH) which in turn stimulates maternal ACTH production and peaks 15-fold during the stress of delivery. Diagnosis of Cushing's syndrome during pregnancy is difficult. The hypothalamic pituitary axis response to exogenous glucocorticoids is blunted during normal pregnancy and makes interpretation of dexamethasone suppression tests for adrenal excess problematic.

Pancreas and Glucose Metabolism

The biochemical profile of the pregnant woman usually reveals a fasting hypoglycemia, postprandial hyperglycemia and hyperinsulinism.[27] Despite a rise in insulin secretion and unchanged degradation of insulin, a diabetogenic effect is prominent due to the counter-regulatory hormones, i.e. estrogen, progesterone, cortisol and human placental lactogen. Pregnant women have higher blood glucose levels after a carbohydrate bolus as compared to non-pregnant women although their insulin levels are higher. In order to accommodate the increased demand for insulin, hypertrophy and hyperplasia of beta cells occurs in the maternal pancreas.

Also demonstrable is enhanced peripheral tissue resistance to insulin. Decreased maternal ability to utilize her own insulin is a protective mechanism to ensure ample glucose supply in order to meet the fetal demands. Maternal insulin does not cross the placenta to the fetus. The fasting blood glucose levels of women during the third trimester are significantly lower than that of non-pregnant individuals. The relative hypoglycemic state results in fasting hypoinsulinemia.[28] Although rare, normal physiologic changes of pregnancy make the woman more prone to ketoacidosis.[18] These physiologic alterations are restored to normal within 24 hours of delivery.

SUMMARY

As the gravid uterus prepares for the growth and birth of the fetus, the mother is subjected to numerous physiological changes. These primarily occur to meet the growing metabolic demands of the fetoplacental unit. Changes occurring in the renal, hepatic, gastrointestinal and endocrine systems have consequences that affect the course of anesthesia.

Owing to increase in renal blood flow and glomerular filtration rate, the serum creatinine and urea levels are decreased as compared to non-pregnant women, hence levels at the upper range of the normal spectrum should prompt the physician to rule out renal dysfunction. Due to decreased reabsorptive capacity of the distal tubules, proteinuria and glycosuria is a normal feature in pregnancy. The upper limit accepted as normal in a 24 hrs urine sample collection is 300 mg of protein and 10 grams of glucose. These values are double that accepted as normal in the non-pregnant state. Change in the axis of the stomach due to upward push by the gravid uterus, increased intragastric pressure and lowered esophageal sphincter tone contribute to acid reflux in the parturient. Use of opioids during labor delays the gastric emptying time and predisposes to Mendelsons syndrome. All women from about 16 weeks gestation are to be considered as full stomach and aspiration prophylaxis is mandatory. The gastrointestinal changes usually revert to normal by 48–72 hrs after delivery.

With regard to liver function tests, serum albumin, transaminases and bilirubin levels may be lower than in the non-pregnant state while alkaline phosphatase levels are usually elevated in the third trimester. Plasma pseudocholinesterase levels decrease from the 10th week of gestation up to 6 weeks postpartum but do not affect neuromuscular blockade in the healthy parturient. However, dosage of succinylcholine may have to be reduced in HELLP syndrome where 60% of these patients can have pseudocholinesterase activity below normal. Hyperplasia of the beta cells of the islets of Langerhans occur in the mother and levels of insulin are usually high. Inspite of this, pregnancy is a diabetogenic state due to relative insulin resistance. The fetus is not dependent on the mother for insulin; rather the fetal insulin levels vary according to the glucose load transferred to it across the placenta. Hence, a good glucose control is necessary in the mother. T4 levels in pregnancy rise as the concentration of thyroid binding globulin increases. Since free T4 and free T3 concentrations are not affected, these assays are recommended during pregnancy.

Key Points

1. Epidural analgesia with local anesthetics does not delay gastric emptying but addition of opioids (by any route including epidural) increases the stomach transit time. All women are to be considered full stomach from about 16 weeks gestation to 72 hours postpartum and should be given aspiration prophylaxis.
2. Serum alanine aminotransferase, aspartate aminotransferase and prothrombin time remain within the range fixed for nonpregnant women and are preferred for routine diagnosis of liver disease in pregnancy.
3. Serum creatinine and urea levels at the upper end of the normal range indicate decreased renal function in pregnancy.
4. Glycosuria and proteinuria can occur in normal pregnancy due to decreased reabsorptive capacity of the distal tubules. In a 24 hr urine sample collection, 300 mg protein and 10 grams of glucose/ day is considered normal.
5. Free T3, free T4 and TSH assays are used as diagnostic and prognostic indicators of maternal thyroid disorders.

REFERENCES

1. Bacq Y. The liver in normal pregnancy. In: Madame Curie Bioscience Database [Internet]. Austin (TX): Landes Bioscience; 2000.
2. Jamjute P, Ahmad A, Ghosh T, Banfield P. LFT and pregnancy. J Matern Fetal Neonatal Med 2009;22:274–83.
3. Shnider SM. Anesthesiology 96:335,1965.
4. Steven Gabbe, Jennifer R Niebyl, Henry L Galan, Eric Jauniaux, Mark Landon, Joe Leigh Simpson. Maternal Physiologyin Obstetrics: Normal and Problem Pregnancies, 6th ed, Elsevier Saunders.
5. Bailey RR, Rolleston GL. Kidney length and ureteric dilatation in the puerperium. J Obstet Gynaecol Br Commonw1971;78:35–61.

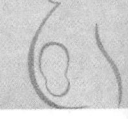

6. Rasmussen PE, Nielsen FR. Hydronephrosis during pregnancy: a literature survey. Eur J Obstet Gynaecol Reprod Biol 1988;27:249–59.

7. Katharine L Cheung, Richard A Lafayette. Renal physiology of pregnancy. Adv Chronic Kidney Dis 2013;20(3):209–14.

8. Edwin Chandraharan and Sir Sabaratnam Arulkumaran. Anatomical and physiological changes in pregnancy. Obstetric and Intrapartum Emergencies: A Practical Guide to Management. Cambridge University Press, 2012.

9. Fischer MJ. Chronic kidney disease and pregnancy: Maternal and fetal outcomes. Adv Chronic Kidney Dis 200;14:132–45.

10. DC Dutta's Textbook of Obstetrics: Including Perinatology and Contraception, 7th ed. Jaypee Brothers; 2014.

11. Davison JH. Edema in pregnancy. Kidney Int Suppl 1997;59:590–6.

12. Lind T, Godfrey KA, Otun H, Philips PR. Changes in serum uric acid concentration during normal pregnancy. Br J Obstet Gynaecol 1984;91:128–32.

13. Weisinger RS, Burns P, Eddie LW, Wintour EM. Relaxin alters the plasma osmolality-arginine vasopressin relationship in the rat. J Endocrinol 1993;137(3):505–10.

14. Unraveling the mysteries of preeclampsia. Am J Obstet Gynecol 2005;193:3–4.

15. Ulmsten U, Sundstrom G. Esophageal manometry in pregnant and nonpregnant women. Am J Obstet Gynecol 1978;132:260–4.

16. Wong CA, McCarthy RJ, Fitzgerald PC, et al. Gastric emptying of water in obese pregnant women at term. Anesth Analg 2007;105:751–5.

17. Ewah B, Yau K, King M, et al. Effect of epidural opioids on gastric emptying in labour. Int J Obstet Anesth 1993;2:125–8.

18. Barash PG, Cullen BF, Stoelting RK, (Eds). Clinical Anesthesia (5th ed). Published by Lippincott, Williams and Wilkins, Philadelphia, USA.

19. ElsterAD, Sanders TG, Vives FS, et al. Size and shape of the pituitary gland during pregnancy and postpartum: measurement with MR imaging. Radiology 1991;181:53.

20. Prager D, Braunstein GD. Pituitary disorders during pregnancy. Endocrinol Metab Clin North Am 1995;24(1):1–14.

21. Zeeman GG, Khan-Dawood FS, Dawood MY. Oxytocin and its receptor in pregnancy and parturition: current concepts and clinical implications. Obstet Gynecol 1997;89:873.

22. Glinoer D. The regulation of thyroid function in pregnancy: Pathways of endocrine adaptation from physiology to pathology. Endocr Rev 1997; 18:404–33.

23. John H. Lazarus: Thyroid function in pregnancy. Journal of Prenatal Medicine 2012;6(4):64–71.

24. Kovacs CS, Kronenberg HM. Maternal-fetal calcium and bone metabolism during pregnancy, puerperium and lactation. Endocr Rev 1997; 18:832–72.

25. Goland RS, Jozak S, Conwell I. Placental corticotrophin-releasing hormone and the hypercortisolism of pregnancy. Am J Obstet Gynecol 171:1287,1994.

26. Chestnut DH, Wong CA, Tsen LC, NganKee WD, Beilin Y, Myhre JM (Eds). Chestnut's Obstetric Anesthesia: Principles and Practice, 5th Edn, 2nd Revision. Published by Elsevier.

27. Kuhl C. Etiology and pathogenesis of gestational diabetes. Diabetes Care 1998;21(Suppl 2):B19–B26.

28. Felig P, Lynch V. Starvation in human pregnancy: hypoglycemia, hypoinsulinemia and hyperketonemia. Science 1970;170:990–2.

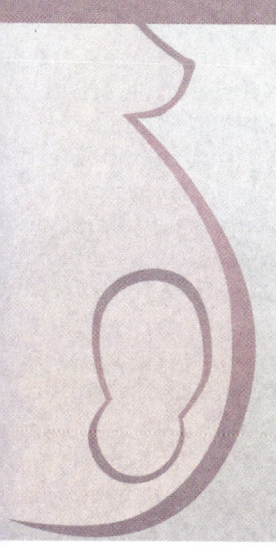

Essentials of Physiological Changes of Pregnancy in Musculoskeletal and Nervous Systems

Rita Wahal

GENERAL CONSIDERATIONS

Rising levels of multiple hormones—estrogen, progesterone, prostaglandins and chorionic gonadotropins, are primarily responsible for the anatomical and physiological changes in early pregnancy. Whereas, increasing size of uterus assumes the responsibility for altering the function of various systems in the later part of pregnancy.

Enlarged uterus causes the body to respond with a shift in the center of gravity backwards, higher on the pelvis and hormonal changes increase the laxity of ligaments hence, increased strain on back muscles leading to low back pain in pregnant women.

Increased sensitivity of the nervous system to anesthetic agents due to hormonal changes and the anatomical changes during pregnancy result in reduced dose requirement of IV anesthetic agents, inhalational anesthetic agents and the local anesthetic agents.

Almost all the anesthetic agents are shown to have effect on the fetal neurodevelopment when administered during 'growth spurt' period in animals and provokes one to think, whether it is safe to administer anesthetic agents in humans during pregnancy.

Impact of physiological changes in the central and peripheral nervous system and the musculoskeletal system will be discussed. Effect of maternal anesthetics on fetal neurodevelopment will be reviewed herewith.

ANATOMICAL CHANGES DURING PREGNANCY IN VERTEBRAL COLUMN

Multiple hormonal changes and the enlarged size of uterus are responsible for the anatomical changes in the vertebral column during pregnancy.

With progression of pregnancy, lordosis increases and the relationship of pelvis to vertebral column changes. Interspinous spaces are narrowed in lordosis, resulting in midline approach difficult for the epidural and spinal anesthesia. The hormonal changes of pregnancy make the perivertebral ligaments and the ligamentum flavum feel softer, which makes identification of the epidural space a little difficult.

Tuffier's line, the line joining the two posterior superior iliac points, shifts cephalad from L4–5 interspace to L3–4 interspace.[1] Apex of the lumbar lordosis shifts caudad and the thoracic kyphosis is reduced. These changes make the local anesthetic agent spread higher in the intrathecal space and higher sensory levels are achieved.

Enlarged uterus compresses the inferior vena cava, which causes engorgement of the epidural veins, resulting in increased volume of epidural veins and reduced volume of CSF.[1,2] Trauma to the engorged veins, intra-vascular injections of anesthetic drugs and epidural catheter cannulation of the veins are, therefore, more common in pregnant patients as compared to non-pregnant patients. Vertebral foraminal veins, which are in continuation with the epidural veins, are also engorged and obstruct the foramina, thereby reducing the leakage of anesthetic drug and resulting in higher spread of anesthetic drug in the intrathecal space. This further results in reduced requirement of the dose of anesthetic drug in pregnant patients. CSF specific gravity is also reduced during pregnancy, further reducing the dose requirement of local anesthetic agent.[3]

Lumbar epidural pressure is positive in lateral position in pregnant patients as compared to non-pregnant patients, it further increases in supine position and during labor due to increased blood flow.[4] The epidural pressure returns to normal levels within 12 hours postpartum. CSF pressure in the pregnant patient remains the same as that of non-pregnant patient.

CHANGES IN NERVOUS SYSTEM

Sensitivity of both central and peripheral nervous systems is increased during pregnancy.

Requirement of thiopental is reported to decrease in human during pregnancy by 17%.[5] Concentration of inhalational anesthetic agent required to produce loss of consciousness is also reduced by 28% for isoflurane in pregnant patients.[6] Increased sensitivity was also observed in human nerve fibers to local anesthetics.[7] A recent study has shown increased sensitivity of the pregnant nerve fiber to bupivacaine.[8] Progesterone levels are raised 10-20-fold and have sedative effect, which may be responsible for these changes.[9,10] Progesterone or one of its active metabolites may be responsible for the observed increased sensitivity of the peripheral nerve fibers to local anesthetics during pregnancy, as rabbit nerve fibers show increased sensitivity when chronically treated to exogenous progesterone.[11] Beta-endorphin levels are also raised, but not until active labour,[98] so not involved in reducing the MAC value.

CHANGES IN SYMPATHETIC NERVOUS SYSTEM

Sympathetic activation is reported in early pregnancy in a recent study,[12] and this activity remains increased throughout the pregnancy to maintain the hemodynamic stability, and peaks at term.[13]

Another study has shown that sympatho-vagal balance shifts progressively from a higher vagal modulation towards a higher sympathetic modulation, and the sympathetic activity is increased in late pregnancy[14] to prepare the parturient to meet the stress of pregnancy.

ALTERATIONS IN MUSCULOSKELETAL SYSTEM DURING PREGNANCY

Weight gain, enlarged size of uterus and hormonal changes that occur during pregnancy are collectively responsible for the biomechanical alterations in the musculo-skeletal system.

Enlarged uterus and weight gain of over twenty pounds result in lordosis to compensate for the body changes. Lumbar lordosis and rotation of pelvis on the femur[15] further cause anterior flexion of the cervical spine. As a safety measure to prevent instability, the center of gravity shifts higher and back over the pelvis, resulting in increased strain on the muscles and ligaments supporting the vertebral column.[16] Laxity in the anterior and posterior longitudinal ligaments of the lumbar spine creates instability in the lumbar spine and increase the muscle strain.

Stretching, weakness and separation of abdominal muscles further increase the strain on paraspinal muscles. Pelvis is tilted anteriorly with increased strain on extensor muscles of hip, abductors and plantar flexor muscles.

Sacroiliac joints and pubic symphysis joint are widened and the mobility of the joint is also increased to prepare the birth canal for passage of fetus.

Fluid retention causes compression on nerves.

Relaxin, hormone produced by the corpus luteum and placenta, is responsible for remodeling of pelvic connective tissue. The concentration peaks during the first trimester with placental implantation. Later in pregnancy, relaxin contributes to separation of the symphysis pubis.[17]

Laxity in the joints of the extremities appears to be due to other factors as is shown in a study, in which 19 of 35 women (54%) demonstrated a $\geq$10% increase in wrist laxity from the first to the third trimester, but the increase did not correlate with relaxin levels.[18] Subjective joint pain was associated with increased estradiol and progesterone levels, but not with elevated relaxin concentrations.[18]

PAIN AND ANALGESIA DURING PREGNANCY

Low Back Pain

50 to 70% pregnant women complain of low back pain, that is pain in the lumbar spine area.[19–22] In most cases, back pain is due to hormonal and mechanical factors. Muscle weakness, joint laxity, and fluid retention within connective tissue are the common causative factors.[23] The L4 to L5 level is vulnerable for spondylolithiasis in pregnant women.[24] There is no evidence of disk herniation as the cause of back pain during pregnancy.[25]

History of back pain is most prevalent in the second half of pregnancy. The pain is aggravated by activity and relieved by rest. It occurs in the lower back, radiate down the back of the thighs or anterior thighs.[26] The pain is often worse at night and may interfere with sleep.

About 80% of patients recover in six months after delivery.[27]

Pelvic Girdle Pain

Pelvic girdle pain is related to the sacroiliac joint. Low back pain, obesity, young maternal age, multiparity, low educational level, heavy physical work, and cesarean delivery are the factors responsible for sacroiliac pain.[28–31]

Pelvic girdle pain is of stabbing nature that occurs between the posterior iliac crest and the gluteal fold, radiate to the posterior thigh.[32] Pelvic floor tenderness may be present[33] but pelvic floor function does not appear to be affected.[34]

Relaxin level increases by 10-folds during pregnancy, is responsible for softening of ligaments and pelvic joint laxity. The extent of instability and joint laxity correlate with maternal serum levels of relaxin and severity of back pain during pregnancy.[35]

Recovery from pelvic girdle pain may be delayed-up to two years.[36]

Pelvic joint pain during pregnancy is treated by standard treatment along with acupuncture[37–39] and stabilizing exercises.[40,41] One trial randomly assigned 386 pregnant women with PGP to standard treatment or standard treatment with stabilizing exercises or acupuncture.[39] The addition of acupuncture or stabilizing exercises to standard treatment resulted in significantly lower pain scores at six weeks.[40,41] However, another randomized trial that compared standardized therapy alone to standardized treatment plus stabilizing exercises or standardized treatment plus acupuncture found no differences in recovery among the three treatment groups.[37] Stabilizing exercises are targeted to the muscles supporting the pelvic girdle under supervision of a physiotherapist.[43] A brace or girdle provides stability to the sacroiliac joints and is useful for management of posterior pelvic pain.[42]

Cesarean delivery is associated with higher rates of persistent pelvic pain in postpartum.[31]

Knee Pain

Knee pain is common in pregnant women during latter half of pregnancy due to postural changes, increase in weight and increased laxity of ligaments. Significant improvement occurs by four months postpartum.[44]

Leg Pain

Leg cramps are fairly common complaint during the latter half of pregnancy especially at night due to painful muscle contractions, secondary to a buildup of lactic and pyruvic acids leading to involuntary contraction of the affected muscles.[45]

A Cochrane review found that the placebo-controlled trial of calcium treatment showed no benefit in the treatment of leg cramps, but placebo controlled trials of magnesium supplementation suggested a possible benefit.[45] This was a small trial of 69 pregnant women with persistent leg cramps. The drug used was magnesium lactate/citrate 5 mmol in the morning and 10 mmol in the evening.[46]

Regular exercises—calf strengthening and stretching exercises, are effective preventive measures. Non-pharmacologic methods recommended are—warm tub bath, ice massage, increased hydration and proper foot gear.

Meralgia Paresthetica

Compression of the lateral femoral cutaneous nerve as it penetrates the tensor fascia lata at the inguinal ligament causes dysesthesias in the upper and middle part of the lateral thigh. It is a sensory neuropathy, also known as meralgia paresthetica, and is caused by the expanding abdominal wall and increased lumbar lordosis. Symptoms occur late in pregnancy, rarely need treatment and resolve within 3 months postpartum.

Carpal Tunnel Syndrome

Carpal tunnel syndrome is relatively common during pregnancy, with an incidence reported between 5 and 35%.[47,48] The increased incidence in pregnant women is thought to be due to fluid retention leading to compression of the nerve in the carpal tunnel and hormonal changes affecting the musculoskeletal system.[49] Symptoms tend to occur during the last trimester, but can occur at anytime.[48,50] In most cases, symptoms resolve over a period of weeks after delivery; however, can be prolonged for months in women who are breastfeeding.[51] Recurrence in subsequent pregnancies is common.

Pharmacologic Treatment of Pain during Pregnancy

Acetaminophen: It is the safest drug for treating pain at all stages of pregnancy in standard therapeutic doses. Two studies have shown association between attention-deficit/hyperactivity disorder and in utero exposure to acetaminophen[52,53] which was reported to inconclusive by the 2015 US Food and Drug Administration Drug Safety Communication on the basis of available evidence.[54] There is no strong evidence of congenital anomalies or neurodevelopmental damage in humans.[55,56] Studies have reported small but statistically significant association between cryptorchidism in offspring of woman who used acetaminophen during pregnancy.[57–59] Therefore, it is reasonable to avoid its prolonged use in pregnancy, until more data are available.

Aspirin: Aspirin inhibits platelet function and can contribute to maternal and fetal bleeding,[60] but not associated with other congenital anomalies.[61] Overall, large trials demonstrate low-dose aspirin's relative safety and generally positive effects on reproductive outcome.[62]

NSAIDs: The risks and benefits of using non-steroidal anti-inflammatory drugs for treatment of pain depend on the dose, gestational age, and duration of therapy (up-to-date). No studies have shown consistent evidence of increased teratogenic effects in either humans or animals following therapeutic doses during the first trimester. However, even short-term use of NSAIDs in late pregnancy is associated with a substantial increase in the risk of premature ductal closure.[63]

Opioids: There is limited information on the effects of long-term opioid use during pregnancy. Neonatal withdrawal syndrome is reported.[64,65] Studies have reported an association between maternal opioid use in early pregnancy and central nervous system malformations (neural tube defect) in offspring.[66,67]

A 2015 US Food and Drug Administration Safety Announcement stated further investigation of this issue is needed for evidence to support the presence of an increased risk of neural tube defects related to opioid exposure in early pregnancy.[67] However, data from an animal study support an association.[68] Further study is needed. In the meantime, during the first month of embryonic development when neural tube development occurs, a small potential increase in incidence of neural tube defects needs to be balanced with the needs of women with moderate to severe pain, given the frequent lack of effective alternative analgesics.

Fentanyl patch: In the literature, only case reports are available. In one report, a high-dose fentanyl patch (i.e. 125 µg/h) was used throughout pregnancy, the newborn infant showed mild withdrawal symptoms at 24 to 72 hours after birth.[69] In the other, a lower dose of the fentanyl patch was used, where infant manifested no adverse effects.[70]

Medications used in therapeutic doses to relieve pain appear to be relatively safe in pregnancy. To minimize fetal risk, lowest effective dose should be started especially in late pregnancy, after careful review of medical and drug history of the parturient. NSAIDs should be avoided after 32 weeks' gestation, owing to the possibility of anti-platelet effect or prolonged bleeding. Opioids should also be used with caution, especially in higher doses in late pregnancy when the infant should be observed carefully in the neonatal period for any signs of withdrawal.

IMPACT OF MATERNAL ANESTHESIA ON FETAL NEURODEVELOPMENT

Historically, most of the elective surgeries are delayed till second trimester of pregnancy to avoid the teratogenic effects of anesthetic agents in the first trimester. Second trimester was considered a safe period as embryogenesis completes by this time. However, evidence from animal studies suggests that anesthetic agents when administered during the 'growth spurt' period of early brain development, result in neurodegenerative changes and learning abnormality. This provokes one to think whether it is safe to administer anesthetics in human during second trimester. To understand the neurodegenerative effects of anesthetic agents, it is necessary to know the fetal brain development, mechanism of action of anesthetic agents on brain cells, timing of surgery and the safe anesthetic agents.

Fetal Brain Development

The development of the human nervous system consists of neurogenesis, neuronal migration and synaptogenesis. Neurogenesis starts in the fetus at 5 weeks gestation with differentiation and neuronal migration and peaks at 25 weeks in utero, followed by establishment of synaptogenesis at 10 weeks. Neuronal migration completes between 30 to

36 weeks, while synaptogenesis continues even after birth.[71,72] Both neurogenesis and neuronal migration reach a peak during and after the second trimester.[73] The formation of synapses is dependent on electrochemical activity, and involves the activation of calcium channels.[72] Neurogenesis and synaptogenesis are activity-dependent: "Neurons that form together, are the ones which synapse together".[71] Generation of supporting glial cells, astrocytes and oligodendrites occurs between 20 and 40 weeks. The peak period of myelination occurs during the first two years after birth, during which period the brain structure drastically changes its biochemical composition.[74]

The brain's ability to learn, remember, forget, recover from injury and re-organize is called cerebral plasticity.[71] The developing brain has the greatest potential for recovery from any injury because of an overproduction of neurons in the fetus and the overproduction of synapses after birth.[71]

Neuronal migration is guided by cell-intrinsic mechanism as well as humoral mediators such as GABA (gamma-amino-butyric acid) and N-methyl–D-aspartate-NMDA-subtype glutamate.[75,76] Pharmacological interventions on these neuro-modulator systems induce long-lasting impairment of fetal brain development, mainly by impaired neurogenesis and altered neuronal migration.[77,78]

Mechanism of Action of Anesthetics on the Brain

The majority of anesthetic agents work in two basic mechanisms in the brain: an increase in inhibition via the gamma-aminobutyric acid (GABA) receptors, e.g. benzodiazepines, barbiturates, propofol, etomidate, isoflurane, enflurane and halothane,[80] and a decrease in excitation through the N-methyl-D-aspartate (NMDA) receptors, e.g. ketamine, nitrous oxide (N_2O) and xenon.[81,82] Dexmedetomidine is the exception to these mechanisms. It is a

potent α_2-adrenergic receptor agonist, has sedative, analgesic and anxiolytic properties.[83]

Recent findings indicate that drugs that act by inhibition of either the GABA or the NMDA receptors induce widespread neuronal apoptosis in the immature rat brain when administered during synaptogenesis.[84] Apoptosis is increased, if the neurons are exposed to a combination of GABA agonists and NMDA antagonists.[79] Neuronal exposure to anesthetics during a critical neurodevelopmental period triggers an unknown chain of events, causing translocation of BCL2-associated X protein to mitochondria, followed by mitochondrial membrane disruption and permeability, resulting in the leakage of cytochrome c into the cytosol.[79]

ANESTHETIC-RELATED DEVELOPMENTAL NEUROTOXICITY

Long-term neurobehavioral deficits after anesthesia exposure, including extensive neuroapoptosis is evident from animal studies.[85] All clinically-used general anesthetic agents are potentially neurotoxic to the developing brain in animals. Single exposure to general anesthetics, during the peak period of synaptogenesis, can result in significant increase of both neuronal and glial cell apoptosis in neonatal animals.[85]

Evidence

Infant rats exposed to commonly used anesthetic agents—N_2O, isoflurane and sevoflurane, have shown widespread apoptotic neurodegeneration and learning impairments.[86,87]

Single exposure to 1.4% isoflurane for 4 hrs during second trimester caused long-lasting impairment of spatial working memory in the rodent offspring.[88] Currently, it is unknown if these behavioral abnormalities are due to impaired neurogenesis, altered neuronal migration or cell death.[89] They further showed that 1.3% isoflurane for 4 hours in midgestational period caused memory impairment and maternal isoflurane activated apoptotic mechanism with decreased number of synapses in hippocampal region.[90] A study investigated fetal exposure to an anesthetic combination during all the three trimesters in pregnant guinea pigs reported significant apoptotic changes and neuronal death in the first and second trimester, but not in third trimester.[91]

Sevoflurane anesthesia in pregnant mice can induce acute neurotoxicity, including increases in IL-6 levels and reductions in synapse marker PSD-95 and caspase-3 activation, in the brain tissues of fetal mice.[86] These results suggest that sevoflurane anesthesia in pregnant mice may induce neuro-inflammation, caspase activation, and synaptic loss, leading to long-term learning and memory impairment.[86]

Intravenous anesthetics—propofol, ketamine, midazolam and thiopentone all have shown neuronal apoptosis in rodents.[92] 24 hrs exposure to ketamine has shown persistent neurocognitive deficit in monkeys also after several years.[87]

In humans, only retrospective studies evaluating neurocognitive functions are published. A study by Mayo clinic published in 2009 concluded that there was no evidence of harm on learning disabilities of children under 5 years after obstetric anesthesia.[93] In another study, authors concluded that multiple exposures to anesthesia in children under the age of 4 years may cause learning disabilities in reading, written language and mathematics.

The mechanisms of anesthetic-induced neurotoxicity seem to involve altered expression of ligand-gated ion channels, disturbance to intracellular calcium homeostasis, and mitochondria-mediated apoptotic pathway. In addition, the anesthetic exposure during the neonatal period is associated with persistent structural and chemical dysfunction of brain cells which may lead to learning and memory (hippocampus-dependent) impairment in adult animals.[86] However, due to high-grade brain plasticity in young animals, persistent neuronal cell loss was not observed, unless repeated and prolonged courses of anesthesia were administered in neonates.[86]

Recent studies have suggested that inhibition of excessive NMDA-mediated excitatory pathway, prevention of reactive oxygen species accumulation, and improvement of perianesthesia neuro-inflammation can all ameliorate anesthetic-associated cognitive impairment in animal models.[87,97] Advances in the understanding of stem cell biology and neuroscience have opened up research avenues for investigating early-life anesthetic-induced neurotoxicity and developing prevention strategies against such neuronal injuries. Human embryonic neural stem cells model might serve as a bridging platform to provide the most expeditious approaches toward decreasing the uncertainty in extrapolating preclinical data to the human condition.

Neuroprotection

Hypothermia is known to improve the neurological outcome in many neonatal studies with hypoxic–ischemic encephalopathy.[71] However, other studies have shown harmful effects of hypothermia on newborns.[95]

Erythropoietin, antidepressants and lithium are all reported to help in recovery from neuronal injury.[71,85]

Melatonin is known to reduce the severity of anesthesia-induced apoptotic neurodegeneration in the developing rat brain in dose-dependent manner.[96] Melatonin results in up-regulation of the anti-apoptotic protein and a decrease in anesthesia-induced cytochrome c release. Melatonin also reduces anesthesia-induced activation of caspase-3 and neuronal apoptosis.

Dexmedetomidine is shown to improve neurocognitive deficit induced by subanesthetic dose of isoflurane, by reducing neuronal apoptosis in dose-dependent manner.[85] This was shown by blocking the α-2 adrenoceptor, indicating that this effect is mediated through these receptors.

FUTURE DEVELOPMENTS

Several international research groups are focusing on the long-term neurodevelopmental outcome and neurobehavioral defecit after anesthetic exposure.

- PANDA study (Pediatric Anesthesia Neuro-Development Assessment study) is comparing the neurodevelopment of children exposed to anesthesia and those not exposed to anesthesia.
- GAS study—international multicentre randomized controlled study focusing on the long-term effects of general anesthesia and spinal anesthesia on the neurodevelopmental outcome.
- MASK study—the study compares performance of children with no anesthetic exposure to those with single or multiple exposure.

NCTR (National Centre for Toxicological Research, USA) is studying in rodents and primates the mechanism, long-term deficit and strategies to prevent/decrease neurotoxicity with clinically-relevant anesthesia.

SUMMARY

- Anatomical changes in the vertebral column and increased sensitivity of the nervous system during pregnancy result in reduced dose requirement of inhalational anesthetic agents, intravenous anesthetic agents and local anesthetic agents.
- Increasing size of uterus and rising levels of hormones during pregnancy are associated with physiological changes in musculo-skeletal system, resulting in joint laxity and lordosis. Changes in musculoskeletal system are responsible for low back pain, pelvic girdle pain, leg cramps and carpal tunnel syndrome during pregnancy.
- Conservative and non-pharmacological interventions are recommended as treatment for these ailments. If medication is required, acetaminophen is considered to be safe and effective choice.
- Animal studies have shown that almost all the anesthetic agents have detrimental effect on early brain development. Human studies are limited and lacking evidence of vulnerable effect on the fetal brain. Sufficient evidence is not available to withhold the use of analgesics, sedatives and anesthetics in pregnant patients. Multicenter international studies will hopefully delineate the risk of anesthetic exposure to fetus.

REFERENCES

1. Hirabayashii Y, Shimizu R, Fukuda H, et al. Soft tissue anatomy within the vertebral canal in pregnant women. Br J Anaesth 1996;77:153–6.
2. Hogan QH, Prost R, Kulier A, et al. Magnetic resonance imaging of cerebrospinal fluid volume and the influence of body habitus and abdominal pressure. Anesthesiology 1996;84:1341–9.
3. Richardson MG, Wissler RN. Density of lumbar cerebrospinal fluid in pregnant and non-pregnant humans. Anesthesiology 1996;85:326–30.
4. Messih MN. Epidural space pressures during pregnancy. Anaesthesia 1981;36:775–82.
5. Gin T, Mainland P, Chan MTV, Short TG. Decreased thiopental requirement in early pregnancy. Anaesthesiology 1997;86:73–786.
6. Gin T, Chan MTV. Anaesthesiology 1994;81:829–32.
7. Butterworth JF, et al. Pregnancy increases median nerve susceptibility to lidocaine. Anesthesiology 1990;72:962.
8. Datta S, et al. Differential sensitivies of mammalian nerve fibers during pregnancy. Anesth Analg 1983;62:1070.
9. Datta S, Hurley RJ, Naulty SJ, et al. Plasma and cerebrospinal fluid progesterone levels in pregnant and nonpregnant women. Anaesth Analg 1986;65:950–4.
10. Hirabayashi Y, Shimizu R, Saitoh K, Fukuda H. Cerebrospinal fluid progesterone in pregnant women. Br J Anaesth 1995;75:683–7.
11. Flanagan HL, et al. Effect of exogenously administered progesterone on susceptibility of rabbit vagus nerves to bupivacaine (abstract). Anesthesiology 1988;69:676.

12. Sara S, et al. Sympathetic activation during early pregnancy in humans. The Journal of Physiology, 15(vol 590):3535–3543.

13. Assali NS, Prystowsky H. Studies on autonomic blockade. J Clin Invest 1950;29,1354–66.

14. Matsuo H, et al. Change of autonomic nervous activity during pregnancy and its modulation of labor assessed by spectral heart rate variability analysis. Clin Exp Obstet Gynecol 2007;34(2):73–9.

15. Hartmann S, Bung P. Physical exercise during pregnancy-physiological. Journal of Perinatal Medicine 1999;27(3):204–15.

16. Wang TW, Apgar BS. Exercise during pregnancy. American Family Physician 1998;57(8):1846–52.

17. Ivell R. Endocrinology. this hormone has been relaxin too long! Science 2002;295:637.

18. Marnach ML, Ramin KD, Ramsey PS, et al. Characterization of the relationship between joint laxity and maternal hormone in pregnancy. Obstet Gynecol 2003;101:331.

19. Wang SM, Dezino P, et al. Low back pain during pregnancy; prevalence, risk factors and outcomes Obstet Gynecol 2004;104:65.

20. Thorell E, Kristansson P. Pregnancy related to aerobic fitness? A longitudinal cohort study. BMC Pregnancy Childbirth 2012;12.

21. Kovacs FM, Garcia E, Royuela A, et al. Prevalence and factors associated with low back pain and pelvic girdle pain during pregnancy: a multicenter study conducted in the Spanish National Health Service. Spine (Phila Pa 1976) 2012;37:1516.

22. Mogren IM, Pohjanen, et al. Low back pain and pelvic pain during pregnancy. Spine 2005;30:983.

23. MacEvilly, Back pain and pregnancy a review. Pain 1996;64:405.

24. Sanderson PL, Fraser RD. The influence of pregnancy on the development of degenerative spondylolisthesis. J Bone Joint Surg Br 1996;78:951.

25. Chan YL, Lam WW, Lau TK, et al. Back pain in pregnancy—magnetic resonance imaging correlation. Clin Radiol 2002;57:1109.

26. Weinreb JC, Wolbarsht LB, Cohen JM, et al. Prevalence of lumbosacral intervertebral disk abnormalities on MR images in pregnant and asymptomatic nonpregnant women. Radiology 1989;170:125.

27. Bjelland EK, Stuge B, et al. The effect of emotional distress on persistent pelvic girdle pain after delivery: a longitudinal population study. BJOG 2013;120:32.

28. Bjelland EK, Eskild A, Johansen R, Eberhard-Gran M. Pelvic girdle pain in pregnancy: the impact of parity. Am J Obstet Gynecol 2010;203:146.e1.

29. Bjelland EK, Eberhard-Gran M, Nielsen CS, Eskild A. Age at menarche and pelvic girdle syndrome in pregnancy: a population study of 74973 women. BJOG 2011;118:1646.

30. Bjelland EK, Stuge B, Engdahl B, Eberhard-Gran M. The effect of emotional distress on persistent pelvic girdle pain after delivery: a longitudinal population study. BJOG 2013;120:32.

31. Bjelland EK, Stuge B, Vangen S, et al. Mode of delivery and persistence of pelvic girdle syndrome 6 months postpartum. Am J Obstet Gynecol 2013; 208:298.e1.

32. Vleeming A, Albert HB, Ostgaard HC, et al. European guidelines for the diagnosis and treatment of pelvic girdle pain. Eur Spine J 2008; 17:794.

33. Fitzgerald CM, Neville CE, Mallinson T, et al. Pelvic floor muscle examination in female chronic pelvic pain. J Reprod Med 2011;56:117.

34. Stuge B, Sætre K, Brækken IH. The association between pelvic floor muscle function and pelvic girdle pain—a matched case control 3D ultrasound study. Man Ther 2012;17:150.

35. Aldabe D, Ribeirio DC, et al. Pregnancy-related pelvic girdle pain and its relationship with relaxin levels during pregnancy: a systematic review. European Spine Journal 2012;21:1.

36. Vøllestad NK, Stuge B. Prognostic factors for recovery from postpartum pelvic girdle pain. Eur Spine J 2009;18:718.

37. Elden H, Hagberg H, Olsen MF, et al. Regression of pelvic girdle pain after delivery: follow-up of a randomised single blind controlled trial with different treatment modalities. Acta Obstet Gynecol Scand 2008;87:201.

38. Wang SM, Dezinno P, Lin EC, et al. Auricular acupuncture as a treatment for pregnant women who have low back and posterior pelvic pain: a pilot study. Am J Obstet Gynecol 2009;201:271.e1.

39. Elden H, Ladfors L, Olsen MF, et al. Effects of acupuncture and stabilising exercises as adjunct to standard treatment in pregnant women with pelvic girdle pain: randomised single blind controlled trial. Br Med J 2005;330:761.

40. Richardson CA, Snijders CJ, Hides JA, et al. The relation between the transversus abdominis muscles, sacroiliac joint mechanics, and low back pain. Spine (Phila Pa 1976) 2002;27:399.

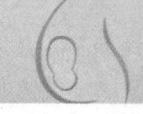

41. Richardson CA, Jull GA. Muscle control-pain control. What exercises would you prescribe? Man Ther 1995;1:2.

42. Ostgaard HC, Zetherström G, Roos-Hansson E, Svanberg B. Reduction of back and posterior pelvic pain in pregnancy. Spine (Phila Pa 1976) 1994;19:894.

43. Stuge B, Laerum E, Kirkesola G, Vøllestad N. The efficacy of a treatment program focusing on specific stabilizing exercises for pelvic girdle pain after pregnancy: a randomized controlled trial. Spine (Phila Pa 1976) 2004;29:351.

44. Dumas GA, Reid JG. Laxity of knee cruciate ligaments during pregnancy. J Ortho Sports Phys Ther 1997;26:2.

45. Young GL, Jewel D. Intervention for leg cramps in pregnancy, Cochrane Database Syst Rev 2002.

46. Dahle LO, Berg G, Hammer M, et al. The effect of oral magnesium substitution to reduce pregnancy-induced leg cramps. Am J Obst Gynae 1995;173–5.

47. Mabie WC. Peripheral neuropathies during pregnancy. Clin Obstet Gynecol 2005;48:57.

48. Meems M, Truijens S, Spek V, et al. Prevalence, course and determinants of carpal tunnel syndrome symptoms during pregnancy: a prospective study. BJOG 2015;122:1112.

49. Padua L, Aprile I, Caliandro P, et al. Symptoms and neurophysiological picture of carpal tunnel syndrome in pregnancy. Clin Neurophysiol 2001;112:1946.

50. McLennan HG, Oats JN, Walstab JE. Survey of hand symptoms in pregnancy. Med J Aust 1987;147:542.

51. Wand JS. Carpal tunnel syndrome in pregnancy and lactation. J Hand Surg Br 1990;15:93.

52. Liew Z, Ritz B, Rebordosa C, et al. Acetaminophen use during pregnancy, behavioral problems, and hyperkinetic disorders. JAMA Pediatr 2014;168:313.

53. Thompson JM, Waldie KE, Wall CR, et al. Associations between acetaminophen use during pregnancy and ADHD symptoms measured at ages 7 and 11 years. PLoS One 2014;9:e108210.

54. FDA Drug Safety Communication: FDA has reviewed possible risks of pain medicine use during pregnancy. US Food and Drug Administration, 2015.

55. www.Reprotox.org (Accessed on July 01, 2009).

56. Feldkamp ML, Meyer RE, Krikov S, Botto LD. Acetaminophen use in pregnancy and risk of birth defects: findings from the National Birth Defects Prevention Study. Obstet Gynecol 2010;115:109.

57. Kristensen DM, Hass U, Lesné L, et al. Intrauterine exposure to mild analgesics is a risk factor for development of male reproductive disorders in human and rat. Hum Reprod 2011;26:235.

58. Snijder CA, Kortenkamp A, Steegers EA, et al. Intrauterine exposure to mild analgesics during pregnancy and the occurrence of cryptorchidism and hypospadia in the offspring: the Generation R Study. Hum Reprod 2012;27:1191.

59. Jensen MS, Rebordosa C, Thulstrup AM, et al. Maternal use of acetaminophen, ibuprofen, and acetylsalicylic acid during pregnancy and risk of cryptorchidism. Epidemiology 2010;21:779.

60. Werler MM, Mitchell AA, Moore CA, Honein MA. Is there epidemiologic evidence to support vascular disruption as a pathogenesis of gastroschisis? Am J Med Genet A 2009;149A(7):1399–1406.

61. Østensen M, Förger F. Management of RA medications in pregnant patients. Nat Rev Rheumatol 2009;57:382–90. 90 Epub 2009 Jun 9.

62. James AH, Brancazio LR, Price T. Aspirin and reproductive outcomes. Obstet Gynecol Surv 2008;63(1):49–57.

63. Koren G, Florescu A, Costei AM, Boskovic R, Moretti ME. Nonsteroidal antiinflammatory drugs during third trimester and the risk of premature closure of the ductus arteriosus: a meta-analysis. Ann Pharmacother Epub 2006 Apr 25.

64. Kellogg A, Rose CH, Harms RH, Watson WJ. Current trends in narcotic use in pregnancy and neonatal outcomes. Am J Obstet Gynecol 2011;204:259.e1.

65. Hadi I, da Silva O, Natale R, et al. Opioids in the parturient with chronic nonmalignant pain: a retrospective review. J Opioid Manag 2006;2:31.

66. Broussard CS, Rasmussen SA, Reefhuis J, et al. Maternal treatment with opioid analgesics and risk for birth defects. Am J Obstet Gynecol 2011;204:314.e1.

67. Yazdy MM, Mitchell AA, Tinker SC, et al. Periconceptional use of opioids and the risk of neural tube defects. Obstet Gynecol 2013;122:838.

68. Geber WF, Schramm LC. Congenital malformations of the central nervous system produced by narcotic analgesics in the hamster. Am J Obstet Gynecol 1975;123:705.

69. Regan J, Chambers F, Gorman W, MacSullivan R. Neonatal abstinence syndrome due to

prolonged administration of fentanyl in pregnancy. BJOG 2000;107(4):570–2.

70. Einarson A, Bozzo P, Taguchi N. Use of a fentanyl patch throughout pregnancy. J Obstet Gynaecol Can 2009;31(1):20.

71. Holt RL, Mikati MA. Care for child development: basic science rationale and effects of interventions. Pediatr Neurol 2011;44:239–53.

72. Palanisamy A. Maternal anesthesia and fetal neurodevelopment. Int J Obstet Anesth 2012; 21:152–63.

73. de Graaf –Peters VB, Hadders-Aigra M. Ontogeny of the human central nervous system; what is happening when? Early Hum Dev 2006;82: 257–66.

74. Matsuzawa J, Matsui M, Konishi T. Age-related volumetric changes of brain gray and white matter in healthy infants and children. Cereb Cortex 2001;11:335–4.

75. Belvindrah R, Lazarini F, et al. postnatal neuro-genesis from neuroblast migration to neuronal integration. Rev Neurosci 2009;20,331–40.

76. Heng JL, Moonen G, Nguyen L. Neurotrans-mitters regulate cell migration in the telence-phalon. Eur J Neurosci 2007;26:537–46.

77. Uban K A, Sliwowska JH, et al. prenatal alcohol exposure reduces neurons and glia in hippo-campus in female rats. Horm Behav 2010;58; 835–43.

78. Manent JB, Jorquera I, et al. Fetal exposure to GABA–acting antiepileptic drugs generates hippocampal and cortical dysplasia. Epilepsia 2007;48:684–93.

79. Hays SR, Deshpande JK. Newly postulated neurodevelopmental risks of pediatric anesthesia. Curr Neurol Neurosci Rep 2011;11:205–10.

80. Franks NP, Lieb WR. Molecular and cellular mechanisms of general anaesthesia. Nature 1994;367:607–14.

81. Lodge D, Anis NA. Effects of phencyclidine on excitatory amino acid activation of spinal inter-neurones in the cat. Eur J Pharmacol 1982;77: 203–4.

82. Jevtovic-Todorovic V, Todorovc SM, Mennerick S. Nitrous oxide (laughing gas) is an NMDA antagonist, neuroprotectant and neurotoxin. Nat Med 1998;4:460.

83. Bhana N, Goa KL, McClellan KJ. Dexmedeto-midine. Drugs 2000;59:26.

84. Ikonomidou C, Bosch F, Miksa M. Blockade of NMDA receptors and apoptotic neurodegene-ration in the developing brain. Science 1999;283: 70–4.

85. Stratmann G. Neurotoxicity of anesthetic drugs in the developing brain. Anesth Analg 2011;113:1170–9.

86. Zhaowei Zhou, Daqing Ma. Anaesthetic-induced Neurotoxicity in Developing Brain: An Update on Preclinical Evidence, Brain Science, 2014.

87. Nemergut ME, Aganga D, Flick RP. Anesthetic neurotoxicity: what to tell the parents? Ped Anesth 2014;24:120–6.

88. Palanisamy A, Baxter MG, Keel PK, et al. Rats exposed to isoflurane in utero during early gestation are behaviorally abnormal as adults. Anesthesiology 2011;114:521–8.

89. Palanisamy A. Maternal anesthesia and fetal neurodevelopment. International Journal of Obstetric Anesthesia 2012;21:152–62.

90. Kong F, Xu L, He D, Zhang X, Lu H. Effects of gestational isoflurane exposure on postnatal memory and learning in rats. Eur J Pharmacol 2011;670:168–74.

91. Rizzi S, Carter LB, Ori C, Jevtovic-Todorovic V. Clinical anesthesia causes permanent damage to the fetal guinea pig brain. Brain Pathol 2008;18: 198–210.

92. Sanders RD, Davidson A. Anaesthetic-induced neurotoxicity of the neonate; time for clinical guidelines? Ped Anesth 2009;19;1141–6.

93. Sprung J, Flick RP, Wilder RT, et al. Anesthesia for cesarean delivery and learning disabilities in a population-based birth cohort. Anesthesiology 2009;111:302–10.

94. Hui Zheng, Yualin Dong, et al. Anaesthesiology 2013;3(vol.118):516–26.

95. Laptook A, Salhab W, et al. Admission tempe-rature of low birth weight infants: predictors and associated morbidities. Pediatrics 2007;19:643–9.

96. Yon JH, Carter LB, et al. Melatonin reduces the severity of anaesthesia-induced apoptotic neuro-degeneration in the developing rat brain. Neurobiol Dis 2006;3:522–30.

97. Jevtovic–Todorovic V, Hartman RE, et al. Early exposure to common anesthetic agents causes widespread neurodegeneration in the developing rat brain and persistent learning defects. J Neurosci 2003;23:876–82.

98. Steinbrook RA, et al. Dissociation of plasma and cerebrospinal fluid beta-endorphin-like immuno-activity levels during pregnancy and parturition. Anesth Analg 1982;61:893.

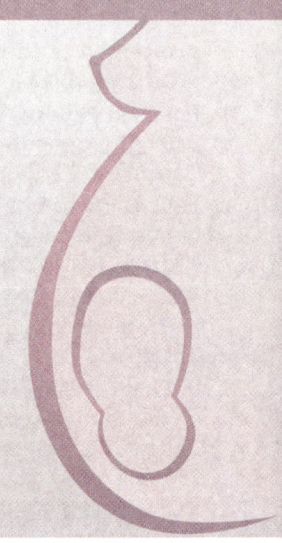

CHAPTER 6

Essentials of Physiological Changes of Pregnancy in Hematological and Coagulation System

Pardnya Bhalerao

INTRODUCTION

Normal pregnancy is characterized by profound changes in almost every organ system to accommodate demands of the fetoplacental unit. Changes in hematological indices are seen in this complex physiological phenomenon. Change in the indices is influenced by factors like seasonal variation, lactation, general health during pregnancy, nutritional status and access to medical care.[1] Hematological indices in turn have an effect on pregnancy and its outcome.

HEMATOLOGICAL CHANGES (Table 6.1)

Blood Volume

Blood volume begins to increase as early as 6 weeks of gestation and increases to more than 50% of the prepregnant state.[2] The change in plasma volume during pregnancy is due to increased plasma renin activity and reduced atrial natriuretic peptide levels. These hormonal changes occur due to pregnancy-induced systemic vasodilatation and increase in vascular capacitance.[3] After delivery, the plasma volume gradually comes to prepregnant values as a result of diuresis.

Table 6.1: Hematological changes[7]		
	Parameter	Change in Pregnancy
Blood volume	Total blood volume	Increase by 45%
	Plasma volume	Increase by 50%
Blood cells	RBC volume	Increase by 30%
	WBC volume	Increase
	Hematocrit	Decrease by 15%
	Hemoglobin	Decrease by 15%

Maternal blood volume begins to increase as early as six weeks, continues to rise by 45–50% till 34 weeks of gestation, returning to normal by 10–14 days postpartum. This physiological hypervolemia helps to maintain blood pressure in presence of decreased vascular tone, facilitates maternal and fetal exchange of respiratory gases, nutrients and metabolites. Besides it protects the mother from hypotension, reducing the risks associated with hemorrhage at delivery.[4,5] Increased fetal and maternal production of estrogen and progesterone also contribute to the rise in plasma volume. Progesterone enhances aldosterone production. Both estrogen and aldosterone increase plasma renin activity. This in turn enhances renal sodium absorption and causes water retention via the renin-angiotensin-aldosterone system.[5] The rise in concentration of plasma adrenomedullin, a potent vasodilating peptide during pregnancy, correlates significantly with blood volume.[6] Around one liter of blood is contained within the uterus and maternal blood spaces of the placenta. Therefore, increase in blood volume is more marked in multiple pregnancies and in iron deficient states.

Hemoglobin, Red Blood Cell, and Plasma Volume

At the outset, no change in the hemoglobin concentration is seen. But after the 16th week, there is a steady fall until the second trimester as a result of expansion of plasma volume. Similar changes are seen in the packed cell volume (PCV) and red blood cell count (RBC). The increase in red cell and hemoglobin (Hb) mass is reported to be maximum at 12–28 weeks of pregnancy.[8] There is little change in red blood cell indices during pregnancy. The underlying cause of anemia during pregnancy is hemodilution, i.e. rise in plasma volume more as compared to increase in the red cell mass (40% vs 20% respectively).[3] After delivery, hemoglobin and hematocrit increases on day 1, is reduced on day 3 and 5, then rises in such a way that by day 42, the normal non-pregnant value is achieved.[9] RBC volume decreases during the first 8 weeks, increases to the pre-pregnancy level by 16 weeks, and undergoes a further rise to 30% above the pre-pregnancy level at term. This rise is due to elevated erythropoietin concentration and a furthur effect of erythropoietin on progesterone, prolactin and placental lactogen.[8]

The resulting hemodilution leads to physiological anemia of pregnancy.[8] The decrease in blood viscosity due to lower hematocrit values reduces resistance to blood flow, as a compensatory mechanism. However, if the Hb concentration falls <10 gm/dL, other causes of anemia should be considered.[8]

Changes in White Blood Cell (WBC) Count

The other prominent change during pregnancy is leukocytosis which is due to physiological stress. This rise occurs early in pregnancy and remains elevated throughout pregnancy. The WBC count during healthy pregnancy varies from 6000 to 9000/cumm hours after delivery.[10] It takes 4 weeks for WBC count to come back to normal postpartum.

Leukocytosis, occurring during pregnancy, is as a result of physiologic stress due to increased inflammatory response to normal pregnancy, which could be a consequence of selective immune tolerance, immunosuppression and immunomodulation of the fetus.[2] Amongst leukocytes, there is a preponderance of the neutrophils, which is due to impaired neutrophilic apoptosis in pregnancy. Neutrophil counts during pregnancy can be twice its postpartum values. Besides this, there is an increase in the oxidative metabolism in neutrophils. Monocytosis also occurs in this state, but the other cells in differential count, i.e. lymphocytes, eosinophils and basophils decline in number. There is evidence of bone marrow hyperplasia with neutrophilic leukocytosis during the last trimester of pregnancy.[11]

Pearl

A blood loss of 1 liter after cesarian section and 500 mL after normal delivery is tolerable because of hemodilution.

Pearls

- Avoid unnecessary use of antibiotics postpartum.
- Correlate leukocyte count to clinical findings.
- Immature myelocytes and metamyelocytes may be seen in the peripheral blood smear of healthy pregnant women.
- Monocytosis is helpful as it prevents fetal allograft rejection by infiltrating the decidual tissue (7th to 20th week) and causes PGE_2 mediated immunosuppression.

Leukocyte and neutrophil count increase significantly on day one postpartum, but start decreasing until the fifth day, to return back to normal.[2]

Platelets

After anemia, the most common hematological abnormality during pregnancy is thrombocytopenia.[12] The average platelet count decreases in pregnancy and there is an increase in platelet aggregation especially during last 8 weeks of gestation. A significant fall in platelet count can occur from 32 weeks of gestation. Increased consumption of platelets as well as decrease in their lifespan in the uteroplacental circulation has been suggested to be the explanation for the reduction in number of circulating platelets during pregnancy. Platelet count as well as other hemostatic factors return to normal 6 weeks postpartum.[2]

'Gestational thrombocytopenia' is partly due to hemodilution and partly due to increased platelet activation and accelerated clearance.[11] However, other etiologies, like megaloblastic anemia, thrombotic microangiopathic syndromes, immune thrombocytopenia, eclampsia and liver disorders, must be excluded before labeling the patient as gestational thrombocytopenia.[12]

Additional evidence of *in vivo* platelet activation in late pregnancy is the increased concentration of β-thromboglobulin and thromboxane A_2 derivatives.[2]

Pearls
- Gestational thrombocytopenia requires no specific treatment and corrects itself spontaneously after delivery.
- Gestational thrombocytopenia is not associated with adverse outcomes to either the mother or fetus.
- Regional anesthesia is generally considered at values >75,000/cumm

COAGULATION FACTOR CHANGES (Table 6.2)

Normal pregnancy is associated with major changes in hemostasis, all contributing to maintain placental function during pregnancy and to prevent excessive bleeding during delivery. Most changes in blood coagulation and fibrinolysis create a state of hypercoagulability.

Table 6.2: Overview of coagulation changes during pregnancy[13]	
Factor	Change in pregnancy
II	Unchanged
VII and fibrinogen	Increased
VIII, IX, X, XII	Increased
XI	Reduced
Protein S	Reduced
Protein C and AT-III	Unchanged
Plasminogen	Increased
D-dimer	Increased

Pearl
This phenomenon protects the woman from hemorrhage during delivery but predisposes her to thromboembolism both during pregnancy and in puerperium.

Changes in Various Factors

1. The concentrations of coagulation factors VII, VIII, IX, X, XII and von Willebrand factor rise significantly, accompanied by a relevant increase in the concentration of plasma fibrinogen.
2. Plasma fibrinogen often increases to over 600 mg/dL in late pregnancy. Factor VII may increase as much as tenfold.
3. The von Willebrand factor and factor VIII are elevated in late pregnancy, when coagulation activity is about twice that in the non-pregnant state.
4. The increase in factors IX and XI concentration is small.

5. After an initial increase, factor XIII falls gradually, reaching 50% of the normal non-pregnant value at term.

6. Factors II and V do not change significantly.

7. Protein C activity appears to be unaffected by gestation. Protein C antigen levels, however, tend to increase in the second trimester but values are within the normal non-pregnant range. Activated protein C (APC) sensitivity is reduced during pregnancy. At term, 45% of pregnant women have an APC sensitivity ratio below the normal range for non-pregnant women of similar age. About 50% of the healthy women develop APC resistance, which reaches its lowest value by the second trimester. This is often called 'acquired' APC resistance.[13]

8. Neutrophil activation is known to trigger endothelial thrombomodulin (TM) proteolysis and to increase TM plasma levels in the third trimester of pregnancy. The TM levels have been found to increase continuously during pregnancy, with a rapid decrease postpartum.

9. A fall in free protein S levels occurs. It may contribute to the hypercoagulable state of pregnancy and increased incidence of thromboembolism.

10. Total protein S has been reported to fall progressively with increasing gestation.

11. Heparin cofactor II, a natural coagulation inhibitor, increases in plasma during pregnancy.

12. Protein Z is a vitamin-K-dependent plasma glycoprotein. It inhibits the activation of factor X. A progressive increase in protein Z levels with gestational in normal pregnancies protects from thrombosis. Return to normal levels around 6 to 12 weeks postpartum has been noted.[14]

Fibrin

Plasma fibrinolytic activity is reduced during pregnancy, continues to be low during labor and delivery, and returns to normal early after placental delivery. Tissue plasminogen activator (t-PA) activity decreases during pregnancy. This occurs due to the gradual increase in plasminogen activator inhibitor-1 (PAI-1) and plasminogen activator inhibitor-2 (PAI-2) both. PAI-1 values increase during pregnancy and normalize at 5 weeks postpartum. Villous cells are the source of PAI-2, so changes in the amount of placental tissue may influence its level in plasma. Thus, a positive correlation is found between PAI-2 concentrations and placental weights. The concentration of PAI-2 also varies with birth weights indicating that it depends not only on the quantity and quality of the placental tissues but also on fetal growth.

Pearls

- The increase in D-dimer makes the use of this parameter in the exclusion of venous thromboembolism in pregnant patients with clinical suspicion difficult.
- Attempts to establish protein S normal levels during pregnancy are not recommended.
- Protein Z deficiency has been reported in women with unexplained early fetal losses, and antibodies to protein Z can contribute to adverse pregnancy outcomes.[14]

  aPTT is usually shortened, by up to 4 seconds in the third trimester largely due to hormonally influenced increase in factor VII. No marked increase in PT or TT occurs.

Changes in Coagulation and Fibrinolysis after Delivery

1. The increase in clotting activity at the time of delivery is most likely related to expulsion of the placenta and release of thromboplastic substances at the site of separation.

2. The changes in the hemostatic mechanism during the puerperium are the same as those observed after extensive surgery.

3. The mean platelet count decreases slightly at the time of placental delivery and starts to increase on days 2–5 postpartum. In high-risk patients where thrombopro-

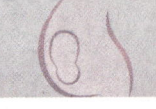

phylaxis is indicated postpartum, the difference in reactive thrombocytosis postpartum, due to operative delivery, should be considered.

4. Plasma antithrombin levels significantly rise after normal delivery for at least 2 weeks postpartum.

5. A rise in protein C level has been shown immediately after delivery and till 3 days postpartum.

6. The level of total and free protein S increases significantly after delivery from the first day of the puerperium; whereas total protein S normalizes in the first week postpartum, free protein S does not normalize even at 5 weeks postpartum. The free fraction of protein S does not appear to reach the non-pregnant value within 8 weeks postpartum, which might be taken into consideration when evaluating thrombotic risk.

> **Pearls**
> - Three weeks after delivery, blood coagulation and fibrinolysis has generally normalized.
> - The state of compensated, accelerated intravascular coagulation may be necessary for maintenance of the uterine placental interface and preparation for the hemostatic challenge of delivery.
> - The peak in clotting and platelet activity seems to occur immediately after placental delivery, whereas the peak of fibrinolytic activity is seen during the first 3 hours postpartum, as reflected by an increase in D-dimer levels.
> - Coagulation factors become normal maximum by the 8th to 12th week.

Other Coagulation Changes

Microparticles

Microparticles (MP) are membrane vesicles shed from various cellular surfaces.

The mechanisms that can result in microparticle formation are cell activation and apoptosis. Microparticles are associated with thrombotic and inflammatory complications. Endothelial cells produce these when the cells are exposed to cytokines, such as interleukin-1 and tumor necrosis factor. Circulating platelet microparticle concentration is a marker of platelet activation.

Normal pregnancy is characterized by increased levels of platelet and endothelial MP compared to non-pregnant healthy women. But the prevalence and role of MP in vascular complications remain controversial.[15]

Homocysteine

Hyperhomocysteinemia is a strong independent risk factor for venous thromboembolism

> **Pearls**
> - The hypercoagulability of blood during pregnancy has been confirmed with thromboelastography (TEG) and is thought mainly due to the increased production of factor VII and fibrinogen.
> - Coagulation factors are increased during pregnancy; none to the extent of factor VII and fibrinogen.
> - The risk of developing a venous thromboembolism increases about 100-fold when a parturient is admitted to a hospital and also seems to be worse during the third trimester.
>   This is thought to be due to changing hormonal levels, particularly increased estrogen as pregnancy progresses.[17]
> - It is important to note that the classic Virchow's triad favors thrombus formation in pregnancy with increased venous stasis, increased coagulation factors, and increased endothelial damage.
> - Risk of venous thromboembolism in pregnancy increases with the following additional risk factors: obesity, smoking, multiple gestations, advanced maternal age, increased parity, cesarean section and presence of a concomitant thrombophilia.[18]
> - There is some evidence to suggest that the body creates a level of homeostasis by increasing fibrinolysis. During pregnancy, we see increase in plasma activity of plasminogen, alpha 2-antiplasmin and elevated concentrations of D-dimer, which suggests increased fibrinolytic activity and restriction of fibrin formation.[19]
> - Thus despite all the factors favoring a hypercoagulable state in pregnancy, venous thromboembolism is relatively rare.
>   Unfractionated heparin and low molecular weight heparin are the modalities of choice for anticoagulation during pregnancy.

and is associated with adverse pregnancy outcomes like pre-eclampsia, placental abruption, early pregnancy loss and neural tube defects. Studies have reported that homocysteine is lower in normal pregnancy than in the non-pregnant state. Although the exact mechanism of homocysteine lowering during pregnancy is not well understood (even if the physiological increase in glomerular filtration rate plays a role), it may protect women from pregnancy complications and thromboembolism, thus maintaining homeostasis in hemostasis. Mean total homocysteine concentrations were found to be lower in pregnant women taking folic acid supplements than in those did not.[16] During the third trimester, total levels were significantly higher in pregnant women with a history of miscarriage than in women with no previous history.

CHANGES IN PROTEINS

Hemoglobin decreases to 12 g/dL, clotting factors (I, VII, VIII, IX, X, XII) are elevated, anticoagulants (S) are decreased and amino acids increase by the second trimester. There is a significant decrease in most fasting maternal amino acid concentrations in early pregnancy prior to the accretion of significant maternal or fetal tissue. There is a 15% increase in protein synthesis during the second trimester and a further increase in the third trimester by about 25%.

Plasma Proteins (Table 6.3)

During the first 20 weeks of pregnancy, the plasma protein concentration is reduced as a result of a rise in plasma volume. This leads to lowered osmotic pressure and edema of the lower limbs especially seen in late pregnancy.

Plasma protein concentration is said to fall from 7 to 6 gm% due to hemodilution. This results in diminished viscosity of the blood and reduced colloid osmotic pressure because of marked fall in albumin level by about 30%. There is a marginal rise in globulin, mainly alpha-globulin.

Significant changes in plasma protein composition in turn affect drug binding and subsequent drug response. The extent of these changes is governed by the stage of gestation.

Both albumin and alpha 1-acid glyco-protein fractions are reduced. Consequently, the binding of both acidic and basic drugs may be affected.

The degree of binding to plasma proteins is an important determinant of drug disposition and response.

Normal pregnancy is associated with changes in concentration of plasma proteins, free fatty acids and other endogenous substances interfering with drug binding.

An associated change in plasma binding capacity, therefore, needs to be considered.

For many drugs, differences have been demonstrated in the degree of protein binding between maternal and cord plasma. This probably causes a marked difference in total drug concentration between maternal and fetal plasma at the time of delivery.

Table 6.3: Plasma protein changes			
Protein	Non-pregnant	Pregnancy and near term	Changes
Total protein (gm)	180	230	Increased
Plasma protein concentration (gm/100 mL)	7	6	Decreased
Albumin (gm/100 mL)	4.3	3	Decreased
Globulin (gm/100 mL)	2.7	3	Slightly increased
Ratio	1.7: 1	1: 1	Decreased

Pearls

- The plasma protein binding of a number of drugs is decreased during pregnancy, particularly during the last trimester. Drugs whose unbound fraction increases during pregnancy include diazepam, valproic acid, phenytoin, phenobarbitone, salicylic acid, pethidine, lignocaine, dexamethasone, sulphafurazole and propranolol.
- Hemodilution and low colloid osmotic pressure (decrease up to 18% of prepregnant levels) predispose the patient to pulmonary edema.
- Pseudocholinesterase levels may fall by 20–25%.

IMMUNE SYSTEM (Table 6.4)

Pregnancy is a state of relative immuno-suppression. It is characterized by anti-inflammatory cellular responses that promote tolerance to fetal antigens. Reversal of these changes during the postpartum period may result in overt clinical manifestations of otherwise quiescent or latent infections.

During pregnancy, unique immunological changes are seen. It is characterized by anti-inflammatory responses which is critical for maintenance of pregnancy.

Th2 (T-helper cells 2) and Th3 responses which support pregnancy are enhanced and Th1 cytokines which are potentially detri-mental to the foreign fetus are suppressed.[20]

Other hormones including progesterone, cortisol, norepinephrine and 1, 25-dihydroxy-cholecalciferol play a major role in modulating immune response during pregnancy.

The shift in the maternal immunology towards Th1 postpartum may be associated with an enhanced proinflammatory response.

Besides this, the immunological system is altered to actively tolerate the semiallogenic fetus. These include changes in the local immune responses in the uterine mucosa. After implantation, the endometrium is rapidly infiltrated by fetal trophoblast cells, which then develops into decidua and ensures anchorage of the placenta and proper fetal nutrition.

Local decidual immune cells, like uterine natural killer cells and macrophages, are important regulators of this balance between tolerance of fetal trophoblasts and limitation of their invasion.

Pearls

Worsening of an existing infection, flaring up of a dormant one and activation of autoimmune responses is often seen postpartum.

SUMMARY

The hematological changes in pregnancy are important to maintain the milieu interior conducive for the growing fetus and protection of the mother.

The relative anemia of pregnancy along with plasma volume expansion guards against blood loss and facilitates fetomaternal gas exchange.

Table 6.4: Immunological changes[20]

Cellular immunity		
Innate	Monocytes and granulocytes	Increased levels
	Natural killer cells	Downregulation
Adaptive	T cells	Enhanced Th2 and Th3, suppressed Th1
	B cells	Increased Th2, induced B cell activity
Humoral immunity		
Innate	Complement	Increased C3, C4
	Acute phase reactants	Increased reactants like fibrinogen and ceruloplasmin
Adaptive	T cells	Increased T cell-mediated immunoglobin production

Gestational thrombocytopenia does not warrant any treatment.

The change in the leukocyte count with rise in neutrophils and monocytes along with immunological changes prevent rejection of the fetus.

Pregnancy is a procoagulant state. However, a converse increase in fibrinolytic activity aids in prevention of thrombo-embolism.

REFERENCES

1. Ichipi-Ifutor PC, Jacob J, Ichipi-Zfukor RN, Ewrhe OL. Changes in the haematological indices in pregnancy. Physiology Journal 2013;1–4.

2. Kaur S, Khan S, Nigam A. Hematological profile and pregnancy: A review. Int J Adv Med 2014;1(2):68–70.

3. Dennen F, Ocaña J, Karasik S, Egan L, Paredes N, Flisser A, et al. Comparison of hemodynamic, biochemical and hematological parameters of healthy pregnant women in the third trimester of pregnancy and the active labor phase. BMC Pregnancy Childbirth 2011;11:33.

4. Grewal A. Anaemia and pregnancy: Anaesthetic implications. Indian J Anaesth 2010;54:380–6.

5. Birnbach DJ, Browne IM. Anesthesia for Obstetrics. In: Miller RD, Eriksson LI, Fleisher LA, Wiener-Kronish JP, Young WL (Eds). Miller's Anesthesia, 7th ed. USA: Churchill Livinstone Elsevier; 2010,p. 2204–6.

6. Hayashi Y, Ueyama H, Mashimo T, Kangawa K, Minamino N. Circulating mature adrenomedullin is related to blood volume in full-term pregnancy. Anesth Analg 2005;101:1816–20.

7. Cheek TG, Gutsche BB. Maternal physiologic alterations. In: Hughes SC, Levinson G, Rosen MA (Eds). Shnider and Levinson's Anesthesia for Obstetrics, 4th ed. Philadelphia, Lippincott: Williams & Wilkins, 2002, p 3.

8. Gaiser R. Physiologic changes of pregnancy. In: Chestnut DH, Polley LS, Tsen LC, Wong CA (Eds). Chestnut's Obstetric Anesthesia: Principles and Practice, 4th ed. USA: Mosby Elsevier 2009, pp. 21–3.

9. Ramakers C, van der Woude DA, Verzijl JM, Pijnenborg JM, van Wijk EM. An added value for the hemoglobin content in reticulocytes (CHr) and the mean corpuscular volume (MCV) in the diagnosis of iron deficiency in postpartum anemic women. Int J Lab Hematol 2012; 34(5):510–6.

10. Chandra S, Tripathi A, Mishra S, Amzarul M, Vaish A. Physiological changes in haematological parameters during pregnancy. Indian J Haematol Blood Transfus 2012;28(3):144–46.

11. Verma A, Chaudhary H. Study of hematological parameters in advanced pregnancy. Int J Recent Trends Sci Technol 2013;7(1):16–9.

12. Khellaf M, Loustau V, Bierling P, Michel M, Godeau B. Thrombocytopenia and pregnancy. Rev Med Intern 2012;33(8):446–52.

13. Prisco D, Ciuti G, Falciani M. Hemostatic changes in normal pregnancy. Haematologica Reports 2005;1(10):1–5.

14. Quack Loetscher KC, Stiller R, Roos M, Zimmermann R. Protein Z in normal pregnancy. Thromb Haemost 2005;93:706–9.

15. Bretelle F, Sabatier F, Desprez D, Camoin L, Grunebaum L, Combes V, et al. Circulating microparticles: a marker of procoagulant state in normal pregnancy and pregnancy complicated by preeclampsia or intrauterine growth restriction. Thromb Haemost 2003;89:486–92.

16. Holmes VA, Wallace JM, Alexander HD, Gilmore WS, Bradbury I, Ward M, et al. Homocysteine is lower in the third trimester of pregnancy in women with enhance folate status from continued folic acid supplementation. Clin Chem 2005;51:629–34.

17. Sultan AA, West J, Tata LJ, Fleming KM, Piercy CN, Grainge MJ. Risk of first thrombo-embolism in pregnant women in hospital: population based cohort study from England. Br Med J 2013;347:60–99.

18. Armstrong EM, Bellone JM, Hornsby LB, Treadway S, Phillippe HM. Pregnancy—Related Venous Thromboembolism. J Pharm Pract 2014; 27(3):243–52.

19. Uchikova EH, Ledjev I. Changes in haemostasis during normal pregnancy. Eur J Obstet Gynecol Reprod Biol 2005;119(2):185–8.

20. Singh N, Perfect JR. Immune reconstitution syndrome and exacerbation of infections after pregnancy. Clinical Infectious Diseases 2007; 45(9):1192–9.

CHAPTER 7

The Placenta

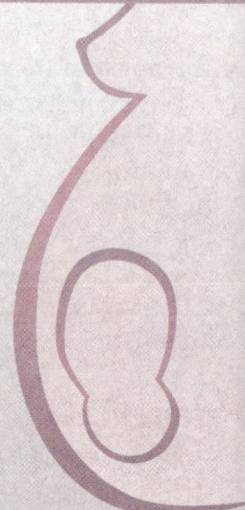

Amit Padvi, Namita Padvi, Namrata Padvi

The name placenta (Greek, *plakuos* = flat cake) is on the basis of this organs appearance. It begins developing at the site of implantation of blastocyst. The placenta is formed as a result of interactions between the invading blastocyst and the tissue of the uterine wall. Morphologically, the placenta is an accessory fetal structure that brings fetal and maternal circulation to close relationship. This is partially of fetal origin (trophoblast from fetus) and partly of maternal origin (transformation of maternal uterine mucosa).

> **Clinical pearl**
> Placenta and placental blood at birth in recent times has been seen as novel source for stem cells for bone marrow replacement and transplant therapy for many diseases.

EMBRYOLOGY AND ANATOMY

The placenta develops as a blastocyst, syncytiotrophoblasts erode the surrounding deciduas and maternal blood circulates around the blastocyst. On the basis of histological structure, human placenta is classified as hemochorial, place where chorion comes in close contact to maternal blood. Its main role is embryonic nutrition. In early placental development, the form of initial transfer of nutrition from mother to embryo is described as histiotrophic nutrition and later blood-borne nutrition is called as hemotrophic nutrition.[1]

Early Placental Anatomy

Important Terminologies

- **Primary villi** (at week 2) are first stage in chorionic villi (Fig. 7.1) developmental process. Trophoblastic shell cells (syncytiotrophoblasts and cytotrophoblasts) form finger-like projections in maternal decidua. Trophoblasts are seen at about day and implanting egg in uterine mucosa is due to proteolytic process which occurs at days 6 to 7. This consists of inner cellular layer, cytotrophoblast, and outer syncytial layer, known as syncytiotrophoblast.
- **Secondary villi** (at week 3) develop in second stage of chorionic villi development, extraembryonic mesoderm grows in villi and covers full surface of chorionic sac.
- **Tertiary villi** depict third stage of chorionic villi developmental process, mesenchyme

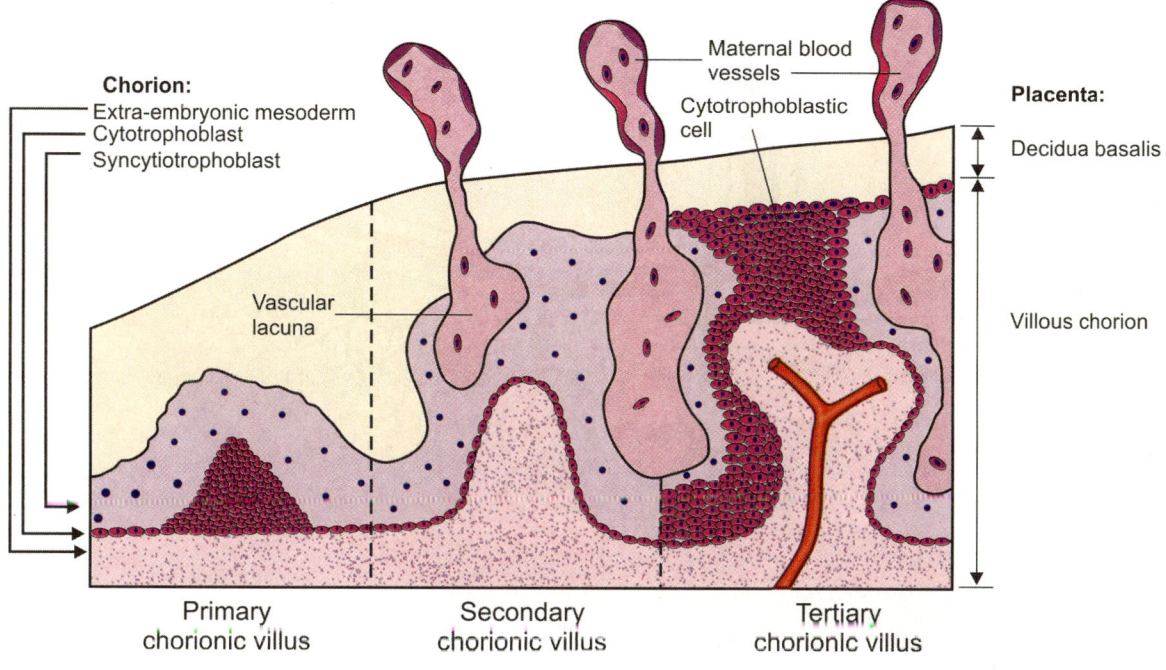

Fig. 7.1. Chorionic villi

forms by differentiation into blood vessels and cells, forms arteriocapillary network, which fuse with placental blood vessels, developing into connecting stalk.

- **Stem villi** also known as anchoring villi are cytotrophoblastic cells attached to maternal tissue.
- **Branched villi and terminal villi** grow from all the sides of stem villi, it is the region of main exchange as surrounding maternal blood flows into intervillous spaces.
- **Terminal villi** are passive extensions induced by capillary vessel coiling because of growth produced by fetal capillaries within mature intermediate villi (in third trimester).
- **Chorionic plate** is a region of membrane at base of villi through which placental arteries and vein pass.
- At birth, placenta is discoid in shape which measures around 20 cm in diameter and 3 cm thick (at term) and weighs 500–600 gm.

- **Umbilical cord** is a connecting stalk which anastomoses in chorion. It extends maternally toward chorionic villi and embryonically into the sinus venosus vessels and dorsal aorta. It is 1–2 cm thick in diameter, 30–90 cm long and covered with **amniotic membrane** attached to **chorionic plate**. It contains paired arteries which carry deoxygenated blood (of dorsal aorta) and waste products into placental villi and two veins, initially. In due course of time, only one is left in embryonic period to carry oxygenated blood to embryo (sinus venosus).
- **Cotyledons** form cobblestone appearance, they are originally placental septa forming grooves. It is covered with maternal decidua basalis.

Clinical pearl

The maternal and embryonic surfaces are both delivered at parturition and their retention may cause postpartum hemorrhage.

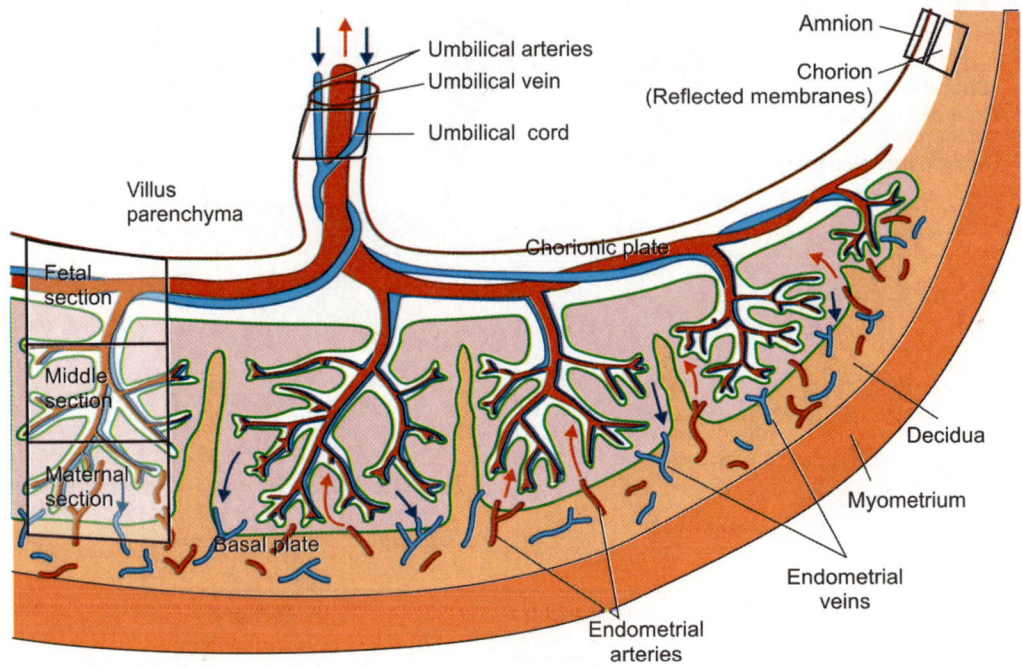

Fig. 7.2. Regulation of placental blood flow

DEVELOPMENT OF VASCULATURE IN THE PLACENTA (Fig. 7.2)

1. At the first month, the placenta has some single blood vessels into villus.

2. At second month, the vascular core has developed.

3. After 4 months, villus has rich vasculature and with thin coat because of disappearance of cytotrophoblast. This is in contrast to villus of second month.

4. At full term, large blood vessels follow villus core to basal plate, and vascular trunks into anchoring villi which give rise to capillary blood vessel network that are involved in all the branches of villi.

5. The placenta at term may show a few large, persistent cytotrophoblastic areas (particularly on the maternal plate), but, as term nears, the cytotrophoblast vanishes in this region as well and is replaced by a fibrinoid layer.

6. As a result of numerous branching, the villus has become comparable to a 'bushy tree'. Its branches form a tangled mass in whose meshes the maternal blood circulates.

7. Formation of the decidua results from the changes in the uterine mucosa that accompany pregnancy.

8. Intervillous space is limited on the maternal side by the basal plate whereas on the fetal side it is limited by the chorionic plate. It is incompletely limited laterally by the decidual septa.

9. The complex division of the villi affects the rate of fetal–maternal exchange.

10. Fetal circulation is comparable to pulmonary circulation of adult in a way that desaturated blood enters fetal arteries and oxygenated blood returns by veins. Blood comes from two umbilical arteries that are branches of iliac arteries of fetus. This is dispersed in highly dense network

that penetrates smallest villus division available. Blood is returned from umbilical vein and it ultimately reaches inferior vena cava of fetus. Fetal circulation is closed circuit of vascular system where average pressure is near about 30 mm Hg that is much higher than that seen in intervillous space, i.e. 10 mm Hg. The difference in pressure prevents the collapse of the villus vessels.

11. Maternal circulation: The blood comes to uterus by branches of uterine artery and it spreads into intervillous spaces, and circulates into branches of villus trees. Blood is returned by branches of uterine veins. Flow in two circulations is extremely high, about 500 mL/minute that favors fetal and maternal blood exchange. Maternal circulation results from difference in pressures that is very high in artery (about 70 mm Hg) and relatively low in intervillous space (which is about 10 mm Hg). Blood spurts into chorionic plate, and then comes toward basal plate and which is taken up by uterine veins where pressure is much lower than which is found in the intervillous space.

EXTRAEMBRYONIC CAVITIES AND MEMBRANES

In the developing embryo, there are number of membranes and cavities, which serve important role in the maintenance of the growing fetus. The amniotic cavity develops as an ectodermally lined space that will eventually surround the fetus. The primary yolk sac forms when the blastocoel becomes lined with extraembryonic endoderm. This then develops into the secondary or definitive yolk sac as acellular mesenchyme and then extraembryonic mesoderm which spreads along the basal lamina of the endoderm. The definitive yolk sac plays an important role in the first trimester. Its circulation (the vitelline circulation) is the first component of the blood vascular system to develop in the embryo.

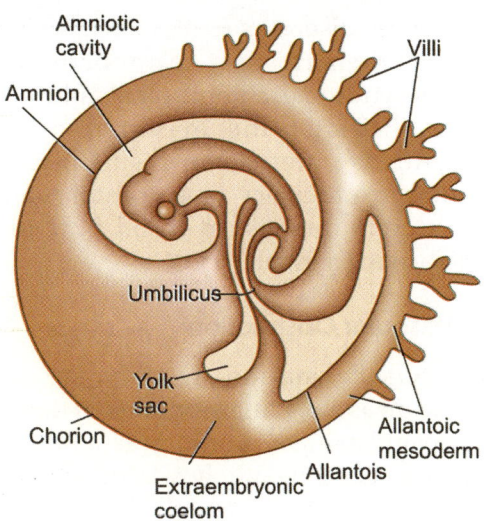

Fig. 7.3. Extraembryonic cavities and membranes

Vitelline veins deliver nutrients from the yolk sac to the embryo, via the hepatic portal system. In addition, the best evidence is that the first hematopoietic cells differentiate in association with the yolk sac. The allantois forms as a diverticulum from the cloaca (Fig. 7.3).

PLACENTAL PATHOLOGY

Maternal Vascular Underperfusion[2]

Systemic maternal diseases, such as severe heart disease, diabetes mellitus, chronic or pregnancy-induced hypertension and pre-eclampsia/eclampsia, thrombophilias (factor V Leiden mutation, deficiency of antithrombin III, protein C or S deficiency, hyper-homocysteinemia, prothrombin mutation),

---

Clinical pearls
- Placental malperfusion results in a chronically underperfused placental bed with decreased fetoplacental growth (small placenta and IUGR).
- The placental underperfusion can also result in a thin umbilical cord, which is predisposed to injury, and underperfusion can lead to oligohydramnios with potential adverse effects on normal fetal lung development.

autoimmune disorders (particularly systemic lupus erythematosus), antiphospholipid antibody syndrome, chronic renal failure, and abnormalities of the maternal arteries supplying the uterus can result in utero-placental insufficiency or placental malperfusion due to diminished blood flow to the uteroplacental vascular bed.

Fetal Vascular Obstruction[3–5]

Thrombus formation within the fetal vasculature as a result of endothelial damage, hypercoagulable states, or turbulent flow with stasis is dictated by Virchow's triad.

FUNCTIONS AND TRANSPORT MECHANISM OF PLACENTA

The placenta acts as an organ of respiration, excretion, and digestion for the fetus. It also plays a major role in the synthesis and regulation of hormones. Placenta synthesizes glycogen, cholesterol, fatty acids, etc. Trans-portation of almost all materials across placental membranes is by simple diffusion, facilitated diffusion, active transport and pinocytosis.

> **Clinical pearl**
>
> The exchange across the placenta is inversely proportional with thickness of placental membranes and which increases progressively during gestation reaching to maximum before normal full term (Fig. 7.4).

Factors Governing Placental Exchange

1. **Size:** Smaller-sized drugs with MW <500 Daltons cross the placenta, while larger-sized drugs with MW >1000 Daltons do not cross placenta, e.g. heparin, protamine and insulin.

> **Clinical pearl**
>
> Succinylcholine (highly ionized) and non-depolarizing NMBDs (high molecular weight) are not able to cross the placenta.

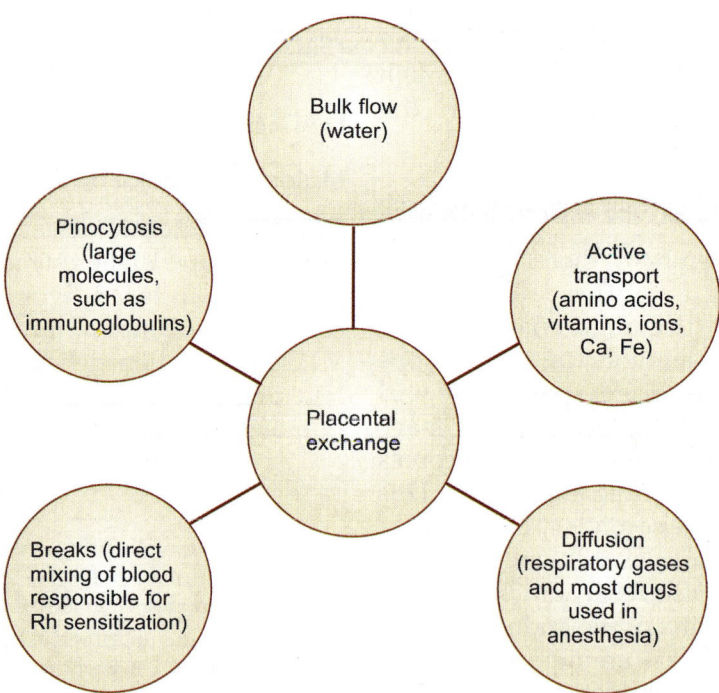

Fig. 7.4. Placental exchange can occur by one of the five mechanisms

Table 7.1: Placental transfer of various elements

Elements	Remarks
Gases: Oxygen, carbon dioxide, carbon monoxide	1. Cross by simple diffusion 2. Near term, uterus extracts 20–35 mL oxygen/minute from maternal blood
Nutrients	1. Water is exchanged freely; water-soluble cross-faster compared to fat-soluble) 2. Little to no transfer of maternal cholesterol, triglycerides, or phospholipids
Hormones	1. Unconjugated steroid hormones have free passage 2. Protein hormones do not cross in large amounts
Electrolytes	Freely exchanged
Antibodies	Provide fetus some amount of passive immunity due to gamma globulin (7S, IgG) which reach the fetus
Wastes	CO_2, urea, uric acid, bilirubin, etc. freely cross placenta
Drugs	Most of them (and their metabolites) cross placenta by diffusion
Infectious agents	Rubella and coxsackie viruses and viruses associated with variola, varicella, measles, encephalitis, and polio cross placenta

2. **Charge:** Non-ionized drugs cross the placenta more freely than ionized drugs; however, the fetus usually has a lower pH than the mother, leading to 'ion trapping'.

3. **Protein binding:** Traditionally, it was taught that protein-bound drugs do not cross the placenta, however, as these medications exist in equilibrium with non-bound versions, it appears contrary.[6]

4. **Lipophilicity:** Liphophilicity generally favors placental transfer, but extreme lipophilicity (e.g. sufentanil) may impede transfer as highly lipophilic substances can accumulate in the placenta.

Anesthetic Drugs Implications

All inhalational agents and most intravenous agents freely cross the placenta.

Intravenous agents: They readily cross the placenta and can be detected in the fetal circulation. Fetal side effects are limited by drug distribution, metabolism, and possibly placental uptake except benzodiazepines.

Opiates: They readily cross the placenta, but their side effects on neonate at birth vary considerably. Morphine causes maximal respiratory depression, while fentanyl the least. Remifentanil too has potential to produce respiratory depression though it is rapidly metabolized in the neonate.

Muscle relaxants: They are highly ionized which hampers placental transfer, resulting in minimal effects on the fetus.

Local anesthetics: They are weakly basic drugs which are primarily bound to α1-acid glycoprotein. Placental transfer of LA depends upon:

1. pKa,
2. Maternal and fetal pH
3. Degree of protein binding.

Acidosis in fetus produces higher and faster fetal-to-maternal drug ratios due to binding of hydrogen ions to non-ionized forms causing trapping of local anesthetic into fetal circulation. Highly protein-bound agents poorly diffuse across placenta; due to greater protein binding of bupivacaine and ropivacaine as compared to lidocaine, leading to lower levels in fetal blood. Chloroprocaine is least transferred as it is rapidly broken down by plasma cholinesterase in maternal circulation.

Anesthetic adjuncts, like ephedrine, antihistamines (H_1 and H_2 blockers), metoclopramide, vasodilators, adrenergic blockers (labetalol and esmolol), phenothiazines, given to mother, are transferred to fetus freely. Atropine and scopolamine cross but not glycopyrrolate. Glycopyrrolate has a quaternary ammonium (ionized) structure that results in limited transfer.

> **Clinical pearls**
> - Inhalational agents cause minimal fetal depression when given in limited doses (<1 MAC) and baby birth occurs within 10 minutes of the induction of anesthesia.
> - Epidural and intrathecal opiates cross to lesser extent and generally produce minimal neonatal respiratory depression.
> - Thiopental, propofol, benzodiazepines, and ketamine all cross the placenta, although only benzodiazepines are noted to produce significant fetal side effects.

Specific Use of Anesthetic Agents

Specific use of anesthetic agents is briefly given in Table 7.2.

Teratogenicity of Anesthetic Drugs

Drugs Associated with Teratogenicity

Timing of exposure is a major deciding factor. During the first 15 days of human gestation, an all-or-nothing phenomenon occurs: the embryo is typically lost or preserved fully intact. The risk of major congenital malformations is increased with exposures between days 13 and 60 in human embryos.[7]

Multiple studies show risk for birth defects in the children of women who had exposure to anesthesia during pregnancy. Overall no study has conclusively shown a higher rate of birth defects in children of women who underwent surgery during pregnancy. At the same time, they have shown a small increase in risk of miscarriage or abortion and premature delivery.[8,9]

Nitrous oxide affects DNA synthesis and has teratogenic effects in animals. Studies have suggested an association between occupational exposure to nitrous oxide in early pregnancy with miscarriage and birth defects. There is a higher risk of spontaneous abortion with exposure to unscavenged nitrous oxide. Modern scavenging techniques can reduce exposure to nitrous oxide by more than 90%.

Most anesthetic medications, including propofol, barbiturates, opioids, neuromuscular blocking agents, and local anesthetics, are generally safe for use during

Table 7.2: Summary of placental transfer of used anesthetic drugs	
Drugs which do not cross the placenta	All muscle relaxants
	Glycopyrrolate, insulin, heparin
Drugs which cross the placenta	
Potentially dangerous	Opiates (morphine, fentanyl in doses of more than 1 µg/kg)
	Benzodiazepines, ephedrine (increased metabolism)
	Local anesthetics, atropine, β-blockers
Drugs which cross the placenta	
Safe	Propofol, thiopental, ketamine, fentanyl at <1 µg/kg
	Epidural opiates (fentanyl, sufentanil)

pregnancy. Evidence for anesthetic-induced neuronal apoptosis is less clear to humans.

REFERENCES

1. Burton GJ, Watson AL, Hempstock J, Skepper JN, Jauniaux EJM. Uterine glands provide histiotrophic nutrition for the human fetus during the first trimester of pregnancy. Clin Endocrinol Metab 2002;87(6):2954–9.

2. Redline RW, et al. Maternal vascular under-perfusion: nosology and reproducibility of placental reaction patterns. Pediatr Devel Pathol 2004;7:237–49.

3. Kraus FT, Acheen VI. Fetal thrombotic vasculopathy in the placenta: cerebral thrombi and infarcts, coagulopathies, and cerebral palsy. Hum Pathol 1999;30:759–69.

4. Parast MM, et al. Placental histologic criteria for umbilical blood flow restriction in unexplained stillbirth. Human Pathol 2008;39:948–53.

5. Gogia N, Machin GA. Maternal thrombophilias are associated with specific placental lesions. Pediatr Dev Pathol 2008;11:424–9.

6. Pacifici GM, Nottoli R. Placental transfer of drugs administered to the mother. Clin Pharmacokinet 1995;28(3):235–69.

7. Tuchmann DH. The teratogenic risk. Am J Ind Med 1983;4:245–58.

8. Shnider SM, Webster GM. Maternal and fetal hazards of surgery during pregnancy. Am J Obstet Gynecol 1965;92:891–900.

9. Czeizel AE, Pataki T, Rockenbauer M. Reproductive outcome after exposure to surgery under anesthesia during pregnancy. Arch Gynecol Obstet 1998;261:193–9.

Principles in
Management of Obstetric Anesthesia

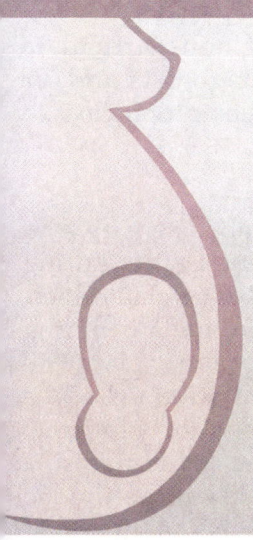

Anesthesia Management in Early Pregnancy Complications

Anita Malik, Namisha Malik

A thorough understanding of the physiological changes of early pregnancy, the specific issues associated with each pathologic condition and their anesthetic implications is essential in the anesthetic management of early pregnancy complications.

PHYSIOLOGICAL CHANGES OF EARLY PREGNANCY

Respiratory Changes[1]

The increased oxygen demand and carbon dioxide production of the growing placenta and fetus cause minute ventilation to be increased more than non-pregnant values in the first trimester and for the remainder of the pregnancy. The sensitivity of the respiratory center to carbon dioxide is increased by elevated progesterone concentrations which stimulate the respiratory efforts in pregnancy. Increase in tidal volume with a little increase in respiratory rate (physiological hyperventilation) results in respiratory alkalosis with maternal arterial partial pressure of carbon dioxide ($PaCO_2$) decreasing to 30–33 mm Hg by 10–12 weeks gestation. Partial compensation by decreased bicarbonate concentration leads to a maternal pH that is slightly above normal (approximately 7.44). Maternal room air PaO_2 is more than 100 mm Hg in early pregnancy because of the presence of hyperventilation and the associated decrease in alveolar CO_2. The minute ventilation is increased by at least 15% at 12 weeks gestation and by 25% at 20 weeks gestation. Thus an increase in minute ventilation is advisable for pregnant woman requiring mechanical ventilation in early pregnancy.

Cardiovascular Changes

At 18 to 20 weeks gestation, the uterine fundus reaches the umbilicus and is large enough to cause aortocaval compression whenever the patient assumes the supine position[2] so a left uterine tilt is required and should be attained by elevating the right hip with a wedge. In the presence of multiple gestation, polyhydramnios, or gestational trophoblastic disease, the need for a left uterine tilt occurs earlier in gestation. Maternal intravascular fluid volume begins to increase in the first trimester secondary to the increasing progesterone (from the gestational sac) induced changes in the renin-angiotensin-aldosterone system promoting sodium absorption and water retention.[3] Due to a reduction in systemic vascular resistance, systemic blood pressure decreases in an uncomplicated pregnancy. Systolic, diastolic, and arterial blood pressure may all decrease 5–20% by 20 weeks gestational age, though they may be affected by positioning and parity. During the first half of pregnancy, a blood loss of 500 to 1500 mL rarely requires blood transfusion (provided that the blood loss is replaced with an adequate volume of crystalloid or colloid) because a pregnant women has an expanded blood volume, and can tolerate such an amount of blood loss.[4]

Gastrointestinal Changes

During the first trimester, the tone of the lower esophageal sphincter is decreased due to increased progesterone levels. At 15 weeks gestation, the fasting gastric volume is approximately 30 mL in both pregnant and non-pregnant women and this volume can be reduced to 50% by metoclopramide 10 mg, intravenously 15 to 30 minutes prior to anesthesia.[5] The movement of uterus out of the pelvis at 18 to 20 weeks gestation leads to anatomic and intragastric pressure changes that contribute to gastroesophageal reflux. For all these reasons, pregnant women who require general anesthesia as early as 12 to 14 weeks gestation should be intubated apart from the women in early pregnancy who are at increased risk of gastric content aspiration (e.g. history of gastroesophageal reflux, morbid obesity, food ingestion within 6 to 8 hours) and those with a suspected difficult airway or a history of a difficult airway. Sodium citrate, an H2-receptor antagonist, and/or metoclopramide prophylactically reduce the risk of aspiration pneumonia further. A recent Cochrane review states that a combination of antacids plus H2 antagonists is more effective than no pharmacologic intervention and better than antacids alone in decreasing gastric acidity.[6] Current American Society of Anesthesiologists (ASA) guidelines for obstetric anesthesia state, "the timely administration of non-particulate antacids, H2 receptor antagonists and/or metoclopramide for aspiration prophylaxis."[7]

Neurologic Changes

The nervous system is more sensitive to general and local anesthetic agents during early pregnancy. The MAC of a volatile anesthetic is reduced by 28% in humans during the first trimester of pregnancy.[8] The minimum alveolar concentration (MAC) is approximately 30% lower with halothane, enflurane, and isoflurane. Presumably, a reduction in MAC also occurs with desflurane and sevoflurane. As early as the first trimester, the local anesthetic dose requirement is decreased for neuraxial block before significant aortocaval compression or other mechanical or pressure-related changes occur.[9]

ECTOPIC PREGNANCY

Clinical Presentation

Most ectopic pregnancies occur in the fallopian tube. Ectopic pregnancies outside the fallopian tubes are more likely to be associated with massive hemorrhage, especially with abdominal pregnancies, when the placenta is removed. Classic clinical signs of impending rupture or a ruptured tubal pregnancy include abdominal or pelvic pain (95%), delayed menstruation (75 to 95%), and vaginal bleeding (60 to 80%).[10]

Sudden collapse may occur, if the tube ruptures (caused by reflex vagal activity or hypovolemia, if bleeding is severe, or both). Physical findings include abdominal tenderness with or without rebound (80 to 95%), a uterus that is smaller than expected for dates (30%), and a tender adnexal mass (30 to 50%).[4]

Diagnosis

Transvaginal ultrasonography is the current modality of choice because it can detect an intrauterine gestational sac as soon as 21 days after conception (when beta-hCG concentrations are greater than 1400 mIU/mL with use of the International Reference Preparation [IRP] standard). Transabdominal ultrasonography visualizes an intrauterine pregnancy when the serum beta-hCG concentrations are higher than 6000 to 6500 mIU/mL IRP.[11] Serial beta-hCG concentrations that show a change in the form of a decrease, plateau, or a subnormal rise (less than 53% over 48 hours) indicate a nonviable pregnancy usually which may be either an ectopic pregnancy or an impending abortion.[12] A slower decline is suggestive of an ectopic pregnancy. Beta-hCG concentrations greater than 100,000 mIU/mL are usually associated with viable intrauterine pregnancies.[13]

Problems/Special Considerations

The main risk of ectopic pregnancy is sudden severe hemorrhage, which may be intra-abdominal and thus concealed until rapid decompensation and collapse occur. However, even at this early stage of pregnancy, there may be features of the physiological changes of pregnancy.

Anesthetic Management

Operative management usually involves laparoscopy unless there is severe hemodynamic instability, in which case a laparotomy is performed. Patients with an unruptured tubal pregnancy usually have a normal intravascular volume and little bleeding before and during surgery. The anesthetic and surgical risks are low. Anesthetic aspects of the procedure itself are as for any other laparoscopic operation.

Ruptured ectopic pregnancy may be associated with significant preoperative blood loss as women typically present late with significant hemoperitoneum and/or hypovolemic shock. General anesthesia is preferred in cases in which significant bleeding has occurred (e.g. ruptured tubal

pregnancy) or is likely to occur (e.g. cervical, interstitial, cornual, prior cesarean scar, or abdominal ectopic pregnancy). Large-bore intravenous catheters should be placed as soon as possible. Adequate units of blood products should be immediately available.

General Considerations

Blood typing and antibody screening is usually done. Aspiration prophylaxis is provided, if the patient has a full stomach. Routine non-invasive monitors (electrocardiogram, blood pressure cuff, pulse oximeter, temperature probe, and nerve stimulator) are attached. One wide bore peripheral intravenous catheter with crystalloid solution is started. If major bleeding has occurred or is expected to occur (e.g. ruptured tubal, interstitial, cervical, uterine scar, or abdominal ectopic pregnancy) two or more intravenous catheters are inserted. Bladder catheterization is done to monitor urine output.

General Anesthesia

If the patient has a good airway but a full stomach, rapid-sequence induction with cricoid pressure application is planned. Induction is done with thiopental or propofol (ketamine or etomidate should be considered, if patient is hemodynamically unstable). Muscle relaxant is used and endotracheal intubation is performed with end-tidal carbon dioxide monitoring. Maintenance is provided with oxygen, nitrous oxide, opioid and a volatile anesthetic agent or a propofol infusion as tolerated. Placement of an oro-/nasogastric tube is done. Post-surgery, reversal of muscle relaxant is done and extubation is performed once the patient is awake and responds to verbal commands.

Neuraxial blockade

In hemodynamically stable patients with a low likelihood of significant hemorrhage (i.e. unruptured tubal pregnancy), neuraxial anesthesia may be considered. Prehydration with 1000 mL of crystalloid solution, supplemental oxygen, and minimal sedation with midazolam is advised. Subarachnoid block may provided with bupivacaine 12 to 15 mg with fentanyl 25 μg, to achieve a T4 sensory blockade.[4]

ABORTION AND INTRAUTERINE FETAL DEMISE

Clinical Presentation

Abortion refers to a pregnancy loss or termination, either before 20 weeks gestation or when the fetus weighs less than 500 g. It can be spontaneous or can be performed electively for personal or medical reasons. A threatened abortion is defined as uterine bleeding without cervical dilation before 20 weeks gestation. Bleeding may be accompanied by abdominal cramps or backache. After the confirmation of diagnosis, the patient's activities are restricted until symptoms resolve. An inevitable abortion is defined as cervical dilation or rupture of membranes without expulsion of the fetus or placenta. Spontaneous expulsion of the uterine contents usually occurs, but infection can be a complication.

A complete abortion is defined as a total, spontaneous expulsion of the fetus and placenta. Partial expulsion of the uterine contents (i.e. an incomplete abortion) is more common after 8 weeks gestation.[14] Signs of an incomplete abortion are persistent bleeding and cramping after expulsion of tissue. Recurrent or habitual abortion refers to the occurrence of three or more consecutive spontaneous abortions in the same patient. In a patient with a missed abortion, fetal death may go unrecognized for several weeks. Intrauterine fetal demise may remain undiagnosed for several days, but if this situation arises, it is potentially life-threatening, since the mother is at a risk of developing disseminated intravascular coagulation and sepsis more likely when the fetus dies at an advanced gestational age. Tissue thromboplastin, a trigger factor for disseminated intravascular coagulation, is not released from the fetus until 3–5 weeks after intrauterine death, but it may be released from the placenta following placental separation. Intrauterine infection may also act as a trigger for developing a coagulopathy.

Anesthetic Management

An incomplete abortion usually requires a dilation and evacuation procedure to remove any remaining fetal or placental tissue. Several factors to be considered before planning anesthetic management include dilation of cervix, the presence of significant blood loss, sepsis and full stomach. The physiological changes of pregnancy, the psychological state of the woman and the need for routine preoperative assessment of the patient are considered important. Assessment of blood loss may be difficult as a fit young women may lose a significant proportion of their blood volume without becoming hypotensive. Tachycardia indicates possible hypovolemia. Signs of sepsis should be sought, and prophylactic antibiotics may be considered.

If the cervix is not dilated, anesthesia is usually necessary as dilation of the cervix is relatively painful and may be accomplished with a paracervical block and sedation, or with spinal, epidural, or general anesthesia. Sensory blockade to T10 is necessary for neuraxial anesthesia. If the cervix is dilated, intravenous analgesia with fentanyl and sedation with midazolam or propofol with or without a paracervical block may suffice as suction and curettage are less painful.

In the presence of significant bleeding, appropriate restoration of intravascular volume is required and a paracervical block with sedation may provide adequate analgesia, however, if the patient has significant discomfort after a paracervical block, general anesthesia may be instituted.

Ketamine may be an ideal agent for induction of general anesthesia. Large doses (1.5 to 2.0 mg/kg) of ketamine may be advantageous in patients who require evacuation of the uterus as uterine tone is increased.[15] Dose-dependent relaxation of uterine smooth muscle is produced by volatile anesthetic agents[16] and is associated with increased uterine bleeding.[17] In in vitro experiments, volatile halogenated anesthetics including sevoflurane and desflurane have a dose-dependent association with uterine atony but no clinical differences in blood loss with doses up to 1 MAC have been observed. However, oxytocin appears to successfully diminish these volatile effects up to 1.5 MAC.[18] The risk of uterine perforation may be increased during relaxation of the uterus provided with a volatile anesthetic agent. So administration of a volatile agent during dilation and evacuation/curretage procedures should be avoided. Spinal or epidural anesthesia should be avoided in such patients.

If significant bleeding is not there, general anesthesia is commonly maintained with oxygen, nitrous oxide, an opioid (with or without a small dose of benzodiazepine) and propofol infusion or a low concentration (less than 0.5 MAC) of a volatile agent. However, the volatile agent should be avoided or discontinued, if there is any evidence of uterine atony. Spinal anesthesia has also been advised with a single injection bupivacaine 7.5 mg with fentanyl 20 µg, to achieve T8 sensory blockade[4] as an anesthetic level of T10 is insufficient to prevent pain occurring when the uterine fundus is manipulated or curetted.

INCOMPETENT CERVIX

Incompetent cervix is defined as the inability to sustain a pregnancy to full term and may be an inherent or traumatic deficiency in the structure or function of the uterine cervix. Recurrent second trimester pregnancy losses may be accompanied with painless cervical dilation, herniation followed by rupture of the fetal membranes and a short labor with delivery of a live, immature fetus.

Obstetric Management

Cerclage placement is useful in women with a singleton pregnancy, a short cervix, and a history of cervical insufficiency.[19,20] Modified Shirodkar cerclage[21] and the McDonald cerclage[22] are the commonly performed transvaginal cerclage procedures. A ligature is placed at or near the level of the internal cervical os around the cervix. A transabdominal cerclage may be performed in a failure of previous transvaginal cerclage, congenital or traumatic cervical shortening, severe cervical laceration[23] and most of these patients undergo cesarean delivery. Contraindications to a cerclage procedure are vaginal bleeding, preterm labor, chorioamnionitis, rupture of membranes, placental abruption, fetal anomalies and fetal death. The clinical management guidelines from the American College of Obstetricians and Gynecologists suggest that though the data available on the efficacy of cerclages is limited, an elective cerclage should be performed at 13–16 weeks of gestation in patients with a viable fetus and a history of three or more otherwise unexplained second trimester pregnancy losses or preterm deliveries.[24]

Rupture of the membranes during the performance of emergency cerclage is the greatest risk. As uterine relaxation is essential, administration of a volatile anesthetic agent or a tocolytic drug is required. Steep Trendelenburg position is used for gravity assistance. Immediate complications are rupture of the fetal membranes, hemorrhage, and preterm labor while delayed complications include infection, cervical lacerations and uterine rupture (if labor proceeds with the cerclage in place) and cervical stenosis secondary to scarring.

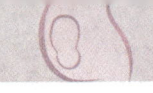

Anesthetic Management

Both regional and general anesthesia techniques are considered acceptable choice for cervical cerclage.[25] Choice of anesthesia technique is influenced by the degree of cervical dilation.

If the cervix is not dilated, general anesthesia, neuraxial blockade may be administered. Because both the cervix (L1 to T10) and vagina and perineum (S2 to S4) require anesthesia, sensory blockade from T10 through the sacral dermatomes is necessary. Adequate anesthesia may not be provided by pudendal block in many patients. Paracervical block is avoided because of the potential adverse effects on uteroplacental perfusion.

If the cervix is dilated and especially if the fetal membranes are bulging, the choice of anesthesia requires prevention of an increase in intra-abdominal and intrauterine pressure that may cause further bulging and possible rupture of the fetal membranes, leading to fetal death subsequently. Thus, general anesthesia may be preferred in the patient with a dilated cervix and bulging fetal membranes. Replacement of the bulging membranes and placement of the cerclage is facilitated by a decrease in intrauterine pressure. During induction and maintenance of general anesthesia, endotracheal tube-induced coughing should be avoided, which might raise intrauterine pressure. Volatile anesthetic agents (isoflurane or sevoflurane) relax uterine smooth muscle and thereby decrease intrauterine pressure. An antiemetic agent should be given as vomiting significantly raises intrauterine pressure.

Administration of neuraxial anesthesia obviates the need for endotracheal intubation and the possibility of coughing on the endotracheal tube. Spinal anesthesia is provided with bupivacaine 7.5 mg with fentanyl 20 µg, to achieve a T8 to T10 sensory blockade.[4] A reduction in placental blood flow due to raised intrauterine pressure subsequent to replacement of bulging membranes and closure of the cervix may require a tocolytic agent to help reduce intrauterine pressure.

GESTATIONAL TROPHOBLASTIC DISEASE

Trophoblastic tissue forms the placenta in normal pregnancies while proliferation of abnormal trophoblastic tissue results in gestational trophoblastic disease (GTD). Hydatidiform mole and malignant gestational trophoblastic neoplasia (GTN) are the two main groups which constitute the gestational trophoblastic disease.

Clinical Presentation and Diagnosis

Hydatidiform mole: Patients present with vaginal bleeding after a period of amenorrhea. There may be history of passing hydropic vesicles. Diagnosis of hydatidiform mole is suggested by the absence of fetal cardiac activity, a uterus large for gestational age, and a marked elevation of beta-hCG concentration. Associated findings may be large ovarian cysts, hyperemesis gravidarum, and an early onset of pregnancy-induced hypertension, anemia, hyperthyroidism, DIC, and infection. Ultrasonography may show characteristic multiechogenic areas representing hydropic villi or hemorrhagic foci. Medical complications occur in about 25% of patients with uterine size of more than 14 to 16 weeks gestation which include ovarian theca-lutein cysts, hyperemesis gravidarum and pregnancy-induced hypertension (PIH).[26–34]

The syndrome of PIH consists of hypertension with proteinuria, edema, and/or hyperreflexia.

Because blood loss may occur gradually, the patient may have a normal intravascular volume despite the presence of severe anemia. Hyperthyroidism may be due to marked elevation of hCG, which can have a thyrotropin-like effect or due to some other thyrotropic substance produced by the neoplasm.[35] Thyroid storm (sinus tachycardia, atrial fibrillation, hyperthermia, cardio-vascular collapse) can be precipitated by anesthesia or surgery.

In patients with a uterine size of 16 weeks or greater, a higher risk of cardiopulmonary complications has been noticed[36,37] like chest pain, cough, tachycardia, tachypnea, hypoxemia, diffuse rales, and evidence of bilateral pulmonary infiltrates in chest radiograph. The etiology of cardiopulmonary distress in more than half the cases is suggested to be trophoblastic embolization, while other causes include high-output cardiac failure from thyrotoxicosis, pulmonary congestion from severe anemia, PIH, aspiration pneumonitis, and iatrogenic fluid overload.[37,38] Symptoms usually develop within 12 hours of uterine evacuation and may subside within hours, however, some patients may require invasive hemodynamic moni-toring and mechanical ventilation. If massive embolization or adult respiratory distress syndrome develops, mortality is high.[39]

Anesthetic Management

Evaluation of specific complications of molar pregnancy, like PIH, hyperemesis gravi-darum, anemia, and thyrotoxicosis, holds an important place in preoperative assessment. Although convulsions rarely occur in PIH patients, prophylactic administration of magnesium sulfate is advisable. An antihyper-tensive agent (hydralazine, labetalol) is required to reduce blood pressure. Significant electrolyte disturbances and volume depletion can be manifested due to hyperemesis gravidarum, and should be corrected before anesthesia.

Invasive hemodynamic monitoring is required in the presence of cardiopulmonary distress before evacuation of the uterus. Two large gauge intravenous catheters for intra-venous access should be established and immediate availability of blood products is required as blood loss may be significant

during evacuation of the uterus and patient may be anemic already due to gradual blood loss through vaginal bleeding.

General anesthesia is preferred because of the anticipated significant blood loss during evacuation of the uterus. As marked hypo-tension in hypovolemic patients may be caused by thiopental, propofol and marked tachycardia in hyperthyroid patients by ketamine,[40] the drug of choice is etomidate. Maintenance of anesthesia involves adminis-tration of oxygen, nitrous oxide, a benzo-diazepine, and an opioid with avoidance of volatile anesthetic agents (increased risk of blood loss and uterine perforation). Spinal anesthesia has been reported for a dilatation and evacuation procedure in a patient with a hydatidiform mole and associated hyper-thyroidism, but with an advise of essential careful attention to blood loss and the ability to rapid transfusion.[41]

Oxytocin facilitates safe curettage and reduced blood loss due to uterine contraction. The patient should be monitored closely postoperatively, for any evidence of uterine hemorrhage or cardiopulmonary distress.

HYPEREMESIS GRAVIDARUM

Hyperemesis gravidarum is a persistent, severe form of nausea and vomiting in pregnant women. There may be evidence of malnutrition and/or dehydration, with associated biochemical and metabolic derangement including renal and particularly hepatic impairment and mineral/vitamin deficiency, e.g. Wernicke's encephalopathy. The muscle bulk is virtually always reduced in severe cases and there may be fetal growth retardation.

Anesthesiologists may be asked to assist in establishing peripheral or central venous access for fluid replacement and/or nutrition, involved in providing analgesia or anesthesia for delivery or, for termination of pregnancy rarely, if hyperemesis is very severe. There are many other conditions that should also

Table 8.1: Conditions to be considered in severe vomiting in pregnancy[4]

Infective	Gastroenteritis, urinary tract infection, hepatitis
Surgical	Intra-abdominal pathology
Neurological	Increased intracranial pressure, migraine
Metabolic	Diabetes, hypercalcemia, uremia
Drug-related	Antibiotics, analgesics, alcohol
Others	Severe reflux esophagitis, acute fatty liver of pregnancy, psychogenic

be considered in severe vomiting in pregnancy (Table 8.1).

Problems/Special Considerations

In cases where dehydration is apparent, intravenous rehydration is required; use of glucose-containing solutions may provide a small amount of caloric intake but excessive administration may result in hyponatremia. Correction of electrolyte abnormalities and pharmacologic antiemetic therapy are indicated. Vitamin and mineral supplementation is advisable, especially with thiamine. Parenteral nutrition may be required in very severe cases.

CORPUS LUTEUM CYST

A persistent corpus luteum is a normal component of pregnancy. It usually appears as a small cystic structure on ultrasonographic imaging, with smooth borders and a fluid center. It may sometimes contain debris, such as clotted blood, which suggests endometriosis or a simple cyst with bleeding into it. The corpus luteum of pregnancy can reach 10 cm in size. Most functional cysts resolve by the early second trimester.[42,43] Cysts more than 10 cm in size are usually resected due to increased risk of malignancy, rupture or torsion. The incidence of ovarian torsion rises 5-fold during pregnancy to approximately 5 per 10,000 pregnancies.[44] Its most common cause in pregnancy is a corpus luteum cyst, which usually regresses spontaneously by the second trimester.[45] Ovarian torsion,

therefore, occurs most frequently in the first trimester, occasionally in the second, and rarely in the third.[46] Delaying surgery until 16–18 weeks' gestation prevents unnecessary surgery by allowing resolution of functional cysts and may also decrease the rate of miscarriage from potential disruption of the corpus luteum and prevents exposure of the fetus to anesthesia during organogenesis, which is typically complete by the end of the first trimester. Ovarian cyst which ruptures, or undergoes torsion or if it shows evidence of malignancy, requires immediate surgery, irrespective of the period of gestation.[47]

Clinical Manifestations and Diagnosis

Ovarian torsion can sometimes be difficult to diagnose in pregnancy. The most common clinical presentation is acute onset of severe, colicky unilateral pelvic pain that is usually unremitting but can wax and wane in cases of incomplete, intermittent torsion. Fall in blood pressure and heart rate is another common response to visceral and deep somatic nociception.[48]

Ultrasound is the diagnostic modality of choice and will most often reveal a unilateral ovarian enlargement that appears solid, cystic, or complex, with or without fluid collections in the pouch of Douglas. Color Doppler sonography often depicts an enlarged ovary without perfusion of the parenchyma.[49] Because the second trimester is a time when the risks of both first trimester loss and preterm labor can be avoided, it is viewed as the ideal window of opportunity for intervention.[50] In the non-pregnant patient and during the first trimester of pregnancy, ovarian torsion can usually be approached laparoscopically.[51] In the first trimester, when ovarian torsion most often occurs in pregnancy, the risk of fetal loss is the smallest with modern anesthetic techniques.[52] Regional anesthesia should be used whenever possible to decrease postoperative pain and the subsequent release of catecholamines, which can stimulate uterine contractility.[53] If the patient is hemodynamically unstable, general anesthesia is preferred.

SUMMARY

The anesthetic management of the patient with early pregnancy complications requires the considerations of the physiological changes of early pregnancy, the psychological state of the woman and the importance of routine preoperative assessment. At 18 to 20 weeks gestation, the uterine fundus reaches the umbilicus and is large enough to cause aortocaval compression whenever the patient assumes the supine position, thus a left uterine tilt is required and should be attained by elevating the right hip with a wedge. The movement of uterus out of the pelvis at this time leads to anatomic and intragastric pressure changes that contribute to gastro-esophageal reflux. As early as the first trimester, the local anesthetic dose requirement is decreased for neuraxial block before significant aortocaval compression or other mechanical or pressure-related changes occur. In ectopic pregnancy, sudden collapse may occur, if the tube ruptures (caused by reflex vagal activity or hypovolemia, if bleeding is severe, or both). Dilation of cervix, the presence of significant blood loss, sepsis and full stomach are important factors to be considered before planning anesthesia management for dilation and evacuation procedure in incomplete abortion. In incompetent cervix, during induction and maintenance

of general anesthesia, endotracheal tube-induced coughing should be avoided, which might raise intrauterine pressure. Preoperative assessment in molar pregnancy requires evaluation of associated specific complications like PIH, hyperemesis gravidarum, anemia, and thyrotoxicosis. In hyperemesis gravidarum, there may be an evidence of malnutrition and/or dehydration, with associated biochemical and metabolic derangement including renal and particularly hepatic impairment and mineral/vitamin deficiency, e.g. Wernicke's encephalopathy. Usually, the corpus luteum cyst resolves in early pregnancy but immediate surgery, irrespective of the period of gestation, is required in ovarian cyst which ruptures, or undergoes torsion or if it shows evidence of malignancy.

REFERENCES

1. Crapo RO. Normal cardiopulmonary physiology during pregnancy. Clin Obstet Gynecol 1996;39: 3–16.

2. Marx GF. Aortocaval compression syndrome: Its 50-year history. Int J Obstet Anesth 1992;1:60–4.

3. Flood P, Rollins MD. Anesthesia for obstetrics. In: Miller RD (Ed). Miller's Anesthesia, 18th ed, Elsevier, 2015.

4. Chantigian RC, Chantigian PDM. Problems of early pregnancy. In: Chestnut DH, Polly LS, Tsen LS, Wong CA (Eds). Chestnut's Obstetric Anesthesia: Principles and Practice, Elsevier, 2009.

5. Wyner J, Cohen SE. Gastric volume in early pregnancy: Effect of metoclopramide. Anesthesiology 1982;57:209–12.

6. Paranjothy S, Griffith's JD, Broughton HK, et al. Interventions at cesarean section for reducing the risk of aspiration pneumonitis; Cochrane Database Syst Rev 1:CD004943,2010.

7. American Society of Anesthesiologists Task Force on Obstetric Anesthesia. Anesthesiology 2007;106:843.

8. Gin T, Chan MTV. Decreased minimum alveolar concentration of isoflurane in pregnant humans. Anesthesiology 81:829, 1994.

9. Fagraeus L, Urban BJ, Bromage PR. Spread Anesthesiology 1983;58:184.

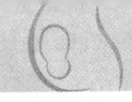

10. Cunningham FG, Leveno KJ, Bloom SL, et al. William's Obstetrics, 22nd ed. New York, McGraw-Hill, 2005;253–72.

11. Fossum GT, Davajan V, Kletzky OA. Early detection of pregnancy with transvaginal ultrasound. Fertil Steril 1988;49:788–91.

12. Seeber BE, Barnhart KT. Suspected ectopic pregnancy. Obstet Gynecol 2006;107:399–413.

13. Stovall TG, Ling FW, Carson SA, Buster JE. Serum progesterone and uterine curettage in differential diagnosis of ectopic pregnancy. Fertil Steril 1992;57:456–7.

14. McNeeley SG Jr. Early abortion. In Sciarra JJ, Dilts PV Jr (Eds). Gynecology and Obstetrics, vol 2. Philadelphia: JB Lippincott, 1992;pp.1–6.

15. Oats JN, Vasey DP, Waldron BA. Effects of ketamine on the pregnant uterus. Br J Anaesth 1979;51:1163–6.

16. Munson ES, Embro WJ. Enflurane, isoflurane, and halothane and isolated human uterine muscle. Anesthesiology 1977;46:11–4.

17. Hall JE, Ng WS, Smith S. Blood loss during first trimester termination of pregnancy: Comparison of two anaesthetic techniques. Br J Anaesth 1997; 78:172–4.

18. Yildiz K, Dogru K, Dalgic H, et al. Inhibitory effects of desflurane and sevoflurane on oxytocin-induced contractions of isolated pregnant human myometrium. Acta Anaesthesiol Scand 2005;49:1355–9.

19. Romero R, Espinoza J, Erez O, Hassan S. The role of cervical cerclage in obstetric practice: Can the patient who could benefit from this procedure be identified? Am J Obstet Gynecol 2006;194:1–9.

20. Berghella V, Roman A, Daskalakis C, et al. Gestational age at cervical length measurement and incidence of preterm birth. Obstet Gynecol 2007;110:311–7.

21. Shirodkar VN. A new method of operative treatment for habitual abortions in the second trimester of pregnancy. Antiseptic 1955;52: 229–30.

22. McDonald IA. Suture of the cervix for inevitable miscarriage. J Obstet Gynaecol Br Emp 1957;64:346–50.

23. Zaveri V, Aghajafari F, Amankwah K, Hannah M. Abdominal versus vaginal cerclage after a failed transvaginal cerclage: A systematic review. Am J Obstet Gynecol 2002;187:868–72.

24. ACOG practice bulletin. Cervical insufficiency. Int J Gynaecol Obstet 2004;85:81–9.

25. Yoon HJ, Hong JY, Kim SM. The effect of anesthetic method for prophylactic cervical cerclage on plasma oxytocin: a randomized trial. Int J Obstet Anesth 2008;17(1):26–30.

26. Soper JT. Gestational trophoblastic disease. Obstet Gynecol 2006;108:176–87.

27. American College of Obstetricians and Gynecologists. Diagnosis and treatment of gestational trophoblastic disease. ACOG Practice Bulletin No. 53. (Obstet Gynecol 2004;103:1365–77).

28. Kohorn E. Practice bulletin No. 53–Diagnosis and treatment of gestational trophoblastic disease (letter). Obstet Gynecol 2004;104:1422.

29. Soper JT, Lewis JL Jr, Hammond CB. Gestational trophoblastic disease. In: Hoskins WJ, Perez CA, Young RC (Eds). Principles and Practice of Gynecologic Oncology, 2nd ed. Philadelphia: Lippincott-Raven Publishers, 1997,pp. 1039–77.

30. Beischer NA, Bettinger HF, Fortune DW, Pepperell R. Hydatidiform mole and its complications in the state of Victoria. J Obstet Gynaecol Br Commonw 1970; 77:263–76.

31. Kohorn EI. Gestational trophoblastic neoplasia and evidence-based medicine. J Reprod Med 2002;47:427–32.

32. Schlaerth JB, Morrow CP, Montz FJ, d'Ablaing G. Initial management of hydatidiform mole. Am J Obstet Gynecol 1988;158:1299–306.

33. Curry SL, Hammond CB, Tyrey L, et al. Hydatidiform mole: Diagnosis, management, and long-term followup of 347 patients. Obstet Gynecol 1975;45:1–8.

34. Berkowitz RS, Goldstein DP. Diagnosis and management of the primary hydatidiform mole. Obstet Gynecol Clin North Am 1988;15:491–503.

35. Amir SM, Osathanondh R, Berkowitz RS, Goldstein DP. Human chorionic gonadotropin and thyroid function in patients with hydatidiform mole. Am J Obstet Gynecol 1984;150:723–8.

36. Cotton DB, Bernstein SG, Read JA, et al. Hemodynamic observations in evacuation of molar pregnancy. Am J Obstet Gynecol 1980;138:6–10.

37. Kohorn EI. Clinical management and the neoplastic sequelae of trophoblastic embolization associated with hydatidiform mole. Obstet Gynecol Surv 1987; 42:484–8.

38. Twiggs LB, Morrow CP, Schlaerth JB. Acute pulmonary complicati onsof molar pregnancy. Am J Obstet Gynecol 1979; 135:189–94.

39. Natonson R, Shapiro BA, Harrison RA, Stanhope RC. Massive trophoblastic embolization and PEEP therapy. Anesthesiology 1979;51:469–71.

40. Kaplan JA, Cooperman LH. Alarming reactions to ketamine in patients taking thyroid medication—treatment with propranolol. Anesthesiology 1971; 35:229–30.

41. Solak M, Akturk G. Spinal anesthesia in a patient with hyperthyroidism due to hydatidiform mole. Anesth Analg 1993; 77:851–2.

42. Mazze RI, Kallen B. Reproductive outcome after anesthesia and operation during pregnancy: a registry study of 5,405 cases. Am J Obstet Gynecol 1989; 161:1178–85.

43. Bernhard LM, Klebba PK, Gray DL, et al. Predictors of persistence of adnexal masses in pregnancy. Obstet Gynecol 1999;93:585–9.

44. Kemmann E, Ghazi DM, Corsan GH. Adnexal torsion in menotropin-induced pregnancies. Obstet Gynecol 1990;76:403–6.

45. Duic Z, Kukura V, Ciglar S, et al. Adnexal masses in pregnancy: a review of eight cases undergoing surgical management. Eur J Gynaecol Oncol 2002;23:133–4.

46. Duic Z, Kukura V, Ciglar S, et al. Adnexal masses in pregnancy: a review of eight cases undergoing surgical management. Eur J Gynaecol Oncol 2002;23:133–4.

47. Hibbard LT: Adnexal torsion. Am J Obstet Gynecol 1985, 152:456–61.

48. Cavun S, Goktalay G, Millington WR. The hypotension evoked by visceral nociception is mediated by delta opioid receptors in the periaqueductal gray. Brain Res 2004;1019:237–45.

49. Van Voorhis BJ, Schwaiger J, Syrop CH, et al. Early diagnosis of ovarian torsion by color Doppler sonography. Fertil Steril 1992;58:215–7.

50. Usui R, Minakami H, Kosuge S, et al. A retrospective survey of clinical, pathologic, and prognostic features of adnexal masses operated on during pregnancy. J Obstet Gynaecol Res 2000;26:89–93.

51. Pan HS, Huang LW, Lee CY, et al. Ovarian pregnancy torsion. Arch Gynecol Obstet 2004; 270:119–121.

52. Visser BC, Glasgow RE, Mulvihill KK, et al. Safety and timing of nonobstetric abdominal surgery in pregnancy. Dig Surg 2001;18:409–17.

53. Hurd WW, Smith AJ, Gauvin JM, et al. Cocaine blocks extraneuronal uptake of norepinephrine by the pregnant human uterus. Obstet Gynecol 1991;78: 249–53.

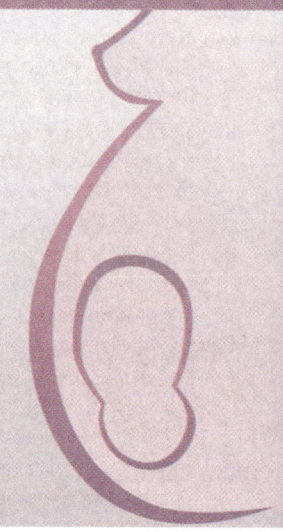

CHAPTER 9

Cardiopulmonary Cerebral Resuscitation in Parturient

Babita Gupta, Antara Gokhale

INTRODUCTION

Cardiopulmonary arrest in a parturient, although a rare situation, is of great significance as it involves two lives—mother and the fetus. According to the Confidential Enquiries into Maternal and Child Health (CEMACH) data published in the UK in 2007, the overall maternal mortality rate was 13.95 per 100,000 maternities. The frequency of cardiopulmonary arrest was calculated at 0.05 per 1000 maternities, or 1:20,000.[1] This shows a rise as compared to the previous reports of incidence of 1:30,000.[2] According to World Health Organization (WHO) published report, it is estimated that of the total maternal mortalities in the world, 17% occur in India, predominantly in rural areas and poor sections of population.[3] Most of the patients are young and healthy, without background medical or surgical problems. Cardiopulmonary arrest may occur in the operating suites, in the labor room, delivery ward or in the emergency room where it is unexpected. Fetal survival largely depends on the maternal survival.[1,5,6]

The altered maternal physiology, involvement of management of two lives and the possibility of need for emergency cesarean section makes the cardiopulmonary resuscitation (CPR) in this situation unique. Hence, a sound knowledge of the altered maternal physiology, awareness of the risk factors for cardiopulmonary arrest and a management protocol of such situations are essential for the practicing anesthesiologist. Involvement of obstetrician and neonatologist early in the arrest is necessary for improved outcome.

The management of cardiac arrest is based on the Basic Life Support (BLS) and Advanced Cardiac Life Support (ACLS) protocols as recommended by American Heart Association (AHA) guidelines published in 2010. It takes into consideration the anatomic and physiologic changes occurring during pregnancy while implementing the basic and advanced life support algorithms. Aggressive resuscitation including perimortem cesarean delivery of fetus in those above 20 weeks of gestation may be warranted, though the reported survival rate is poor. As the number of cases is small, most recommendations are based on case reports and randomized trials are lacking.[1,4]

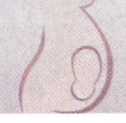

CAUSES OF CARDIOPULMONARY ARREST

The common causes of cardiopulmonary arrest in a parturient are hemorrhage, pulmonary embolism, hypertensive disease, heart disease and amniotic embolism. Hemorrhage is the most common cause of cardiac arrest in developing countries during pregnancy. In the developed countries, pulmonary embolism is now the leading cause.[7]

Cardiac diseases are said to be the most common non-obstetric cause.

BEAU-CHOPS as described in the AHA guideline algorithm on maternal cardiac arrest can be a useful mnemonic for additional etiologies.[1]

B Bleeding/DIC

E Embolism: coronary/pulmonary/amniotic fluid embolism

A Anesthetic complications

U Uterine atony

C Cardiac disease (myocardial infarction/ischemia/aortic dissection/cardiomyopathy)

H Hypertension/pre-eclampsia/eclampsia

O Other: differential diagnosis of standard ACLS

P Placenta abruptio/previa

S Sepsis

Hemorrhage

Postpartum hemorrhage is the commonest cause of maternal death.[7] Concealed or overt hemorrhage can cause hypotension and precipitate cardiac arrest. The various causes of hemorrhage could be placenta previa, abruptio placenta, placenta acreta, increta or percreta. Postpartum hemorrhage and placental atony can occur. Physiological changes occurring during pregnancy may mask the blood loss. A pregnant woman may lose up to 30% of blood volume before tachycardia, hypotension and other signs of hemodynamic instability appear.[8,9]

Early recognition, establishing large-bore intravenous access, intravenous fluid resuscitation, early availability of blood and blood products and if necessary activating the massive transfusion protocol are warranted. Resuscitation must be done in the left lateral position to relieve the aortocaval compression and improve the effectiveness of resuscitation.

Amniotic Fluid Embolism (AFE)

AFE is an important cause of maternal death with the reported incidence of 10–16%. AFE occurs when there is breech between maternal circulation and amniotic fluid. It occurs during labor, delivery and immediate postpartum period. The true incidence is unknown (1:8000–1:80,000) and the diagnosis is by exclusion. Patient presents with breathlessness, cyanosis followed by hypotension and circulatory collapse. Excessive bleeding, disseminated intravascular coagulation (DIC) and coma/seizures may follow.

25% of deaths occur within an hour and mortality is up to 80% with high incidence of neurological deficit in survivors. Treatment is largely supportive. Early, rapid and aggressive resuscitation is required along with oxygen supplementation to prevent additional hypoxemia.[10,11] Emergency cesarean section and perimortem cardiopulmonary bypass have been used to save life in this situation.[12]

Heart Disease

Cardiac causes have been labeled as the leading cause of maternal death according to the confidential enquiry into maternal and child health (CEMACH) data of 2003–2005 published in UK.[13] There is a steady rise in cardiac events during pregnancy with myocardial infarction topping the list. Developed countries, like UK, USA, and Australia, have all shown cardiac causes as the leading non-obstetric cause of mortality.[13,14] There are case series reported from various parts of India showing rheumatic heart disease as the most common cause of cardiac disease causing maternal mortality and morbidity.[15–17]

Myocardial Infarction

Myocardial infarction is likely to occur in women with underlying diabetes mellitus, chronic hypertension, advancing age, obesity and family history.[19] Patients who become pregnant within 6 months of myocardial infarction have a higher incidence of myocardial infarction and mortality.[7, 20] The incidence of acute myocardial infarction is estimated at 0.6–1 per 10,000 pregnancies with a case fatality rate of 5.1 to 37%. Most maternal deaths occur at the time of infarction or within two weeks of infarction, usually in association with labor and delivery. Fetal death occurs in 12–34% of cases, most of which are associated with maternal death. Maternal survival is generally associated with a good fetal outcome.[20]

Interpretation of biochemical markers is somewhat complicated by changes that may occur during normal labor and delivery. There is an increase in the concentration of creatine kinase and its MB fraction by nearly twofold within 30 minutes after delivery. Troponin levels may be elevated in patients with pre-ecalmpsia.[19]

Fibrinolytics are relatively contraindicated in pregnancy, and, therefore, primary percutaneous coronary intervention is the reperfusion strategy of choice to treat ST segment elevation myocardial infarction in the pregnant woman.[20]

Congenital Heart Disease

More women with congenital heart disease are reaching reproductive age due to improvement in surgical and medical management. These patients tend to have higher incidence of pulmonary edema and cardiac failure during the peripartum period especially during labor and immediate postpartum period due to autotransfusion of blood.[1,21,22]

Peripartum Cardiomyopathy

Peripartum cardiomyopathy is a type of dilated cardiomyopathy, occurring with symptoms of heart failure during last month of pregnancy or within 5 months after labor. The mortality is high ranging from 25–35%.[23] Undiagnosed patients developing cardiac arrest immediately after induction of anesthesia have been reported in the literature.[24,25]

Hypertensive Heart Disease
(Pre-eclampsia, eclampsia, essential hypertension)

Pre-eclampsia can progress to severe hypertension which can in turn lead to multiorgan involvement, thus increasing maternal and fetal morbidity and mortality. Pre-eclampsia and its complications account for 20–50% of obstetrical admissions to the intensive care unit and 12–17% of all maternal deaths in the United States.

Anaphylaxis: Anaphylaxis is a severe life-threatening generalized hypersensitive reaction. Maternal IgE does not cross placenta but fetus can suffer due to acidosis, hypotension and hypoxemia. Triggers, like antibiotic administration, anesthetic agents, tocolytics, oxytocin, intravenous iron, or latex, can result in anaphylaxis. The signs and symptoms include pruritus, urticaria, angioedema, bronchospasm, tachycardia and hypotension. Larnygeal/pharyngeal edema, stridor, wheezing and shortness of breath develop over minutes.

Early recognition can avoid precipitation of cardiac arrest. Treatment includes oxygen, IM epinephrine, fluid resuscitation, left lateral tilt, uterine displacement, H1 antihistaminics, inhaled bronchodilators and glucocorticoids.[5]

Complications of tocolytics: Magnesium sulfate toxicity can cause prolongation of QT interval and precipitate cardiac arrest.[1] Patients with renal failure and metabolic disorders can develop magnesium toxicity with relatively low magnesium doses.

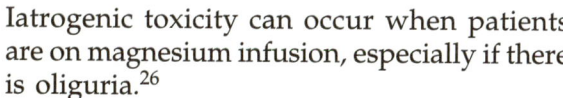
Iatrogenic toxicity can occur when patients are on magnesium infusion, especially if there is oliguria.[26]

Complications of surgical delivery: Uterine atony and postpartum hemorrhage can lead to uncontrolled bleeding and DIC.

Complications of anesthesia: Complications of regional and general anesthesia account for 2% of causes of cardiac arrest.[27] Epidural catheter introduced during labor to provide labor analgesia can migrate into subarachnoid space or a vessel thus causing total spinal anesthesia or systemic toxicity of the local anesthetic respectively. Patient should be instructed to lie in lateral position between examinations and topping up of medication dose to avoid hypotension. The 2010 American Society of Regional Anesthesia (ASRA) practice advisory on the management of local anesthetic systemic toxicity suggests the following infusion of 20% lipid emulsion (values in parenthesis are for a 70 kg patient) as a therapeutic antidote:[28]

1. Bolus 1.5 mL/kg (lean body mass) intravenously over 1 min (100 mL).
2. Continuous infusion at 0.25 mL/kg per min (18 mL/min).
3. Repeat bolus once or twice for persistent cardiovascular collapse.
4. Double the infusion rate to 0.5 mL/kg per min, if blood pressure remains low.
5. Continue infusion for at least 10 min after attaining circulatory stability.
6. Recommended upper limit: approximately 10 mL/kg lipid emulsion over the first 30 min.

Induction of general anesthesia may lead to airway-related issues like loss of airway control, aspiration pneumonia and hypoxemia. During emergence from anesthesia, hypoventilation or airway obstruction can occur. All these can lead to cardiac arrest.

Complications of non-anesthetic medications: Medications, like magnesium, antibiotics particularly accidental bolus doses of vanco-mycin, can cause severe hypotension and cardiac arrest. Cases linking ergot derivatives with cardiac arrest in the parturient are reported in literature.[8,29]

ANATOMICAL AND PHYSIOLOGICAL CHANGES DURING PREGNANCY THAT INFLUENCE THE MANAGEMENT OF CARDIAC ARREST

Pregnant women undergo profound anatomical and physiological changes in order to cope with the increased physical and metabolic demands. Sound knowledge of physiologic and anatomic changes during pregnancy is essential to improve maternal and fetal outcome.

Airway

There is hyperemia of the upper airway under the influence of hormones mainly progesterone. Mucosal edema develops causing symptoms of nasal obstruction and obstructive sleep apnea. The airway becomes friable and bleeds easily. Oral airway must be introduced gently and carefully and introduction of nasopharyngeal airway must be avoided. Laryngoscopy and intubation must be done with utmost care to avoid bleeding. Intubation and mask ventilation may be difficult. It is advisable to choose smaller size endotracheal tubes for intubation. The narrowing of upper airway in third trimester compared to non-pregnant and postpartum females is well documented.[1,30] All intubations in obstetric patients are considered potentially difficult and expert help along with difficult airway cart and failed intubation protocol must be readily available. Besides this, cardiac arrest can occur anywhere and intubating conditions may not necessarily be ideal adding to the difficulty.

The points to remember are:
1. Optimized ventilation and oxygenation with good chest excursion can defer the need for an advanced airway.

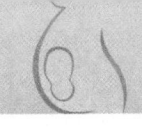

2. Advanced airway placement is difficult in a maternal cardiac arrest. Thorough preparation prior to procedure is important.

3. The most experienced person should secure and manage the advanced airway during a maternal cardiac arrest.[2,5]

Breathing

The changes in the lung volumes and capacities especially the reduced functional residual capacity and residual volume make a pregnant female prone to rapid hypoxia. Arterial blood gases normally show mild alkalosis to facilitate delivery of oxygen to fetus. Partial pressure of oxygen (PaO_2) above 60 mm Hg in maternal blood is adequate to maintain fetal oxygenation provided uterine blood flow is preserved.[8]

The points to remember are:

- Oxygenate well to avoid desaturation
- Avoid hyperventilation to prevent respiratory alkalosis
- Risk of aspiration is high

Circulation

Cardiac output increases by 10–15% after 10 weeks of pregnancy. There is an increase in heart rate by 10–15 beats/min by third trimester and decrease in systolic blood pressure by 10–15 mm Hg. The physiological anemia of pregnancy due to relative increase in plasma volume compared to RBC volume may contribute to misinterpretation of blood loss. Aortocaval compression by the gravid uterus can cause decrease in venous return. Cardiac output can decrease by 30–40% in third trimester in supine position and can precipitate cardiac arrest. The fetal circulation may be compromised due to decrease in uteroplacental blood flow caused by low pressure and vasoconstriction.

The effectiveness of cardiac compression is reduced by the gravid uterus. Left lateral displacement of uterus may help to relieve the compression and improve the blood flow. The left lateral tilt must be as much as possible, but more than 30° tilt causes patients to slip. Some studies have shown that lateral displacement of uterus is equally effective in supine position, while others have shown that aortocaval compression may persist even with 30° tilt.[1]

Various methods to achieve this have been described:

- Placing patient on the rescuers knees
- Placing blankets or pillow
- Use of Cardiff wedge
- Manual displacement of uterus

Effective chest compressions are not easy to perform in left lateral tilt unless patient is on a tilting operation table.

Gastrointestinal System

The lower esophageal sphincter tone decreases as early as 12 weeks of pregnancy. Supine position, gravid uterus and aggressive bag mask ventilation along with cardiac compression increase the chances of regurgitation and aspiration. Hence, intubation must be considered early in the course of the cardiopulmonary arrest.

INTERVENTIONS TO AVOID CARDIOPULMONARY ARREST

If a pregnant patient is in a pre-arrest situation, certain measures can be taken to prevent cardiopulmonary arrest.[1,4]

1. Place the patient in left lateral position or manually displace the uterus.
2. Provide high flow oxygen.
3. Correct hypotension and hypovolemia with IV fluids. Preferably secure large bore cannulas above the level of diaphragm.
4. Secure expert help of obstetrician and neonatologist early during resuscitation.
5. Reevaluate need to administer or withdrawal of any medication.
6. Identify and treat the reversible causes.

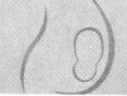

MANAGEMENT OF CARDIOPULMONARY ARREST

The standard algorithm established by the AHA for BLS and ACLS must be followed with certain modification. The 2010 AHA and Emergency Cardiovascular Care (ECC) recommendations for management of cardiac arrest include:

- Immediate recognition of cardiac arrest
- Activation of emergency response team
- Early CPR
- Rapid defibrillation
- Effective advanced life support
- Integrated post-cardiac care

This sequence of events is termed as *chain of survival*.

Basic Life Support

The steps taken on recognition of an unresponsive or gasping pregnant patient are mainly following the CAB, i.e. circulation, airway and breathing sequence:

- Call for help
- Take up to 10 seconds to feel the carotid pulse
- Estimate the approximate gestational age
- If pulses are not felt, place the patient in left lateral position
- Start chest compressions.
- Place the heel of one hand slightly higher on the sternum than the recommended position, i.e. on the centre of the patient's sternum.[1]
- Put the heel of the other hand on top of the first hand.
- Straighten the arms and position shoulder directly above the hands.
- Push hard and fast.
- Push down at least 5 cm with each compression at a rate of at least 100/min.
- Allow the chest to recoil at the end of each compression.
- Minimize interruptions.

Compressions pump the blood in the heart to rest of the body. Chest recoil allows blood to flow into the heart. Chest compression and recoil must be of approximately equal time. The gravid uterus pushes the diaphragm upwards; hence compressions on the sternum must be positioned such that there is no undue pressure on the intra-abdominal organs and uterus causing injury and also the heart is compressed effectively. If there is a single rescuer, **give 30 compression followed by 2 breaths.**

Open the airway for breath using the head-tilt chin-lift maneuver. Push one hand on the patient's forehead and push your palm to tilt the head back. Place the fingers of the other hand on the bony part of the mandible. Lift the jaw to open the mouth. If trauma to head and neck is suspected, use the jaw thrust maneuver. Give mouth to mask breath, or give bag mask ventilation. For one rescuer CPR, stand at the victim's side; place the mask over the victims face to achieve a tight seal using the E-C clamp technique. Place index finger and thumb of one hand along the edge to the mask. Place the thumb of the other hand along the bottom edge of the mask and remaining three fingers along the mandible. Deliver one breath over 1 second to make the chest rise. The breath can be delivered by the rescuer by breathing out into the victims mouth through the mask or with the help of a bag attached to the mask; 100% oxygen must be supplemented whenever available. When **two rescuers** are available, one can continue uninterrupted compressions at minimum rate of 100/min while the other can give breaths at 12/min. Each rescuer gives 5 cycles, i.e. 2 minutes of compression before switching their roles. This is to maintain the effectiveness of the compressions.

The second rescuer on arrival should activate the cardiac arrest code; attach the AED (automated external defibrillator) pads while chest compressions are continued by the first rescuer. If additional help is available, one attendant must maintain the leftward displacement of the uterus to maintain effective venous return.

In the pregnant patient, the position of the pads remains the same at the apex and at the sternum. Placement of the apical pads may become difficult due to the left lateral tilt and enlarged breast. Adhesive defibrillator pads are preferable to paddles in pregnancy. AHA also suggests self-adhesive pads as it reduces the risk of arcing, helps in continuous analysis of the underlying rhythm and helps rapid delivery shock. Standard defibrillation current and position can be used in a pregnant victim, as there is no transthoracic impedance during pregnancy. Also the shock with DC current does not adversely affect the fetus. If the carotid pulse is palpable, continue rescue breaths at 1 breath at 5–6 seconds. If no pulse is palpable, continue with the ACLS algorithm.

The modifications in BLS in case of a parturient include:
- Positioning patient in left lateral position.
- Positioning the hands higher up on the sternum during chest compression.

Advanced Cardiac Life Support

The recommendations of ACLS: Cardiac compressions are continued. The CPR is continued as per the ACLS protocol, i.e.
- Continue chest compressions. Push hard and fast >5 cm deep and >100/min.
- 5 cycles of 30:2 compressions: ventilation without advanced airway.
- Rotate compressors every 2 minutes.
- Assess quality of CPR.

Good quality CPR is indicated by:
- $PetCO_2$ >10 mm Hg
- Intra-arterial pressure. Relaxation pressure (diastolic pressure) more than 20 mm Hg
- CvO_2 >30, if the CVP line is already available.

Due to the increased risk of aspiration, advanced airway needs to be established as early as is feasible.[31] The use of cricoid pressure is not recommended,[31] but it can be used to assist and facilitate intubation. Cuffed endotracheal intubation is preferred as it protects the airway against aspiration and obstruction and maintain effective ventilation. Endotracheal intubation may result in transient interruption in chest compressions. However, the benefits of intubation outweigh this interruption when CPR is continued beyond the BLS level.

Successful placement of endotracheal tube is confirmed by:
- Physical examination—auscultation at 5 points and by observing mist in ETT
- Capnography—quantitative waveform capnography (class I recommendation)
- Non-waveform carbon dioxide detector/colorimetry

After securing the airway, continue continuous waveform monitoring. Administer 100% oxygen for all cardiac arrest patients. The aim is to maintain oxygen saturation above 94%. With the establishment of advanced airway, the ventilation rate is reduced to 8–10 breaths per minute (1 breath every 6 to 8 seconds). The chest compressions are no longer interrupted for ventilation. Ideally the breath should be delivered during chest recoil between compressions but ventilation can be continued without trying to synchronize with compression. Other advanced airway devices like the laryngeal mask airway (LMA) and esophageal-tracheal tube do not prevent aspiration and may cause trauma and bleeding.[31]

The rhythm is analyzed at two minutes interval using ECG/AED. Defibrillate, if it is a shockable rhythm. Ventricular tachycardia or ventricular fibrillation pathway as shown in the chart. Shock energy is the same as per ACLS protocol:
- Monophasic–360 J

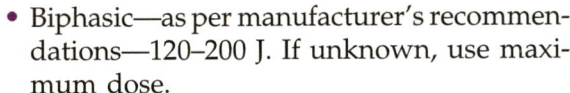

- Biphasic—as per manufacturer's recommendations—120–200 J. If unknown, use maximum dose.

Use adrenaline IV/IO 1 mg every 3–5 minutes, if rhythm is still shockable after 2 minutes of CPR after first shock. A single dose of vasopressin 40 units can replace first or second dose. Alternately amiodarone 300 mg as bolus followed by 150 mg can be used after third shock. At all stages, try to identify and treat the reversible causes, i.e. all Hs and Ts. BEAU-CHOPS as described in the AHA guideline algorithm on maternal cardiac arrest can be a useful mnemonic for additional etiologies related to obstetrics.

ACLS 2010 Modifications in Parturient

The International Liaison Committee on Resuscitation (ILCOR) published the most recent science on maternal resuscitation in 2010. Based on this the AHA and ECC have published guidelines for CPR and the first evidence-based algorithm for cardiac arrest during pregnancy. This algorithm should be the basis for emergency responses during a maternal cardiac arrest for all providers. Highlights of these guidelines include:[1,7,8]

1. Coordinate multiple teams during and after the cardiac arrest.
2. Do not delay usual measures such as defibrillation and the administration of medications.
3. Perform aortocaval decompression maneuvers, preferably manual left uterine dis placement (LUD).
4. Consider the airway difficult, and the most experienced provider should manage the airway.
5. Intravenous access is important but should be placed above the diaphragm.
6. There should be a dedicated timer to document when 4 minutes after the onset of a maternal cardiac arrest have elapsed, in order to make a decision on the need for a perimortem cesarean section (PMCS).

PMCS should be performed by 5 minutes after the onset of a maternal cardiac arrest, if there is no return of spontaneous circulation (ROSC) by 4 minutes with the usual resuscitation measures.

7. Consider an expanded etiology list for the cause of the cardiac arrest; BEAU-CHOPS can be used as a usual mnemonic.
8. If resuscitation remains unsuccessful at the 15th minute, initiate direct cardiac massage when appropriate resources and personnel are available. This is applicable in those centers where cardiovascular surgeons are available.

Electric Interventions in Arrest and Pharmacology of Resuscitation

Defibrillation

Defibrillation and pharmacological therapy during resuscitation of the parturient remains the same as per ACLS protocol and should not be delayed.[1,4] Defibrillation must be performed at doses recommended by the ACLS (level 1C). The placement of leads is the same as in ACLS protocol. Placement of apical lead may be difficult due to lateral position and presence of enlarged breast.

Although there are no studies showing adverse effects of defibrillation on mother and fetus, few case reports indicate that the effect of maternal defibrillation on the fetus can range from no effect to fetal arrhythmias to fetal death a few weeks after defibrillation. Fetal effects possibly depend on the duration and dose of shock delivered. Maximum effect on the fetus is said to occur, if the current flows across the uterus though the amniotic fluid, which like other body fluids, conducts electricity and can precipitate fetal death. Another feared complication is the possibility of electric arcing but this is not documented when current is passed across maternal thorax. If there are any internal or external fetal monitoring devices, they should be removed during maternal defibrillation. It is believed that using gelled pads for defibrillation may reduce the incidence of arcing and reduce the time to deliver shock.[1,4,32–34]

Pharmacological Therapy

The medications used during the resuscitation and the doses used are the same as in a non-pregnant patient.[1,4] Adrenaline and vasopressin are the only vasopressors proved to be of benefit in ROSC. The role of medication is only after delivery of effective chest compression and after delivery of shock. Drug therapy alone has not shown to improve the outcome of the arrest.

Current guidelines (2010) for ACLS recommend a standard dose of 1 mg of epinephrine (IV/IO) every 3 to 5 minutes during adult cardiac arrest (Class IIb, LOE A). Higher doses may be indicated to treat specific problems, such as a beta-blocker or calcium channel blocker overdose.[7]

If the initial arrest rhythm is pulseless electrical activity (PEA) or asystole, the administration of epinephrine is recommended as soon as vascular access is obtained. For VF or pulseless VT, the administration of epinephrine is recommended, after the third shock, and upon the resumption of chest compressions.

Use of vasopressors, adrenaline and vasopressin, has shown to improve survival to hospital admission in non-pregnant patients. Both act by causing peripheral vasoconstriction and diverting the blood from the peripheral organs to the vital organs. This may thus reduce the blood flow from the uteroplacental bed. But in an arrest situation, it is important to keep the mother alive as ultimately fetal survival depends on mother. However, vasopressin has shown to have a better survival rate to hospital admission than adrenaline and hence there is recommendation to replace the first or second dose of adrenaline with vasopressin. Vasopressin has been shown to cause more severe vasoconstriction than adrenaline and is expected to cause more severe compromise in uterine blood flow theoretically.[1,35] Ultrasound at the bedside can be used, if expertise is available to immediately rule out at least certain causes.[1]

Calcium is not the drug mentioned in the ACLS resuscitation protocol. However, it has specific indications in special situation:
1. Reversal of magnesium toxicity.
2. Hyperkalemic cardiac arrest along with glucose-insulin and sodium bicarbonate.
3. Overdose of calcium channel blocker, beta blocker.

Calcium is not used to treat hyperkalemia but to stabilize the cardiac membrane. Both calcium chloride and calcium gluconate can be used. Calcium chloride is preferred over calcium gluconate for a patient experiencing a cardiac arrest because the chloride formulation has approximately 3 times the amount of elemental calcium compared with the gluconate formulation. Usual dosages of calcium chloride are 0.5 to 1 g IV over 2 to 5 minutes. Calcium should be diluted and preferably given via a central line or large peripheral line to avoid potentially harmful effect of its extravasation.[1,36]

Though the circulating blood volume and cardiac output is high during pregnancy, there is no research to show that the amount of medication delivered need to be altered. The AHA recommends no change in the dose of any medication used during resuscitation in cardiac arrest.[1,2,4,5,35]

Peripheral and Central Vascular Access (Intraosseous or Intratracheal Access)

Priority must be given to establish a good venous access early in the course of resuscitation. Large bore venous access is important not only to give fluids rapidly but also to give medications during resuscitation. During a cardiac arrest, the priority is to gain a peripheral venous access using a large bore cannula. The median cubital vein is the preferred site as it is usually large and can readily accommodate large bore cannulas. When intravenous access in upper limbs is difficult, veins on the dorsum of foot or the saphenous vein may be used. But in a pregnant female, the rapidity of delivery of medications may be compromised due to the additional factor of a gravid uterus. The gravid uterus causes a decrease in cardiac output by up to 30% in the supine position by decreasing the venous return. Hypovolemia and hypotension due to fluid loss, blood loss, sepsis, myocardial infarction, anaphylaxis may be the cause of cardiac arrest. Since the gravid uterus may hinder the blood flow, it is recommended that intravenous access be established above the level of diaphragm.

After the injection of the medication, the ACLS protocol recommends to give a fluid bolus of 20 mL normal saline flush to facilitate rapid drug delivery to the heart. Another method recommended in the AHA guidelines is to elevate the limb in addition to deliver the drugs rapidly to the central circulation.[1]

Central venous line insertion in the jugular vein and subclavian vein may be achieved, if peripheral venous access is difficult. The advantages are rapidity of drug delivery and higher levels of drug concentration achieved. These are not recommended as lines of choice during CPR as introduction is time consuming and requires expertise and it may also interfere with the chest compression. In a gravid patient, the insertion of femoral line is difficult. The gravid uterus, possibility of cesarean delivery, and maintenance of left lateral tilt make line insertion technically difficult. Also the gravid uterus may interfere with rapidity of fluid resuscitation.[1,35] Hence, femoral venous access is not preferred in pregnant patients.

Intraosseous route is considered only when intravenous route in not available (Class IIb).[1] The advantages are a short learning curve, ease of insertion, ability to deliver drugs and fluids rapidly and also collect blood sample in all age groups. The tibia is the most preferred site and has high success rate. This non-collapsible venous system not only helps in delivery of medications and fluids but also helps in correction of blood samples. There is no concrete data about the drug level achieved and the effectiveness of the medications given.[1,37–39]

Certain drugs, such as adrenaline, lignocaine, atropine, and naloxone, can be absorbed when delivered through the endotracheal tube. The drug level achieved by these drugs is much lesser than that given by intravenous or intraosseous route. Therefore, endotracheal route is used only if intravenous or intraosseous route is not available.[40,41] Thus in order of priority, two good peripheral large bore cannulas in the cubital fossa are adequate during resuscitation. Central venous access may be considered, if peripheral access is not possible provided there are no contraindications. Intraosseous route may also be used. Last priority is for endotracheal route, if all other routes to gain venous access fail.[1,38–40]

MATERNAL CARDIAC ARREST NOT REVERSIBLE WITH BLS AND ACLS

When a parturient suffers cardiac arrest, resuscitation team leader should activate the protocol for emergency cesarean section.[1–4] An estimate of gestational age can be made by the fundal height. A singleton pregnancy above 20 weeks reaches umbilicus. Some studies indicate that maternal survival improves, if cesarean section is started and baby delivered within 4–5 minutes. Anoxic brain injury occurs within the 4 minutes after a cardiac arrest is identified. Therefore, if team members are unable to achieve ROSC by 4 minutes in a patient that is obviously gravid, and especially if the patient is >20 weeks gestational age, a decision to perform a PMCS should be taken.[1–4] The algorithm for decision-making for perimortem cesarean sections (PMCS) be followed.

Delivery of baby improves the aortocaval compression and helps to improve cardiac output. There are case reports of maternal return of spontaneous circulation (ROSC) after delivery of the baby. Till the surgical preparations are ready, the CPCR should be continued as per ACLS protocol. The PMCS should be performed at the location where the arrest occurs as transporting the mother to an operating room results in significant delays in delivery time. The neonatal team and neonatal resuscitation equipment must be on standby to resuscitate the neonate once delivered.[1,4,5,42–44]

POST-ARREST CARE

The post-arrest (and pre-arrest/unstable) pregnant patient should be placed with left lateral tilt to relieve possible aortocaval compression. Since most studies of hypothermia are in non-parturient, use of therapeutic hypothermia must be decided on a case to case basis. The use of therapeutic hypothermia when appropriate for the non-pregnant patient should be considered in pregnancy. Poor fetal outcome with use of hypothermia was observed in one of the case reports,[45] but there are cases which have reported success as well.[46,47] Therefore, the need for hypothermia is dictated with the aim to save the mother as a priority. If therapeutic hypothermia is not applied, all maternal cardiac arrest patients should be well monitored post-arrest to ensure normothermia and avoid any hyperthermia. The use of therapeutic hypothermia in the bleeding or post-PMCS patient may increase bleeding due to impaired coagulation.[1,48,49]

Fetal monitoring: Patients receiving therapeutic hypothermia should be monitored for fetal bradycardia. Any fetus estimated to be greater than 20 weeks' gestation (i.e. potentially viable) should be observed with fetal tocodynamometry. Initiate early fetal monitoring even if treatment of the mother is not complete. Early signs of fetal distress include tachycardia, loss of beat-to-beat or long-term variability, or late decelerations. The fetus is more sensitive to adverse conditions, and fetal distress could be an indication of impending maternal destabilization.[31]

COMPLICATIONS OF CPR

The most common complications of CPR are:
- Rib fracture with internal injury to lung and heart.
- Development of pneumothorax, pneumomediastinum in those with fracture ribs and ventilation.
- Inability to secure the airway or loss of airway control may occur.
- Aspiration pneumonia—pregnant women are considered full stomach and have high incidence of aspiration. Mask ventilation, loss of lower esophageal sphincter tone, hypoxia, and chest compressions can increase the risk of aspiration.
- Inadequate delivery of compressions can worsen the hypoxemia causing fetal injury.
- Hyperventilation after establishment of definitive airway may decrease venous return and also shift the oxy-Hb curve causing fetal acidosis and hypoxemia.
- Compressions lower on the sternum can cause injury to the stomach and liver and even the uterus causing rupture and internal bleeding.

PREPAREDNESS FOR CESAREAN SECTION

As cardiac arrest is a rare event, preparedness of action plan and regular drills are required so as to act in emergency situations. The emergency department staff as well as those in the delivery suite should be prepared to avoid a panic situation.[1–4,31] The AHA has proposed a protocol to prepare for such an emergency situation. The hospital cardiac arrest team should include an obstetrician with a nurse, neonatologist with assistant and

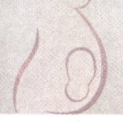

a respiratory therapist. If a hospital does not have an obstetrician and neonatologist, other members should be identified in advance to deal with this situation. The team should be identified and each hospital should have well-planned way of gathering all the team members and equipment at the earliest, in a timely manner without chaos or confusion.

Since the event of cardiac arrest in parturient is rare, situation is often chaotic, the equipment should be ready to perform a cesarean section and receive the newborn. Unfamiliar locations, inadequate illumination, and lack of through asepsis are some of the difficulties encountered.

Studies and questionnaires' carried in various countries in the world have shown inadequate awareness and lack of pre-paredness of the hospital staff in labor rooms and emergency departments to deal with the situation of cardiac arrest. Frequent simulation of all members involved are required to maintain preparedness for such situation.[50–52]

SUMMARY

Cardiac arrest in a parturient is a challenging event which involves 2 lives: the mother and the fetus. Multidisciplinary team is required for the management of the situation. Modifications in the CPCR protocol keeping in line with the changes unique to pregnancy are required. Aggressive resuscitation including cesarean section for rapid delivery after maternal cardiac arrest is becoming widely acceptable technique. Adequate preparedness of the concerned team members and regular simulations are required to improve the co-ordination and outcome in such situation. Ultimately the survival of the fetus depends on the survival of the mother.

Key Points

- Cardiopulmonary arrest in a parturient although a rare situation is of great significance as it involves two lives—mother and the fetus.
- Hemorrhage is the most common cause of cardiac arrest during pregnancy while in the developed countries pulmonary embolism is the leading cause.
- The management of cardiac arrest is based on the Basic Life Support (BLS) and Advanced Cardiac Life Support (ACLS) protocols as recommended by American Heart Association (AHA) guidelines published in 2010.
- The 2010 AHA and Emergency Cardiovascular Care (ECC) recommendations for management of cardiac arrest include: Immediate recognition of cardiac arrest, activation of emergency response team, early CPR, rapid defibrillation, effective advanced life support and integrated post-cardiac care.
- The modifications in BLS in case of a parturient include positioning patient in left lateral position and positioning the hands higher up on the sternum during chest compression.
- Defibrillation and pharmacological therapy during resuscitation of the parturient remains the same as per ACLS protocol and should not be delayed. The medications used during the resuscitation and the doses used are the same as in a non-pregnant patient.
- Aggressive resuscitation including perimortem cesarean delivery of fetus in those above 20 weeks of gestation may be warranted, though the reported survival rate is poor.

REFERENCES

1. Vanden Hoek TL, Morrison LJ, Shuster M, Donnino M, Sinz E, Lavonas EJ, Jeejeebhoy FM, Gabrielli A. Part 12: Cardiac arrest in special situations: 2010 American Heart Association Guidelines for Cardiopulmonary resuscitation and emergency cardiovascular care. Circulation 2010;122(18 Suppl 3):S829–61.

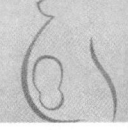

2. Jeejeebhoy FM, Morrison LJ. Maternal cardiac arrest: A practical and comprehensive review. Emerg Med Int 2013;274814.PMC3730371.

3. WHO, UNICEF, UNFPA, The World Bank and the United Nations Population Division. Trends in Maternal Mortality: 1990 to 2013. Estimates by WHO, UNICEF, UNFPA, The World Bank and the United Nations Population Division ISBN: 978 92 4 1507226.

4. Soar J, Perkins GD, Abbas G, Alfonzo A, Barelli A, Bierens JJ, et al. European Resuscitation Council Guidelines for Resuscitation 2010: Section 8. Cardiac arrest in special circumstances: electrolyte abnormalities, poisoning, drowning, accidental hypothermia, hyperthermia, asthma, anaphylaxis. Resuscitation 2010;81(10):1400–33.

5. Zelop CM. Cardiopulmonary arrest in pregnancy. Hepner DL, Ramin SM, Walla RM (Eds). Uptodate 2014.

6. Jeejebhoy FM, Windrim R. Best Pract Res Clin Obstet Gynaecol 2014;28(4):607–18.

7. Rodrigues A, Clode N, Graça L. Cardiac arrest in pregnancy: best practices are needed. Acta Obstet Ginecol Port 2014;8(2):164–8.

8. Dabbous A, Souki F. Cardiac arrest in pregnancy. MEJ. Anesth 2007;19(2):449–68.

9. Walfish M, Neuman A. Wlody D. Maternal hemorrhage. Br J Anaesth 2009;103(Suppl. 1):i47–i56.

10. Rudra A, Chatterjee S, Sengupta S, Nandi B, Mitra J. Amniotic fluid Embolism. Indian J Crit Care Med 2009;13(3):129–35.

11. Baldisseri MR. Amniotic Fluid Embolism Syndrome. Uptodate 2013.

12. Whitey JE. Maternal cardiac arrest during pregnancy. Clinical J Obstet Gynec 2003;45(2):377–92.

13. Lewis G (Ed). The Confidential Enquiry into Maternal and Child Health (CEMACH). Saving mothers' lives: reviewing maternal deaths to make motherhood safer—2003–2005. The Seventh Report on Confidential Enquiries into Maternal Deaths in the United Kingdom. London: CEMACH 2007.

14. Berg CJ, Callaghan WM, Syverson C, Henderson Z. Pregnancy-related mortality in the United States, 1998 to 2005. Obstet Gynecol 2010;116(6):1302–9.

15. Sullivan E, Hall B, King J. Maternal deaths in Australia. 2003–2005, serie 3, Cat No PER 42, Sydney AIHW national perinatal statistics Unit.

16. Konan H, Chaudhari S. Pregnancy complicated by maternal heart disease: A review of 281 women. J Obstet Gynaecol India 2012;62(3):301–6.

17. Koregol M, Mahale N, Nayak R, Bhandary Al. Maternal cardiac diseases and pregnancy. J Turkish-German Gynecol Assoc 2009;10:30–4.

18. Bangal VB, Singh RK, Shinde KK. Clinical study of heart disease complicating pregnancy. IOSR Journal of Pharmacy 2012;2:25–8.

19. Roth A, Elkayam U. Acute myocardial infarction associated with pregnancy. Ann Intern Med 1996;125(9):751–62.

20. Kealey AJ. Coronary artery disease and myocardial infarction in pregnancy: A review of epidemiology, diagnosis, and medical and surgical management. Can J Cardiol. 2010;26(6):e185–e189. PMCID: PMC2903989.

21. Councilman LM. Management of the parturient with cardiovascular disease. American Society of Anaestheiologist Annual Meeting 2011;213:1–4.

22. Dob DP, Yentis SM. Practical management of the parturient with congenital heart disease. Int J Obstet Anaesth 2006;15:137–44.

23. Rashmi HD, Prajwal Patel HS, Shivaramu BT. Peripartum cardiomyopathy—an unsolved mystery to ananesthesiologist. Int J Sci Public Health 2015;4(2):304–6.

24. McIndoe AK, Hammond EJ, Babington PC. Peripartum cardiomyopathy presenting as a cardiac arrest at induction of anesthesia for emergency caesarean section. Br J Anaesth 1995;75(1):97–101.

25. Wake K, Takanishi T, Kitajima T, Hayashi K, Takahashi H, Sakio H. Cardiac arrest during emergency caesarean section due to peripartum cardiomyopathy. Masui 2003;52(10):1089–91.

26. Stephen E. Lapinsky. Cardiopulmonary complications of pregnancy. Crit Care Med 2005;33(7):1616–22.

27. Suresh MS, La Toya Mason C, Munnur U. Cardiopulmonary resuscitation and the parturient. Best Pract Res Clin Obstet Gynaecol 2010;24(3):383–400.

28. Bern S, Winberg J. Local anesthetic toxicity and lipid resuscitation in pregnancy. Curr Opin Anesthesiol.2011;24(3):262–7.

29. ECC Committee, Subcommittees and Task Forces of the American Heart Association. 2005 American Heart Association Guidelines for Cardiopulmonary Resuscitation and Emergency Cardiovascular Care.Cardiac Arrest Associated

with Pregnancy. Circulation 2005;112 (24 Suppl):IV1-203.150–63.

30. Izci B, Vennelle M, Liston WA, Dundas KC, Calder AA, Douglas NJ. Sleep-disordered breathing and upper airway size in pregnancy and post-partum. Eur Respir J 2006;27(2):321–7.

31. Campbell TA, Sanson TC. Cardiac arrest and pregnancy. J Emerg Trauma Shock 2009;39–42. PMCID: PMC2700584.

32. Nanson J, Elcock D, Williams M, Deakin CD. Do physiological changes in pregnancy change defibrillation energy requirements? Br J Anaesth 2001;87(2):237–9.

33. Toongsuwan S. Postmortem caesarean section following death by electrocution. Aust NZJ Obstet Gynaecol 1972;12:265–6.

34. Hrozek D. Intrauterine death of the fetus in a mother shocked by an electric current (case report) [in German]. Zentralbl Gynakol 1963;85: 203–4.

35. Papastylianou A, Mentzelopoulos S. Current Pharmacological Advances in the Treatment of Cardiac Arrest—review article. Emergency Medicine International.Volume 2012. Article ID 815857.

36. Alfonzo A, Isles C, Geddes C, Deighan C. Potassium disorders—clinical spectrum and emergency management. Resuscitation 2006;70:10–25.

37. Gazin N, Auger H, Jabre P, Jaulin C, Lecarpentier E, Bertrand C, Margenet, Combes X. Efficacy and safety of the EZ-IOTM intraosseous device: Out-of-hospital implementation of a management algorithm for difficult vascular access. Resuscitation (2010),doi:10.1016/j.resuscitation.2010. 09.008.

38. Reades R, Studnek JR, Vandeventer S, Garrett J. Intraosseous versus intravenous vascular access during out-of-hospital cardiac arrest: a randomized controlled trial. Ann Emerg Med 2011; 58(6):509–16.

39. Hui D, Morrison LJ, Windrim R, Lausman AY, Hawryluck L, Dorian P, et al. "The American Heart Association 2010 guidelines for the management of cardiac arrest in pregnancy: consensus recommendations on implementation strategies. J Obstet Gynaecol Can 2011;33(8): 858–63.

40. Goldenberg RJ, McClure EM. Maternal mortality. Am J Obstet Gynecol 2011;205(4):293–5.

41. Paxton A, Wardlaw T. Are we making progress in maternal motality? NEJM 2011;364(21):1990–3.

CHAPTER 10

Neurophysiology of Labor Pain

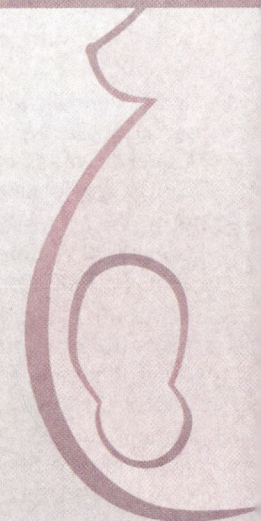

Ekta Rai, Anity Singh

Labor pain[1,2] is a dynamic process that integrates and exemplifies both central and peripheral mechanisms. Pain of first stage of labor is secondary to uterine distension and contractions. These uterine contractions lead to myometrial ischemia and release of noxious metabolites like bradykinin, histamine and serotonin. Pain is transmitted via afferent fibers coursing through paracervical plexus and hypogastric pelvic plexus (inferior, medial and superior) and co-mingle with sympathetic efferent fibers along paravertebral sympathetic chain, to enter the spinal cord at T10 to L1 segments. Near the end of first stage and with the onset of second stage, the mechanoreceptors get stimulated due to the stretching and distension of lower uterine segment, cervix, vagina and perineum. These impulses are transmitted via somatic efferents in pudendal nerve to segments S2 to S4 (Table 10.1).

First Stage of Labor

The pain experienced during this stage is predominantly visceral. This stage is divided into two phases, namely latent phase and phase of maximal dilatation. The latent phase is duration from onset of labor to the point of change of the slope of cervical dilatation. The maximal dilatation begins at 3 cm dilation. This phase can last for 20 hours in nullipara and 14 hours[3] in the multipara. The active phase is entered when contractions appear every 3 min, lasting 1 min with an intrauterine pressure of about 50–70 mm Hg. The cervical dilation proceeds at a rate of 1 cm/hr. The active phase is further

Table 10.1: Pain impulses from different dermatomes and intensity at different phases of labor		
Stages of labor	Dermatomes involved	Intensity of pain
Early first stage	T11–T12	Moderate
Late first stage	T10–L1	Severe
Second stage	T10–S4	Moderate (S2, 3, 4) to severe (T10–L1)
Delivery	T10–S4	Moderate (T10–L1) to severe (S2, 3, 4)

subdivided into acceleration phase, phase of maximum slope and deceleration phase.

Second Stage of Labor

This stage of pronounced somatic pain starts with full cervical dilation and ends with delivery of the baby. It typically lasts for 1–2 hours. The duration can vary as per the parity, with 120–180 minutes for nullipara and 60–120 minutes for the multipara (Table 10.2).

Maternal Considerations[5]

The pain of labor induces various physiological and psychological alterations secondary to the generalized neuroendocrinal stress response. The autonomic nervous system is activated and its over activity influences almost all the systems. Research into this concept has generated considerable evidence, by establishing the elevated levels of adrenaline and noradrenaline in maternal plasma during labor.

Circulatory Effects

The changes in circulatory system secondary to the raised levels of catecholamines are an increase in cardiac output (15–20%), peripheral vascular resistance, blood pressure and decrease in blood flow velocity. This fluctuation in blood flow velocity to vital tissues is especially witnessed during painful contractions.

Respiratory Effects

The hyperventilation associated with painful uterine contractions leads to maternal hypo-carbia (<20 mm Hg) and respiratory alkalosis. The rise in pH of more than 7.55 can lead to two major changes physiologically. Firstly, there is a shift in oxygen dissociation curve to the left, rather than the normal right shift which leads to double Bohr effect, meant to facilitate fetal oxygenation. There is a decrease in transfer of oxygen to tissues. Secondly, eventually there is maternal compensatory renal loss of bicarbonate, contributing to metabolic acidosis. Hypocarbia can also cause hypocalcemia and tetany. This imbalance in acid-base homeostasis and an increase in oxygen consumption lead to hypoxemia in both the mother and fetus.

Obstetric Effects

The uterine activity is under the influence of β receptors, which if stimulated cause uterine relaxation. These receptors are acted upon by elevated level of adrenaline, secondary to the stress response and hence inhibit uterine contractions. The ineffective uterine activity inadvertently prolongs labor and delivery.

Psychological Effects

Historically, women have been lead to believe, in the necessity of experiencing pain of natural childbirth. Any request for pain relief was frowned upon and enveloped them in a sense of low self-esteem and guilt. Various studies have highlighted that; unrelieved pain can lead to long-term emotional and psychological changes. Intense labor pain can aggravate anxiety, phobia, postnatal depression, mania, obsessive–compulsive disorders and sexual aversion.

Table 10.2: Duration of labor				
Stages of labor	Phases	Cervical dilation (cm)	Presentation	Duration of labor (hrs)
First stage	Latent phase	4	+2	8
	Acceleration phase	6		2
	Phases of max acceleration	9		2
	Deceleration phase	10		1
Second stage		10	+4	<1

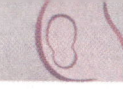

Endocrine-stress Response

The pain of labor is perceived by the body as a stress and thus initiates the stress-response with many hormonal changes. The release of catecholamines from adrenal medulla is accompanied by a rise in other counter-regulatory catabolic hormones like glucagon, cortisol, ACTH, aldosterone and ADH. There is a simultaneous fall in anabolic hormones like insulin, thus leading to enhanced glycolysis, lipolysis, ketogenesis and proteolysis. The associated starvation, ketosis and accumulation of free fatty acids and lactates in the plasma aggravate the acidotic milieu created by a diminished buffering capacity from hyperventilation.

Gastrointestinal Effects

Pain and stress decrease peristalsis, both gastric and intestinal and increase gastric acid secretion as well. Hence, together with a diminished gastric emptying, the maternal gastric pH is low and volume is high, thus predisposing to high-risk of pulmonary aspiration and Mendelson syndrome (Fig. 10.1).[6]

Fetal Consideration

The maternal acid-base environment is reflected in fetus by the increasing acidemia and hypoxemia, but this is not the only potential source of acidosis in fetus. The activated sympathoadrenal system also causes vasoconstriction and decreased blood flow to the uteroplacental unit, which leads to placental hypoperfusion and hence enhanced acidosis. It can cause fetal demise.

PAIN TRANSMISSION AND PERCEPTION

The word pain is derived from the Latin *poena* meaning penalty. The International Association for the Study of Pain (IASP) defines pain as "an unpleasant sensory and emotional experience associated with actual or potential tissue damage or described in terms of such damage". It is a subjective experience and experienced only by the person in pain. The pain of labor is given the highest score on the McGill pain questionnaire (Fig. 10.2)[7] where it just abuts the pain of causalgia.

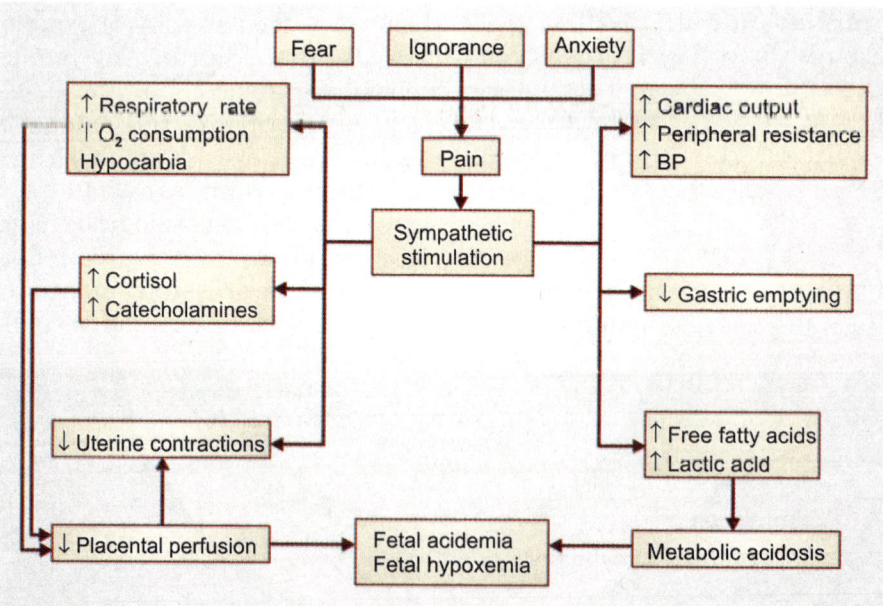

Fig. 10.1. Pain in labor

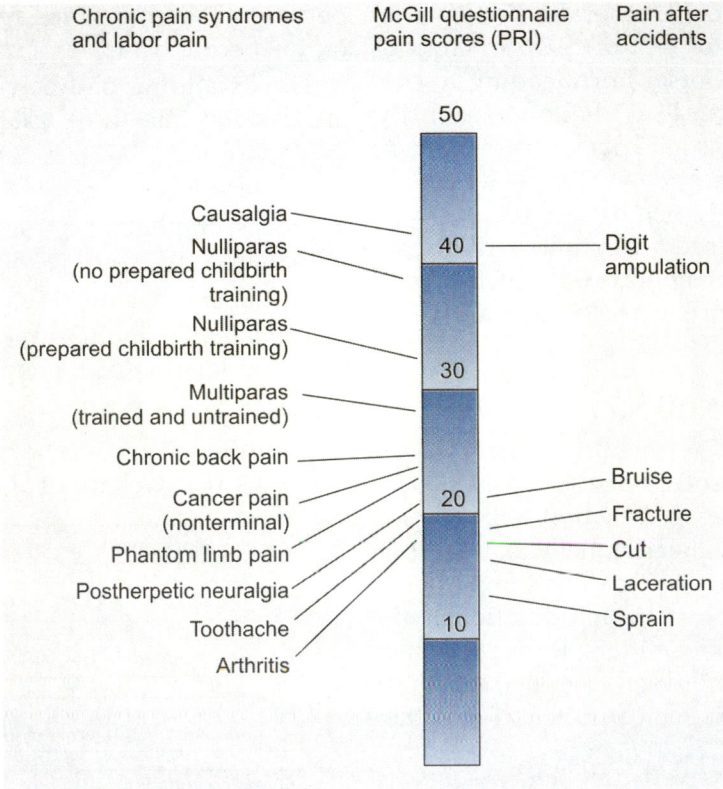

Fig. 10.2. The McGill pain questionnaire

Pain Transmission

Nociceptors

The response generated secondary to a noxious stimuli is initially perceived by the peripheral afferent nociceptors. These receptors respond to tissue damage by thermal, mechanical or chemical injury. They develop from neural crest stem cells and act as sensory neurons located both in somatic and visceral organs, with cell bodies in dorsal root ganglia. The axons from the dorsal root ganglia branch out extensively with peripheral projections, forming the peripheral nervous system. These axons are of two types—the myelinated fast conducting Aδ and unmyelinated slow C fibers.[8]

Peripheral Sensitization[9]

The painful stimuli are perceived by sensory receptors and the stimuli which are above the threshold level generate an action potential, which is transmitted to central nervous system via the axons. Acute pain starts an inflammatory response with release of inflammatory mediators, e.g. bradykinin, prostaglandins, substance P and glutamate from the damage cells. These mediators sensitize the high threshold nociceptors resulting in peripheral sensitisation resulting into functional plasticity of nociceptors. Subsequently, two zones surround the initial injury. The zones are:

1. Primary hyperalgesia: Zone where low threshold stimulus is perceived as painful.
2. Secondary hyperalgesia: Zone surrounding the primary zone and it is this zone where non-noxious stimulus is perceived as painful.

Central Sensitization

When the C-fibers are activated with repeated low-level noxious stimuli of longer duration, they start exhibiting hyperalgesia. This is thought to be due to build-up of action potentials in the dorsal horn leading to the phenomena of 'wind-up'. Following which certain modulations take place centrally such that, subsequent receptive fields get widened, there is abnormally heightened responsiveness and a lowered threshold. All these changes modify perception to stimuli in a way that, even non-noxious stimuli activate nociception.[10]

Pain Pathway (Fig. 10.3)

The axons from the dorsal root ganglia to peripheral nociceptors are the first order neuron. A complex interaction happens at dorsal horn among the peripheral axons, local spinal neurons and descending sympathetic neurons resulting in neuromodulation with the help of neurotransmitters. Rexed laminae contain the dorsal horn cells grouped together with specific physiological function and the

peripheral sensory fibers relay the messages on to specific laminae.

The ascending pathways mediating pain are divided into three tracts:[11]
1. Neospinothalamic tract (lateral spinothalamic tract—pain and temperature)
2. Paleospinothalamic tract (anterior spinothalamic tract—crude touch and pressure)
3. Archispinothalamic tract

The lateral spinothalamic tract is responsible for mediating pain and is presented here.

Lateral spinothalamic tract: It carries pain and temperature sensory modalities to thalamus (Flow chart 10.1).

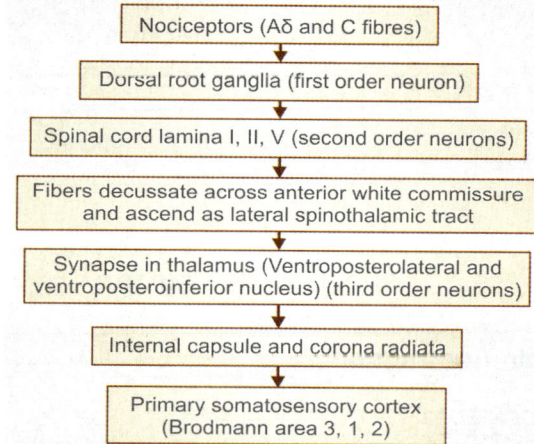

Flow chart 10.1. Pain perception path

Pain Perception

The perception of any painful noxious stimuli is divided into two phases. First phase is when the patient experiences sharp pain, due to stimulation of Aα fibers and second phase is a longer-lasting burning pain carried by C fibers.

To explain the mechanisms involved in pain perception, many theories[15] have been formulated. The three most widely studied ones are:
1. Specificity theory
2. Pattern theory
3. Gate control theory

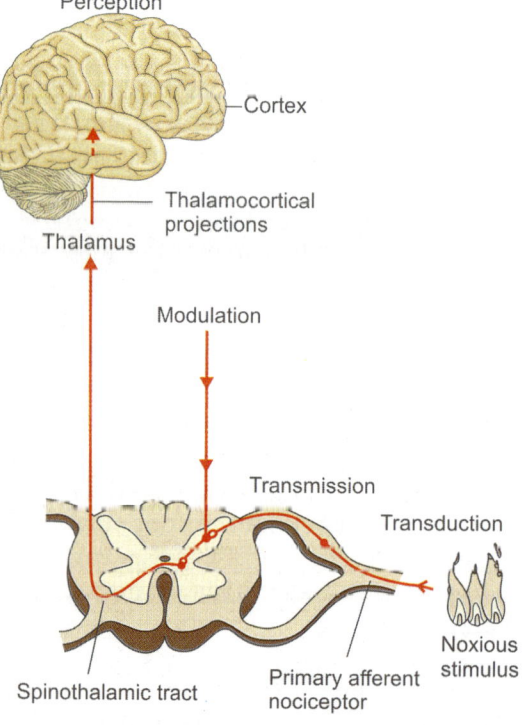

Fig. 10.3. Pain pathway

The specificity theory was given by Von Frey in the year 1895, pattern theory by Goldschneider in 1920 and the most popular gate control theory by Ronald Melzack and Wall in 1965.

Gate Control Theory

This theory as described by Melzack and Wall is the most controversial and widely accepted concept of pain perception. The peripheral nociceptive stimuli are carried by Aβ, Aδ and C fibers to the T cells, located in substantia gelatinosa of the rexed layers of spinal cord. These cells have the ability to inhibit or facilitate transmission of information to higher centers. In the presence of noxious stimuli, the larger Aα fibers which act as the 'hypothetical gate' close and inhibit the relay of transmission from smaller Aδ and C fibers. However, the modulation of pain signals also has a cognitive contribution mediated via T cells (Fig. 10.4).

METHODS OF ANALGESIA

There are various methods of analgesia available for labor pain can broadly be classified into pharmacological and non-pharmacological methods.[16] Pharmacological methods can further classified into systemic and regional.

Non-Pharmacological Methods

These methods are easily available, easy to administer, with limited side effects but unpredictable. These techniques lack the evidence to support them.[17]

Some of the methods are:

- Hydrotherapy—can be useful in first stage of labor pain. But such as there is no evidence to support that hydrotherapy reduces the pain of first stage of labor.
- TENS
- Acupuncture
- Hypnosis and massaging
- Relaxation breathing technique
- Temperature modulation
- Aroma therapy

Acupuncture:[16] Endorphins, metaencephalins and serotonins are documented to be released with the use of technique of acupuncture.

Quality of analgesia is inadequate and also is not predictable.

Transcutaneous electrical nerve stimulation (TENS): TENS involves stimulating electrically on both sides of spinous process at different dermatomal levels for labor analgesia. The basis of this mode of analgesia is stimulation of A fibre and local release of endorphins. Electrodes are placed 2 cm from spinous

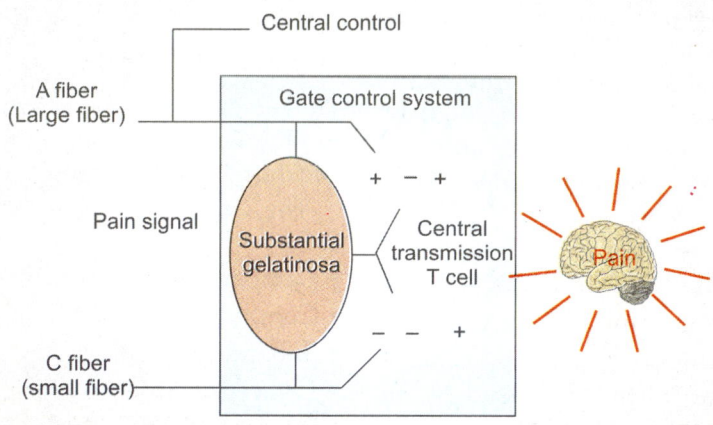

Fig. 10.4. Gate control theory of Melzack and Wall

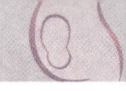

process of T10–L1. Alteration of current intensity can lead to various degrees of analgesia used for labor analgesia.

Pharmacological Methods

Pharmacological methods can be subclassified into systemic and regional.

Systemic Analgesics

Inhalational analgesics: Entonox (50:50 N_2O: O_2) is widely used inhalational agent. Different other inhalational agents, e.g. sevoflurane, desflurane, have been tried but lack of safety has limited their use.[18]

Onset of action of entonox is within 30 seconds and duration of analgesia stays for approx 45 seconds. It relieves the mild to moderate pain consistently. There is concern about the environmental pollution.

Opioids analgesics:

Agonists: Pethidine, remifentanil, alfentanil, sufentanil, fentanyl, morphine and tramadol are used commonly. Pethdine can be harmful to fetus in cervical dystocia.[19]

Routes of administration:
- IV—intermittent, continuous or patient control analgesia (PCA)
- IM

PCA remifentanil is a good alternative available to epidural analgesia. Supplemental oxygen and close monitoring is essential. Easy access to naloxone is suggested. Remifentanil is ultrashort-acting opioid metabolized by plasma and tissue esterases to an inactive metabolite. It crosses placenta but is metabolized by fetus as well.

PCA fentanyl[21] (fentanyl can be used as PCA, if newer drugs are not available).

- Compared to pethidine, fentanyl is 800 times more potent.
- Compared to morphine, fentanyl is 100 times more potent.
- Bolus—25–50 mg IV

- Infusion—0.25 mg/kg/hr
- ADR—nausea and vomiting; itching

Recommended PCA remifentanil[21] is:
- Bolus—20 mg
- Lockout—3 min
- Infusion—0.025 mg/kg/min to 0.15 mg/kg/min.
- ADR—maternal hypoventilation

Agonists antagonists: Agonists antagonists are an alternative. Few examples are nalbuphine (2 mg), butorphenol (2 mg) and buprenorphine (0.3 mg).[16] The side effects have limited the use of this group of analgesics especially in labor analgesia. Butorphenol is 5 times more potent than morphine.

Naloxone: Opioid antagonist for neonatal respiratory effects.

Dose—0.1 mL/kg IV preferred. Though it is not the first step in the management of the neonatal respiratory depression.[22]

Ketamine: The late stage of labor can be benefitted by subanesthetic doses of ketamine. There is always a possibility of psychomimetic side effects.

Ketamine for labor analgesia: Bolus of 10–15 mg can be administered at first stage of labor and then infusion @ 0.5–1 mg/kg/min can be started.

With crowning, another bolus of 0.2–0.4 mg/kg can be given.

Regional Techniques

The regional techniques are the gold standard in the management of the labor analgesia for various obvious reasons.

The various regional techniques available are:
- Lumbar epidural
- Combined subarachnoid epidural
- Subarachnoid block
- Paracervical nerve block
- Pudendal nerve block
- Paravertebral lumbar sympathetic block

EPIDURAL BLOCK

"The delivery of the infant into the arms of a conscious and pain-free mother is one of the most exciting and rewarding moments in medicine". The centrineuraxial blocks were introduced for labor analgesia at the end of the 19th century. Oscar Kreis, a Swiss obstetrician used subarachnoid block for 6 laboring patients with total anesthesia. A German obstetrician, Walter Stoekel, reported caudal epidural for labor pain with decreased incidence of headache. The use of catheter in the caudal epidural space was first introduced by Eugen Bogdan Aburel in 1931. In early 1960, the lumbar epidural analgesia and in 1970 the catheter in lumbar epidural space were introduced. Epidural aims to achieve this state. Epidural block is the gold standard analgesia for the labor analgesia. As it not only keeps the mother free of major pain but also she is wide awake to look after and feed the newborn. The block is placed at lumbar level L2–3/3–4. As the labor progresses, pain shifts from lower thoracic level (first stage) to sacral level (second stage) hence the level of analgesia needs to be modified as per requirement of the mother.

Technique

PAC

Before the epidural is placed in mother, pre-procedure check up is done to rule out any bony abnormality, infection at the site, coagulation disorder, severe degree of fixed cardiac valve lesion, progressive neurological diseases, raised intracranial pressure and then the informed consent has to be taken.

Platelet count of $<80,000/mm^3$ is considered as contraindication for the epidural placement. More than the absolute number of the platelets the trend of the number falling or raising is important.

Raised intracranial pressure from supratentorial tumor is absolute contraindication to epidural block as brain may cause the coning. Epidural should be avoided as there is always a risk of dural puncture while placing epidural block.

Vitals checked and documented: HR, NIBP, SpO_2

Start IV line and connect the fluid for maintenance and correct any fluid deficit, if present.

Position: Sitting (preferred), or left lateral position. Correct position is the most important factor in the successful technique.

"Hamstring stretch position" works to reverse the lordotic spine of the parturient. For this position, the parturient has to sit with extreme knee extended, hip adducted and forward lean. Sitting position should always be supported by the assistant from the front to avoid fall due to orthostatic hypotension or vagal stimulation.

Follow **aseptic precautions**: Handwash after removing the jewellery, cap, mask, gown and gloves.

Skin preparation: Chlorhexidine with alcohol for skin preparation—must dry before placement of needle.

Level: L2–3/L3–4

LOR: Saline is desired for identifying the space as provide more obvious tectile end point. While locating the space too much of saline should not be administered.

Approach: Midline/paramedian

Multiport catheter: 5 cm in space

Aspirate: Rule out intrathecal and vascular placement.

Dressing: Occlusive transparent dressing

Bolus doses: Initiate with 2–3 mL of 0.2% ropivacaine and wait for 5 minutes and then divided doses (5 mL) of ropivacaine should be given. Total of bolus of around 8–12 mL is required followed by infusion.

If ropivacaine is not available, bupivacaine can be given in concentration of 0.1% for the bolus and 0.0625% for the infusion and in the same volume.

Levels to be checked with cold swabs/ice packs after desired bolus is given. Level up to T9–10 should be achieved.

Infusion: 8–12 mL/hr of (0.06–0.1% ropivacaine) along with fentanyl 2 mg/mL should be started.

Complications

1. **Hypotension:** Defined as 20–30% drop from the baseline blood pressure. Since the uterine blood flow is directly dependent on the mother's arterial blood pressure hence the mother's blood pressure should be aggressively treated with both fluids and vasopressors.

   Incidence of hypotension in SAB is approximately 10%.[23]

2. **Pruritus:** Pruritus is the most common side effect of the block.[24] The incidence depends on the dose of opioids and the intrathecal opioids (**58%**) have higher incidence than the epidural opioids (**30%**).[25]

3. **Inadequate analgesia:** Pan et al investigated failure rate with 12,590 neuraxial blocks and found that the failure rate was more with epidural than combined spinal epidural block. The overall failure rate was **12%** whereas for epidural block failure rate was 14%. In the study, **5.6%** of catheters were working in the beginning but had to be reinserted during the course of labor.[26]

4. **Dural puncture:** It is rare complication associated with severe morbidity. The post-dural puncture can grossly limit the mobility of mother and her ability to look after the newborn which is a major concern. Choi et al analysed more than 30,000 obstetric patients and found the incidence of **1.5%** of accidental dural puncture.[27]

5. **Nerve damage:** The incidence of the permanent damage after epidural (0.6/100,000), after SAB (1.5/100,000) and CSEA (3.9/100,000). Overall the incidence of permanent nerve damage is 1.2/100,000.[28] It is important to note that the nerve damage from obstetric cause is approx. 1%.[29]

Trouble Shooting

1. If block is unilateral, pull out the catheter by 0.5–1 cm and give bolus.
2. If block is significantly patchy, rule out subdural block.
3. If desired level is not achieved, further bolus required.
4. If dura is punctured, there are two options:
   - *Option 1:* Leave the catheter is SAB space for 24 hrs, this will reduce the PDPH from 70 to 6%. Labor analgesia can be achieved by this catheter by giving bolus of 0.5–2 mL of low dose epidural mixture for each top up. Remember the dead space for filter is around 1 mL.
   - *Option 2:* Place the epidural catheter in another space and give 10 mL bolus intermittently.
5. If placement of catheter is in vessel, give small boluses and early identification by early signs and symptoms.
6. If pain in second stage of labor, boluses are required to cover sacral dermatomes.

Maintenance of Epidural

Maintenance of epidural can be managed by:
- Continuous infusion
- Intermittent epidural bolus by manual bolus or patient controlled.

Continuous Infusion

Continuous low dose mixtures are started after achieving the target level of analgesia by bolus and then maintained by continuous infusion. Doses recommended are 0.0625% bupivacaine or 0.06–0.1% ropivacaine with 2 µg/mL fentanyl. The total doses required are more in comparison to intermittent boluses technique. We follow in our hospital the continous technique of maintenance analgesia for labor due to constraints of man power.

Intermittent Technique

5 mL bolus after 15 min to reach the level. May require few more bolus. Throughout need monitoring.

PCEA

PCEA is a novel mode of delivery system. In 1988, Gambling et al[30] described patient-controlled epidural analgesia (PCEA) for labor pain which allowed to use minimal local anesthetics thus minimal motor blocks with adequate analgesia along with minimal requirement of the clinician giving the top ups. This method provides the best maternal satisfaction rate.[31] The success of this system depends on the proper explanation of the functioning of the system to the mother and the mother should be encouraged to use it as and when required at slightest pain.

The bolus doses are 3–5 mL. The lockout interval is around 10–20 min. The better mother satisfaction is prediction based on the studies but is not proven. There was no difference between groups in the incidence of obstetrical intervention or neonatal outcome.[32]

Campbell et al analyzed effect of background infusion on 300 women. There were no differences in the obstetrical outcomes, in terms of LSCS, instrumental delivery but significant difference in the clinical top ups required in group who received the basal infusion

Recently, D'Angelo recommended increasing the bolus to 5 mL, reducing the lockout interval to 10 min and adding a 5 mL/h infusion.

Myths Related to Epidural Analgesia

a. **Time of placement of epidural analgesia:** The ACOG and ASA have jointly stated that waiting for the cervix to dilate to 4–5 cm is not required and the epidural should be placed and charged, if the mother request for it.[36]

b. **Epidural has many side effects:** *Fact:*
   - Epidural has minor side effects most of which are self-limiting and transient. The common ones are loss of feeling and weakness which subsides when the epidural drug wears out and strength gets restored.
   - Nausea associated with epidural is mainly due to hypotension and is corrected by fluid bolus and positioning of the mother.
   - Itch is more with CSEA than EA alone and is self-limiting.
   - Spinal headache is rare but needs treatment.

c. **Epidural block needs increasing oxytocin requirements:** With the advent of low dose drugs, it does not hold true.

d. **Epidural increases the operative delivery:** *Fact:* Cochrane database have emphasized that epidural has no significant impact on LSCS. Epidural block may prolong labor by average of 1 hour. The low dose mixtures have reduced the incidence of undesirable side effects, e.g. need of oxytocins, or instrumental delivery.[37]

e. **Epidural is related to long-term back pain post-epidural:** *Fact:* Backache is associated to vaginal birth of baby with or without epidural.[38]

f. **Epidural adversely affects the outcome of the newborn. Leads to more neonatal sepsis work-up:** *Fact:* EA improves the placental circulation and thus should be positively affecting the baby. Epidural analgesia is associated with low degree of pyrexia (<1°C). The exact cause of pyrexia is unknown but prolong labor is cited as one of the factors. Irrespective of the cause, the intrapartum pyrexia should be treated aggressively with fluids, and antipyretics. Neonatal extensive work up is not required, if the temperature is only antepartum and temperature is <1°C.[39]

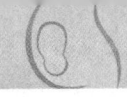

Ultrasound-guided Epidural Block[40]

Ultrasound can guide the performer the location of the midline, the depth of epidural space and also the direction of the needle. The safest way to place the epidural will be real-time ultrasound-guided epidurals.

Combined Spinal Epidural Analgesia

Combined spinal epidural analgesia (CSEA) is a safe technique which follows "the needle in needle" technique and gives a better patient satisfaction with more of ambulatory analgesia. Combined obstetric mobile epidural trial (COMET) showed that low dose epidural analgesia resulted in significant higher vaginal delivery.[41]

Future Scopes

Wong et al worked on the computer integrated epidural analgesia. Computer controls the background infusion based on the patient-controlled demands.[42]

SUMMARY

Labor pain is a dynamic process. It integrates and exemplifies both central and peripheral nervous mechanisms. Pain of first stage of labor is secondary to uterine distension and contractions. These uterine contractions lead to myometrial ischemia and release of noxious metabolites like bradykinin, histamine and serotonin. Pain is transmitted via afferent fibers coursing through paracervical plexus and hypogastric pelvic plexus (inferior, medial and superior), and co-mingle with sympathetic efferent fibers along paravertebral sympathetic chain and further on to spinal cord, thalamus and brain.

REFERENCES

1. Bonica JJ. Obstetric Analgesia and Anesthesia. World Federation of Societies of Anesthesiologists. Seattle, University of Washington Press. As modified by Bonica JJ: The nature of pain in parturition. In: Van Zundert A, Ostheimer GW (Eds). Pain Relief and Anesthesia in Obstetrics. New York: Churchill Livingstone 1996, p 32.

2. Neurophysiology of labour pain, James Eisenach. Anesthesiology and Physiology & Pharmacology, Wake Forest University School of Medicine, Winston-Salem, US, June 12, 2010, European Society of Anaesthesiology.

3. Miller's Anesthesia, 7th Edition, By Ronald D. Miller, MD, Lars I. Eriksson, Lee Fleisher, MD, Jeanine P. Wiener-Kronish, MD and William L. Young.

4. Source:Butterworth JF, Mackey DC, Wasnick JD. Morgan & Mikhail's Clinical Anesthesiology, 5th ed www.accessmedicine.com Copyright–The McGraw-Hill Companies, Inc. All rights reserved.

5. The nature and consequences of childbirth painPeter Brownridge, European Journal of Obstetrics and Gynecology, 59(1995), S9–S15. doi:10.1016/0028-2243(95)02058-Z.

6. Reena, Bandyopadhyay KH, Afzal M, Mishra AK, Paul A. Labor epidural analgesia: Past, present and future. Indian J Pain 2014;28:71–81.

7. The McGill Pain Questionnaire: Major properties and scoring methods. Pain Sept 1975;1(3):277–99.

8. Fein A. Nociceptors: the cells that sense pain, http://cell.uchc.edu/pdf/fein/nociceptors_fein_2012.pdf

9. Handbook of Pain Management: A Clinical Companion to Wall and Melzack's" Textbook of Pain".

10. Miller-Keane Encyclopedia and Dictionary of Medicine, Nursing, and Allied Health, Seventh Edition. © 2003 by Saunders, an imprint of Elsevier, Inc. All rights reserved.

11. NachumDafny. Pain Tracts and Sources, Department of Neurobiology and Anatomy, The UT Medical School at Houston, Chapter 7.

12. Galer B, Gammaitoni A, Alvarez NA: XIV Pain. 11 Neurology. WebMD Scientific American® Medicine Online. Dale DC, Federman DD, Eds. WebMD Corporation, New York, 2002.

13. Fields HL, Basbaum AI. Central nervous system mechanisms of pain modulation. In: Wall PD, Melzack R, (Eds). Textbook of Pain. Edinburgh: Churchill Livingstone; 1999.

14. Purves D, Augustine GJ, Fitzpatrick D, et al. (Eds). Neuroscience. 2nd ed. Sunderland (MA): Sinauer Associates; 2001. The Perception of Pain. Available from: http://www.ncbi.nlm.nih.gov/books/NBK10963.

15. Moayedi M, Davis KD. Theories of pain: from specificity to gate control. J Neurophysiol 2013; 109:5–12.

16. Sunanda Gupta, GS Anand Kumar, Hemesh Singhal. Acute pain—labour analgesia. Indian J Anaesth 2006;50(5):363–9.

17. Smkin PP, O'hara M. Non-pharmacologic relief of pain during labor. Systemic review of five methods. Am J Obstet Gynecol 2002;186:5; S131–59.

18. Rosen MA. Nitrous oxide for relief of labor pain: A systematic review. Am J Obstet Gynecol 2002; 186:S110–26.

19. Sosa CG, Balaguer E, Alonso JG, Panizza R, Laborde A, Berrondo C. Meperidine for dystocia during the first stage labor: A randomised controlled trial. Am J Obstet Gynecol 2004;191: 1212–8.

20. Sunil T Pandya. Labour analgesia: Recent advances. Indian J Anaesth 2010;54(5);400–8.

21. D'Onofrio P, Novell AM, Mecacci F, Scarselli G. The efficacy and safetyof continous intravenous administration of Remifentanyl for birth pain relief:An openstudy of 205 parturients. Anesth Analg 2009;109;1922–4.

22. Chestnut DH. In: Chestnut DH, Polley LS, Tsen LC, Wong CA, (Eds) Chestnut's Obstetrc Anesthesia: Principles and Practice. Phildelphia: Mosby Elsevier; 2009, pp.405–501.

23. Simmons SW, Cyna AM, Dennis AT, Hughes D. Combined spinal epidural verses epidural analgesia in labour. Cochrane database Syst Rev. 2007;3:CD003401.

24. Mardirosoff C, Dumont L, Boulvain M, Tramer MR. Fetal bradycardia due to intrathecal opioids for labour analgesia:A srstemic review. BJOG 2002;109:274–81.

25. Herman NL, Choi KC, Affleck PJ, et al. Analgesia, purities and ventilation exhibit a dose–response relationship in parturients receiving intrathecal fentanyl during labour. Anesth Analg 1999;89: 378–83.

26. Pan PH, Bogard TD, Owen MD. Incidence and characteristics of failures in obstetrics neuraxial analgesia and anaesthesia. A reterospective analysis of 19,259 deliveries. Int J Obstet Anesth 2004;13;227–33.

27. Choi PT, Galnski SE, Takeuchi L, Lucas S, Tamayo C, Jadad AR. PDPH is a common complcaton of neuraxial block in partiurient. A meta analysis of obstetrical studies. Can J Anaesth 2003;50: 460–9.

28. Cook TM, Counsell D, Wildsmith JA. Major complications of central neuraxial: Report on the third National Audit Project of the Royal College of Anaesthesists. Br J Anaesth 2009;102:179–90.

29. Wong CA, Scavone BM, Durgan S, et al. Incidence of postpartum lumbosacral spine and lower extremity nerve inuries. Obstet Gynaecol 2003;101:279–88.

30. Gambling DR, Yu P, Cole C, et al. A comparative study of patient controlled epidural analgesia (PCEA) and continuous infusion epidural analgesia (CIEA) during labour. Can J Anaesth 1988;35: 249–54.

31. Hodnett ED. Pain and women's satisfaction with the experience of childbirth: a systematic review. Am J Obstet Gynecol 2002;186:S160–S172.

32. Ledin-Eriksson S, Gentele C, Olofsson CH. PCEA compared to continuous epidural infusion in an ultra-low-dose regimen for labor pain relief: a randomized study. Acta Anaesthesiol Scand 2003; 47:1085–90.

33. ACOG commetti on obstetric practice. ACOG commetti opinon. No 339: Anagesia and caesarean delivery rate. Obstet Gynecol 2006;107:1487–8.

34. Leighton BL, Halpern SH. The effect of epidural analgesia on labour, maternal and neonatal outcomes. A systematic review. Am J Obstet Gyecol 2002;186:S69–77.

35. Lim Y, Sia AT. Dispelling the myths of epidural pain relief in childbirth. Singapore Med J 2006;47:1096.

36. Leighton BL, Halpern SH. The effect of epidural analgesia on labour, maternal and neonatal outcomes. A systematic review. Am J Obstet Gyecol 2002;186:S69–77.

37. Arzola C, Davis S, Rofaeel A, Carvalho JC. Ultrasound using the transverse approach to lumber spine provides reliable landmarks for labour epidurals. Anesth Analg 2007;104;1188–92.

38. COMET study group UK 2001. Effect of low-dose mobile versustraditional epidural techniques on mode of delivery : A randomised controlled trial. Lancet 2001;358:19–23.

39. Wong CA, Ratliff JT, Sullivan JT, Scavoneb BM, Toledo P, McCarthy RJ. A randomised comparison of programmed intermittent epidural bolus with continous epidural infusion for labour analgesia. Anesth Analg 2006;102;904–9.

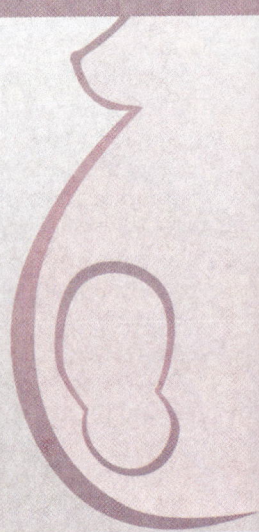

CHAPTER 11

Anesthesia for Cesarean Section

Anjana Sahu, Dinesh K Sahu

The term 'cesarean section' is named after Roman Emperor Julius Caesar (100 BC) as he was born by this technique. In the past, cesarean section (CS) was known to be a type of fatal surgery but now the equation has changed with the advancement of new technologies and modifications. In olden days, ether and chloroform were the only available method of providing anesthesia service for surgery. Now with the knowledge of neuraxial block and advancement in the techniques of general anesthesia, it has become simple, safe and effective. Also obstetricians are able to deal with hemorrhage in a better way, which is most common and leading cause of maternal mortality during cesarean section. With all this advanced knowledge of physiology, anatomy, and techniques of anesthesia, both maternal as well as fetal morbidity and mortality have decreased. In this chapter, we will discuss the various anesthesia techniques for cesarean section and their complications and management.

Indication

Indications for CS are based on maternal and fetal wellbeing. The most common indication for CS is acute fetal distress. Other main indications are maternal hemorrhage, pelvic deformity, prolonged gestation and malpresentation.

PREANESTHETIC EVALUATION

Consent

Consent is an integral part of preanesthetic checkup. It should be informed and obtained in writing from patient. Maternal and fetal condition should be discussed with patient and her close relatives and should be informed about the consequences of it. It is always better to talk to the patient before the procedure as it decreases the anxiety and makes the patient familiar with the environment. She should be informed about the techniques of anesthesia and its complications. Obstetric anesthesiologist in UK and Ireland[1] formed a general consensus that the following neuraxial block which is most common technique of providing anesthesia in CS, the risk factors to be disclosed such as:

- The possibility of intraoperative discomfort and a failed/partial blockade
- The potential need to convert to general anesthesia

- The presence of weak leg
- Hypotension
- Occurrence of an unintentional dural puncture

History

Past medical, surgical and obstetric history should be obtained. Drug history and previous allergic episodes and their cause should be noted. If it is an emergency surgery, general questions should be asked about the comorbid illness such as gestational diabetes and pregnancy-induced hypertension while preparing for the procedure.

Examination

Thorough general examination should be done. In emergency situation, baseline vital parameters, such as pulse rate, blood pressure, respiratory rate, pallor, edema, bleeding gums, icterus, lymphadenopathy and cyanosis, should be noted down. Urine output and its color should also be noted down. Systemic examination should be done to rule out any respiratory and cardiovascular system abnormalities. Auscultation of fetal heart sound gives us an idea of fetal distress. Airway assessment is always mandatory both in neuraxial as well as in general anesthesia, even in case of emergent nature of surgery. Assessment of difficult airway indicators should be performed such as mouth opening, size of tongue, Mallampati classification, thyromental distance, neck mobility, etc.

Blood Products

Generally, CS does not require blood and blood product transfusion but peripartum hemorrhage is always a challenge. Therefore, patient's blood grouping, screening and cross-matching should be done before the procedure and its availability should be confirmed prior to surgery. Coagulation profile should also be checked. Certain high-risk obstetric cases, such as placenta previa, placenta accreta, previous uterine scar, ruptured ectopic pregnancy and ruptured uterus, may need blood transfusion.

Operation Theatre (OT) Preparation

Obstetric OT should be well equipped to deal with routine as well as emergency surgeries. ASA standard monitoring devices, i.e. pulse oximetry, non-invasive blood pressure (NIBP), electrocardiogram (ECG), capnography and temperature monitoring should be checked. Resuscitation equipment and emergency drugs should be available. Difficult airway cart including nasopharyngeal and oropharyngeal airways, classic and intubating laryngeal mask airways, intubating bougie, flexitip laryngoscope, small handle laryngoscope and stylet should be confirmed. Defibrillator should be at hand to manage catastrophic situations. Neonatal resuscitation cart with warmer should be available.

Patient Preparation

Patient should be wheeled to the OT in left lateral position by keeping a wedge under right hip. This prevents aortocaval compression by the gravid uterus, which leads to maternal hypotension and subsequently decreases uteroplacental blood flow. Ideally left lateral position should be maintained till the delivery of baby. Parturients should have a urinary catheter placed *in situ* for urine colour and output monitoring.

Aspiration Prophylaxis

Inhalation of the gastric juice in the pulmonary system in a parturient is known as Mendelson's syndrome. It occurs mostly when gastric acid pH has become <2.5 and volume >25 mL. Acid inhalation causes injury to bronchial mucosa which leads to bronchiolar spasm, peribronchiolar exudates, focal hemorrhages and parenchymal necrosis. Risk of aspiration of gastric content is more in parturients, due to upward shifted diaphragm, reduced esophageal sphincter tone and increased intra-abdominal pressure. Fluctuations in the hormones level make them more vulnerable. Parturients have increased levels of progesterone and decreased levels of motilin hormones, which reduce the gastric tone and motility and hence increases the episodes of nausea and vomiting. In pregnancy towards term, the acid and pepsin secretions are also increased. The use of opioid, ergot derivatives and anesthetic agents (intravenous or inhalational) results into decreased upper airway reflexes and loss of consciousness. Hypotension due to aortocaval compression, hemorrhage or sympathetic block increases the risk of aspiration by triggering the vasomotor centers. Regurgitation can occur in case of raised intra-abdominal and intragastric pressure while giving fundal pressure on the uterus for delivery. To prevent aspiration pneumonitis in the pregnant patients, aspiration prophylaxis is required.

Following methods can prevent aspiration:

1. Reducing intragastric secretion by using H2 blocker
2. Increasing intragastric pH by antacids
3. Increasing lower esophageal sphincter tone by prokinetic agents (metoclopramide and domperidone)
4. Suppressing the vomiting episodes by antiemetic agent (ondensterone)

Histamine Receptor Blocker (H2 Blocker)

Ranitidine (oral 150 mg) is most commonly used histamine blocker to be given a night prior to surgery. It prevents gastric acid secretion, decreases the gastric volume and increases the intragastric pH. It has been proved that a single dose of ranitidine or famotidine administered orally three hours before surgery provides a more effective means to control and neutralize gastric secretion compared to omeprazole in parturients.[2] Intravenous ranitidine in a dose of 50 mg reduces the risk of acid aspiration effectively, if administered 30 minutes prior the surgery.[3]

Antacid

Nonparticulate 0.3 M sodium citrate is effective in raising the intragastric pH >2.5 without affecting gastric volume.[4] It mixes well with gastric juice and causes less pulmonary damage, if aspiration occurs.[5] Intravenous 50 mg ranitidine 30 min prior surgery and 30 mL 0.3 M sodium citrate 15 min before surgery effectively decrease the risk of aspiration both at the time of intubation and extubation.

Physical Means

Placing the nasogastric tube and aspirating the gastric content before induction helps in prevention of aspiration. Cricoid pressure of about 30 Newton (3 kg) prevents aspiration by occluding esophageal opening against cricoid cartilage for which this pressure has to be maintained till endotracheal tube placement.

Fasting

Fasting period should be limited to 6–8 hours in case of elective surgery. Clear fluids (water, fruit juice without pulp, clear tea, black coffee) intake should be allowed only up to 2 hours before induction of anesthesia. Patients in labor should avoid solid food intake, as they may be taken for section any time. Other risk factors for regurgitation and aspiration are morbid obesity, diabetes and difficult airway.

Antibiotic Prophylaxis

Infection is one of the major causes of maternal morbidity and mortality. Antibiotic prophylaxis should be given either before abdominal incision or after umbilical cord clamping, which provides protection against post-cesarean infections, especially endometritis. First generation cephalosporin is recommended for antibiotic prophylaxis by the American College of Obstetrician and Gynecologist (ACOG).[6] Extended-spectrum antibiotic regimen is recommended for active or presumed infection.

Intravenous Fluid

A wide bore intravenous cannula should be secured and non-dextrose containing balanced salt solution started. Crystalloid in a dose of 15–20 mL per kg of body weight should be infused before the neuraxial block as preload. In case of emergency, fluid can be administered simultaneously with neuraxial block as co-load. One should not wait to infuse fixed volume of fluid to prevent hypotension. Either of above technique is effective in preventing hypotension.[7] Vasopressor can be given for its prophylaxis and treatment.[8] Any crystalloid or colloid fluid would be effective to maintain the intravascular volume.[9] The incidence of hypotension is not eliminated with crystalloid or colloid infusion but the severity of hypotension definitely decreases. Type of fluid, volume, rate and timing of infusion are important factors in the prevention and treatment of hypotension. Ripolles et al[10] reviewed and found on meta-analysis that colloid administration significantly reduces the incidence of hypotension associated to spinal anesthesia in elective cesarean section compared with use of crystalloid. Colloid is of advantage when given simultaneously while performing neuraxial block because it stays for a longer time in intravascular compartment. Its disadvantages are that it is expensive, associated with increased risk of pulmonary edema after delivery due to contracting uterus (autotransfusion) and there is risk of anaphylactoid reaction. Non-dextrose-containing balanced salt solution should be infused within 30 minutes of providing anesthesia to maintain intravascular volume. Dextrose-containing fluid may stimulate fetal insulin secretion and will result into fetal hypoglycemia and

hyponatremia. Calcium- or dextrose-containing fluid should not be infused with blood products because of risk of intravascular clotting and clumping of red blood cell.

We prefer preloading or coloading with Ringer's lactate solution over colloid, which effectively reduces the incidence of hypotension. We reserve colloid administration only for those cases, which are at high risk of developing hypotension, or require rapid maintenance of effective intravascular volume.

Monitoring

Standard monitoring includes pulse oximetry, ECG, heart rate (HR), NIBP, temperature, and urine output. Invasive blood pressure monitoring is required in case of severely compromised cardiac disease, refractory hypertension, pulmonary edema or unexplained oliguria, and severe hypovolemic maternal condition. Abnormal ECG is commonly seen in late trimester due to hyperdynamic circulation, circulating catecholamines and altered estrogen and progesterone ratios. Myocardial ischemia may be experienced in small number of patients during CS.[11] Shen et al[12] performed a study on 254 healthy pregnant patients who had undergone spinal anesthesia for cesarean section. They found the incidence of first and second degree atrioventricular block (3.5% each), severe bradycardia (<50 beats/min; 6.7%) and multiple premature ventricular contraction (1.2%). The above increased parasympathetic activity occurred due to blockade of cardiac sympathetic activity post-spinal anesthesia. These types of arrhythmias were transient and resolved spontaneously. Urine output measurement is one of the indicators of systemic perfusion and renal function.

ANESTHESIA TECHNIQUES FOR CS

Type of anesthesia care depends upon the condition of maternal and fetal wellbeing and urgency. General anesthesia is a preferred technique in case of acute fetal distress and in other obstetric emergency (eclampsia, ruptured ectopic pregnancy with unstable hemodynamics or ruptured uterus). Neuraxial anesthesia is the best method of providing anesthesia for other indications of CS.

Neuraxial Anesthesia

Neuraxial anesthesia or regional anesthesia (RA) is the most commonly used method of administering anesthesia for CS. Neuraxial anesthesia includes spinal anesthesia (SA), epidural anesthesia (EA) and combined spinal epidural anesthesia (CSE). Sometimes patient's refusal for neuraxial block may become an indication for general anesthesia. Neuraxial anesthesia allows the mother to remain awake and minimizes or completely avoids the complication associated with airway management like failed intubation and aspiration pneumonitis. It also avoids the neonatal exposure to multiple systemic drugs. Afolabi et al[13] reviewed the Cochrane Pregnancy and Childbirth Group's Trials, 22 out of 29 included studies (1793 women) and compared the effects of RA with those of GA on the outcomes of CS. They found women given either spinal or epidural anesthesia had a lower estimated maternal blood loss. There was a significant difference in terms of maternal satisfaction with anesthetic technique when compared epidural or spinal group to GA. Women in the GA group stated that they would use the same technique again if they needed CS for a subsequent pregnancy (epidural versus GA: risk ratio (RR) 0.80; 95% CI 0.65 to 0.98; one trial, 223 women; spinal versus GA: RR 0.80; 95% CI 0.65 to 0.99; one trial, 221 women). In terms of neonatal Apgar scores and the need for neonatal resuscitation with oxygen, there was no significant difference seen. Staikou et al[14] concluded in their study that the neonatal oxygenation and acid base status values were better preserved in GA as compared to neuraxial technique for

elective CS and Apgar score and neonatal outcomes were not affected by the anesthesia technique. Baraka et al[15] concluded that Apgar score at 1 minute was higher in those cases where the induction delivery interval was less than 10 min and the uterine incision-delivery interval was less than 90 sec and it was not associated with the type of technique used for providing anesthesia.

Lateral or sitting, both the positions can be used for performing neuraxial anesthesia. It also depends upon the preference and skill of the anesthesiologist. Lateral position reduces the incidence of vagal reflexes that includes dizziness, perspiration, pallor, bradycardia and hypotension. Lateral position restricts side to side or front to back movement of patient during needle puncture. Epidural venous plexuses are reduced in size and less engorged in lateral position due to decreased hydrostatic pressure, therefore, there is less incidence of intravascular puncture. Right lateral position is beneficial in relieving the aortocaval compression and maintaining good utero-placental blood flow. In sitting position, the distance from the skin to epidural is less and the spaces are well defined hence one is able to acquire subarachnoid space early. Therefore, in obese patient, sitting position is most preferred position. Some conditions where sitting position cannot be used are fetal head entrapment, umbilical cord prolapse and footling breech presentation.

Order of neuraxial blockade occurs in differential pattern. Autonomic blockade and sympathetic blockade occur first as they are small and myelinated fibers. Autonomic blockade occurs 2–6 dermatome segments higher than sensory block. After autonomic, there is sensory blockade which is 2 segments higher than the motor blockade. Assessment of sensory and autonomic blocks is done by pinprick, light touch and cold stimulation. The motor fibers are thick and last to get blocked. If patient is unable to raise her leg up from hip

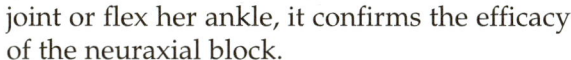

joint or flex her ankle, it confirms the efficacy of the neuraxial block.

Neuraxial block should be supplemented with oxygen. It helps in maintaining maternal as well as fetal oxygenation, especially at the time of fetal distress.[16]

Spinal Anesthesia

Among all the above techniques of neuraxial block, SA is considered as the most simple, safe and reliable technique. In an adult, the spinal cord ends at L1–L2, so SA should be performed at a level lower to this to avoid injury to the spinal cord. SA is most commonly performed at L3–L4 or L4–L5 interspace and the drug is injected into subarachnoid space after confirming the free flow of cerebrospinal fluid (CSF) from the spinal needle. For CS, T4 dermatomal level of anesthesia is required. Level of anesthesia can be achieved with Trendelenburg position of a 15°. More than this should be avoided as it might lead to high spinal. Rapid onset of anesthesia, density of the block, and rapidity at which the procedure can be performed in emergency conditions make it comparatively popular. Spinal anesthesia requires lesser doses of local anesthetic, which decreases the risk of maternal toxicity and there is less transfer of drugs through the uteroplacental circulation to the fetus.

Local anesthetic agents and adjuvant in SA: Choice of local anesthetic agent depends on the expected duration of surgery. Most commonly used local anesthetic agent for CS is hyperbaric 0.5% bupivacaine in a dose of 7.5–12.5 mg. As compare to non-parturient, smaller dose of local anesthetic is required in parturient, reasons being smaller CSF volume, cephaled movement of drug in supine position and greater sensitivity of nerve fibers to the local anesthetic. Low dose 12.5 to 7.5 mg of bupivacaine reduces the chances of hypotension and helps in rapid recovery.[17]

Ropivacaine is less potent than bupivacaine and associated with slower onset, less hypotension and faster recovery; however, FDA does not approve intrathecal ropivacaine and levobupivacaine, therefore, bupivacaine is still a preferred drug for spinal anesthesia.

If the expected duration of surgery is less than 45 minutes, 60–80 mg hyperbaric lidocaine can be used; however, use of this drug is controversial due to its adverse effect of transient neurologic symptoms.

Adjuvant: Adjuvant improves the quality of intraoperative anesthesia and provides longer postoperative analgesia. Opioids, epinephrine and dextrose are commonly used adjuvants. Morphine in a dose of 0.1–0.2 mg is effective but the postoperative monitoring is mandatory as delayed respiratory depression may occur. Fentanyl 10–25 µg augments the spinal anesthesia and also effective in prevention of nausea. Low dose (7.5 mg) hyperbaric bupivacaine with 25 µg fentanyl provides adequate anesthesia, prolongs postoperative analgesia and maintains stable hemodynamics as compared to 10 mg hyperbaric bupivacaine alone.[18] Addition of epinephrine to local anesthetic solution decreases its systemic absorption and prolongs its action. Dextrose makes the local anesthetic hyperbaric so that drug moves in cephalad direction in supine position and adequate level of anesthesia can be achieved.

Epidural Anesthesia

Epidural anesthesia is preferred in surgical procedures of duration >2 hours. It can be given as a bolus injection, top ups or as continuous infusion. Epidural is considered to be safer than spinal anesthesia. Epidural catheter is placed either in L2–L3 or L3–L4 interspace. Epidural anesthesia is most commonly used for providing labor analgesia. For labor analgesia, T8 or T9 dermatome level is required while for CS T4 dermatome anesthesia is needed. If epidural catheter, which has been put for labor analgesia, is already in place, T4 dermatome can be achieved for CS by administering more drug.

The onset and level of anesthesia are achieved slowly in EA and depending upon the duration of surgery it can be maintained for longer time. If initial dose of local anesthetic does not provide significant sensory block, administering more drug through the catheter can increase the height of block. Touhy needle is being used for administering epidural anesthesia. Epidural catheter can be kept for postoperative analgesia. Caudal epidural anesthesia may be used for cesarean section but not very popular due to difficulty in placing the catheter.

Local anesthetic and adjuvant in EA: 2% adrenalized lidocaine is most commonly used local anesthetic in epidural anesthesia. It provides faster onset and additional dose can be given to get adequate height of block. Test dose of 3 mL of 2% adrenalized lidocaine should be given prior to total epidural dose to exclude the intravascular or intrathecal placement of the catheter. Tachycardia within 30 seconds of administration of test dose indicates intravascular placement of epidural catheter. Usually 20 mL volume of local anesthetic agent is sufficient to get the desired T4 level of anesthesia. Other local anesthetic agents are bupivacaine (0.5%), ropivacaine (0.5–0.75%) and 2-chloroprocaine (3%). Bupivacaine has slow onset and longest duration of action. 0.75% bupivacaine used for CS may produce a denser block but this concentration is not preferred in obstetric patients for fear of cardiac arrest owing to accidental intravascular injection.

Sodium bicarbonate increases the pH of local anesthetic solution, therefore, a higher fraction of non-ionized lipid-soluble drug is available for action. Mixing of 2 mL 8.4% of sodium bicarbonate to every 20 mL of lidocaine or 2-chloroprocaine and 0.1 to 20 mL bupivacaine solution is advised.[19] But its disadvantage is rapid development of hypotension and consequently decreased uteroplacental circulation. Hence should be used with caution in high-risk obstetric patient.

Epinephrine, a vasoconstrictor agent, in concentration of 1 in 2,00,000 is added to local anesthetic. It decreases the systemic absorption of local anesthetics thus decreasing the peak blood levels. It intensifies the motor block and prolongs the duration of anesthesia. It is also used as a test dose in concentration of 5 µg/mL with lidocaine to identify intravascular placement.

Epidural opioids, fentanyl 50–100 µg potentiates intraoperative analgesia and decreases nausea and vomiting due to visceral manipulation with no adverse effects on maternal and fetal outcome. Other opioids, such as sufentanil 20–30 µg, morphine 2–5 mg and buprenorphine 90–150 µg, are also used as an adjuvant to local anesthesia. Sufentanil has property of profound analgesia and provides good intraoperative anesthesia. If added to local anesthetic agents. It has minimal maternal side effects and no untoward effects on fetus. Morphine provides effective, safe, prolong and profound analgesia (24 hours) with mild adverse effects. Postoperative monitoring is needed in case of opioid adjuvants.

Position of the patient at the time of induction and effect of gravity influences the quality of block. The epidural catheter should be placed at a proper level of required anesthesia to avert catastrophes of total spinal, convulsion or cardiac arrestcan happen.

Combined Spinal Epidural Anesthesia

Combined spinal epidural (CSE) anesthesia has gained popularity because it has advantages of both spinal as well as epidural anesthesia. It eliminates the individual disadvantages of spinal and epidural anesthesia when used as a sole technique. CSE provides fast onset, extended duration of anesthesia and postoperative pain relief. It causes less hypotension and can be managed easily. CSE can be given through double interspace technique or single interspace technique (needle through needle technique).

In double space technique, an epidural catheter is threaded through epidural needle at L3–L4 interspace once epidural space is confirmed and spinal anesthesia is administered at L4–L5 interspace. Various CSE kits are available but CSE can be performed through 18 G or 16 G Tuohy or Hustead epidural needle and long (12.7 cm or more) 24–26 G pencil point spinal needle (needle through needle technique). Hyperbaric bupivacaine 7.5–12 mg is administered to obtain the adequate level of spinal anesthesia and if required additional drug can be administered later through the epidural catheter to prolong the anesthesia. A study compared 12.5 mg bupivacaine bolus injection of spinal anesthesia with 7.5 mg bupivacaine CSE and found significantly slower onset of hypotension, which could be managed easily.[20]

Sequential CSE: In this technique, low dose of spinal anesthesia is given to have rapid onset of anesthesia and additional dose of local anesthetic is administered through epidural to get required T4 dermatome anesthesia. Two-staged sequential epidural technique provides additional advantage of reducing the incidence and severity of hypotension hence this technique is useful in high-risk medical and surgical condition. Low dose of bupivacaine (5–10 mg) is administered intrathecally to get the desired effective T8–T9 dermatome and increase the height of block to T4 dermatome by administering graded dose of bupivacaine 0.2 to 0.25%.

Complications

Hypotension

Hypotension is a known complication of neuraxial blockade. Hypotension can be defined as a decrease in value of systolic blood pressure by >25% from baseline values or systolic blood pressure <100 mm Hg. Reason for hypotension is sympathetic blockade which leads to decreased systemic venous resistance, increased venous pooling, decreased venous return and decreased cardiac output. Blockade of the sympathetic preganglionic fibers, which innervate the smooth muscle of the arterial and venous vasculature and have significant role in development of hypotension. If hypotension is promptly recognized, it can be treated successfully with fluids, change of table position and vasopressor agent. Main aim of treating the neuraxial block-induced hypotension is to increase the venous return by maintaining adequate hydration. Preloading either with crystalloid or colloid significantly reduces the incidence of hypotension. Head down tilt of 10–15° may help in increasing the venous return but it may cause more cephalad spread of spinal anesthesia; therefore, its role is questionable in preventing hypotension. Leg elevation and leg wrapping may be helpful in increasing the venous return. Left uterine displacement should be maintained as it improves the venous return by eliminating the compression over vena cava and also maintains the uteroplacental flow. Vasopressor agents, such as ephedrine, phenylephrine, mephentermine, and metaraminol, are commonly used for treatment of hypotension. All except phenylephrine improve the uterine blood flow. Ngankee et al[21] reported that ephedrine may cause acidosis in fetus as it depresses fetal pH and base excess due to its metabolic effect, secondary to stimulation of beta adrenergic receptors. Phenylephrine is an effective agent and does not cause acidosis in fetus but as it may depress uteroplacental blood flow. Magnitude of hypotension with EA is lesser than SA and can be easily treated. The WHO Reproductive Health Library (RHL) summarizes evidence-based reviews and says that with spinal anesthesia, the operation could start sooner [weighted mean difference (WMD) 7.91 minutes earlier, 95% confidence interval (CI)-11.59–4.23], but there was an increased risk of hypotension that required treatment (RR 1.23, 95% CI 1.00–1.51).[22]

We recommend blood pressure monitoring every 1 minute for initial 20 minutes of spinal anesthesia and thereafter every 10 minute.

PDPH

PDPH is relatively common and annoying complication of spinal anesthesia. It occurs following puncture of dura mater with a wider bore needle and consequent loss of CSF in spinal anesthesia or accidental dural puncture with epidural needle while performing epidural anesthesia. Time of onset of PDPH is between 24 hours and 3 days of dural puncture. There is a frontal or occipital headache, which worsens in sitting or upright position and gets relieved on lying down. The associated symptoms may be nausea, vomiting, neck pain, dizziness, tinnitus and diplopia. Some patients may also present with hearing loss, cortical blindness, cranial palsies and seizures. Hence, to prevent the incidence of PDPH, smaller-sized spinal needles are preferred. Modification in type of spinal needle and technique decreases the incidence of PDPH. Non-cutting tip needle produces lower incidences of PDPH as compare to cutting bevel tip spinal needle (Quinke).[23] Pencil-tip (Whitacre, Sprotte, Greene) needle separates the dural fibers rather than cutting it and minimizes the incidence of PDPH but it may also cause dural trauma and inflammatory response. Insertion of spinal needle in the perpendicular plane of dural fibers is associated with more incidence of PDPH as compared to parallel plane.[24] Commonly available Quinke needle of smaller gauge with bevel facing to longitudinal plane of vertebral column, however, is used. Different types of needle are available to decrease the PDPH.

Treatment of PDPH includes Trendelenburg position, bedrest, adequate hydration, oral analgesics, caffeine, dextran 40 and autologous epidural blood patch. Intravascular (500 mg) or oral (300 mg) caffeine, oral theophylline (300 mg, sustain release tablets), injection ondansetron (0.15 mg/kg) are some of the drugs effective in treatment of PDPH. Withdrawing 15–20 mL blood from patient's vein (autologous) and injecting immediately through epidural at the site of dural puncture relieves headache in most of the cases. The other alternative therapy to autologous blood is dextran 40 in a volume of 20–30 mL, provides complete relief within 2 hours.[25]

High or Total Spinal, Total Epidural

High or total spinal occurs due to cephalic spread of local anesthetic or accidental injection of local anesthetic into subarachnoid space while performing epidural anesthesia. Clinical features include hypotension, bradycardia, apnea, aphonia, complete sensory and motor blockade, loss of control of airway reflexes and loss of consciousness. Keeping a pillow underneath the shoulder immediately after performing spinal anesthesia prevents the higher spread of local anesthetic and incidence of hypotension. Treatment of high spinal is depending upon the severity of symptoms appeared. It includes 100% oxygen through mask ventilation and management of hypotension with fluids and vasopressor agents. Severe cases require aggressive management with endotracheal intubation and positive pressure ventilation along with circulatory support through vasopressor agents. Patient regains consciousness as soon as the action of local anesthetic agent wears off. Any delay in the management may lead to hypoxic and circulatory insult to the vital organs and may become fatal.

Nausea and Vomiting

Nausea and vomiting are most common intra-operative complications. The causes are hypotension, increased vagal activity, increased uterine bleeding, surgical stimuli and drugs (e.g. inhalational agents, opioids, uterotonic drugs and antibiotic). Hypotension due to sympathetic block causes hypoperfusion of cerebral and brainstem and stimulates medullary vomiting center. Due to gut hypoperfusion, emetogenic substances (e.g. serotonin) are released.[26] Surgical stimulation, such as visceral manipulation, exteriorizing of the uterus, peritoneal traction, can cause visceral pain and subsequently stimulation of vagal fibers leads to nausea and activation of vomiting center. Addition of opioid to local anesthetic reduces the nausea and vomiting induced by visceral pain pathway. Metaclopromide, dimenhydrinate, ondansetron or granisetron are successfully used to treat nausea and vomiting. It has been proved that supplemental oxygen (FiO_2 0.8)[27] has role in reducing nausea and vomiting in non-pregnant patient. Subhypnotic dose (1 mg/kg/hr) of propofol after cord clamping can be used in reducing nausea and vomiting.[28]

Shivering

Shivering is most often encountered intra-operative complication. It is common during neuraxial anesthesia. It can be treated with ondansetron, meperidine and fentanyl. Use of warm blanket and warm fluid administration provide relief to the patients.

Pruritus

Pruritus is commonly occurred due to intra-thecal opioid. This is usually happened after 30–75 minutes of injection. Pruritus may be generalized or localized to nose, face, chest and abdomen. Treatment with opioid antagonist, an opioid agonist/antagonist, a serotonin antagonist ondansetron and low dose propofol are effective.[29] Antihistaminic is ineffective as mechanism of an opioid-induced pruritus is not known and is not due to histamine release.

Neurologic Complication

Peripheral neuropathy can occur due to position. Constant and long-standing elevation of right hip can compress the structure of left hip and may lead to sciatic neuropathy.[30] Transient neurologic symptoms (TNSs) can occur with the use of any local anesthetic agent but it is most commonly associated with the use of intrathecal concentrated lidocaine. Rorarius et al[31] studied neurologic sequelae after cesarean section in 219 patients and reported 17 mothers (8.8%) complained of TNSs lasting mostly 1–2 days, in the buttocks and/or legs during the first three postoperative days. Eleven patients (5.7%) complained of postdural puncture headache. Two patients (emergency cesarean section because of protracted labor in one and elective cesarean section because of previous cesarean section in the other) complained of persisting pain or sensory abnormalities and they concluded women after cesarean section under a spinal block seem to suffer more often from TNSs than non-pregnant women. The persisting neurologic symptoms in two patients might also be due to the obstetric procedure itself but these conclusions are, however, uncertain, as they had no control group operated on under other than spinal anesthesia. TENs usually resolve within 1 week. Cauda equina syndrome has been reported in some patients after spinal anesthesia. The incidence is very less about 0.1 per 10,000. Reason being direct exposure of lumbosacral spinal nerve roots to large doses of local anesthetic, high concentration local anesthetic, prolonged exposure to a local anesthetic through a continuous catheter.

General Anesthesia

General anesthesia is advocated for high-risk emergencies and cases where neuraxial anesthesia is contraindicated or has failed. Severe eclampsia, ruptured uterus and acute fetal distress are some of the commonly encountered high-risk obstetric emergencies. Pregnancy with known medical disease (cardiac and neurological), spine disorders, lumbar disk disease, infection and coagulo-pathies are some non-emergent cases, where GA is planned. Advantages of general anesthesia are rapid onset of anesthesia, better control of airway, stable hemodynamics and

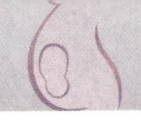

good relaxation of abdomen. Patient with high level of anxiety may refuse to undergo neuraxial anesthesia. Maheshwari et al[32] found GA as preferred choice of anesthesia by the highly anxious patients (72.7%) for elective CS.

Advocating GA to a pregnant patient requires effective aspiration prophylaxis, plan for failed intubation and avoidance of factors that may cause fetal depression. Histamine H_2 blocking agents like IV cimetidine or IV ranitidine are useful in preventing aspiration when given 45–60 min prior to induction. Omeprazole, a proton pump inhibitor, decreases gastric acidity but it requires at least 40 min for onset of its action. As discussed in regional section, non-particulate 0.3 M sodium citrate 15–30 mL in one dose, 10–15 min prior to induction is preferred and effective antacid in obstetric cases. Metaclopromide 10 mg is preferred for its prokinetic action, by enhancing gastric emptying and increasing gastroesophageal sphincter tone. Generally, rapid sequence induction is preferred technique of providing GA. Here cricoid pressure or Sellicks maneuver should be performed to prevent aspiration. In this method, an assistant gives pressure over the cricoid to occlude the esophageal lumen against the cricoid cartilage and maintains this pressure until the endotracheal tube is secured. Initially cricoid pressure of 10 N (1 kg) is applied and then this magnitude is increased to 30 N (3 kg) once patient has lost consciousness. Patient should be ventilated with not >2–3 puffs and smaller tidal volume before intubation. Rapid endotracheal intubation should be performed and patient should be extubated the patient when fully awake and able to protect her airway. These measures can help to reduce the risk of aspiration.

Airway assessment should be done prior to any regional or general anesthesia. Mallampati class III and IV are considered to be difficult for laryngoscopy. Mucosal edemas due to increased progesterone level especially oropharyngeal and laryngeal edemas are common presentation in obstetric cases, which increase the incidence of difficult airway. Increased body mass index with short neck and pendulous breast are significant predictors of difficult airway. Proper planning can reduce the incidence of failed intubation. Call for help is a must, if one is unable to secure the airway. Repeated attempts at intubation may lead to edematous cords and injury to oral and pharyngeal structures making it more difficult to secure the airway. Maternal hypoxia should be avoided. Prolonged induction to delivery interval may result in low Apgar score in neonate.

Technique

Patient should be shifted to OT in left lateral position by keeping a wedge under the right hip to prevent maternal hypotension. Try to maintain this left lateral position till the delivery of the baby. Routine monitors, include pulse oximetry, ECG, non-invasive blood pressure and capnography, should be attached. Wide bore IV line should be secured and non-dextrose containing balanced salt solution should be started. Antiemetic and antacid prophylaxis should be given, if not given earlier. Ideal time is 40 minutes prior induction of anesthesia. Sniffing position (discussed in failed intubation) should be given. Preoxygenation (denitrogenation) with 100% oxygen should be initiated and continued for 3 minutes with tight fitting mask or patient should be asked to take 4 maximal vital capacity breadths within 30 seconds.[33] This prevents incidence of maternal hypoxia in apneic period of induction and intubation. Maternal oxygen consumption in pregnant is 20% greater than non-pregnant at term and their functional residual capacity (FRC) is also reduced by 20% due to upward shift of diaphragm.[34] Their vital capacity, total lung capacity and chest compliance are also reduced. Work of breathing is increased due to increased pressure of abdominal content against the diaphragm. Therefore, pregnant patients are prone to develop hypoxia rapidly during induction of anesthesia. To reduce fetal exposure to multiple drugs, the surgeon should be asked to prepare and drape the patient's abdomen before starting induction of anesthesia. Avoid positive pressure ventilation with mask to prevent unintentional insufflation of stomach, which can provoke regurgitation. Ask the assistant to give cricoid pressure of 10 N to occlude esophagus. Patient should be induced preferably with thiopental (4–5 mg/kg) as it causes less neonatal depression as compared to propofol (2–2.5 mg/kg). Other agents can be used depending on the maternal condition. Ketamine (1 mg/kg) and etomidate (0.3 mg) are preferred agents in hemodynamically unstable patient. As soon as patient is unconscious, cricoid pressure is increased to 30 N and short-acting muscle relaxant succinylcholine (1–1.5 mg/kg) is given to facilitate rapid endotracheal intubation. Pretreatment with smaller dose of non-depolarizing muscle relaxant for defasciculation is not recommended in parturient, which may delay the onset of action of succinylcholine. Conditions where succinylcholine is contraindicated such as malignant hyperthermia, myotonic dystrophy, hyperkalemia and spastic paraparesis, rocuronium (0.6–1 mg/kg) can be of choice for acquiring rapid intubation. In case of difficult airway, role of rocuronium is questionable due to prolong duration of action, which would be deleterious, if one was unable to intubate the patient. Because of the fear of total paralysis and increased risk of aspiration, priming preinduction with non-depolarizing muscle relaxant is not recommended in pregnant patient. Vecuronium (0.08–0.1 mg/kg) or atracurium (0.5 mg/kg) can be used for muscle relaxation during induction, if airway is normal. Endotracheal tube of smaller size 6.5–7.0 mm should be used and secured under vision. Difficult airway algorithm should be followed, if one is unable to intubate the patient. Air entry to the chest should be confirmed by auscultation bilaterally. Patient should be auscultated over epigastrium as well to detect inadvertent esophageal intubation. Capnography is most confirmatory sign of endotracheal intubation. Bilateral visible movement of thorax with each positive pressure ventilation is also a good indicator of presence of endotracheal tube in trachea. Patient should be maintained on oxygen (with or without 50% N_2O) and with or without halogenated agent till the delivery of baby. At 50% N_2O with low concentration of halogenated agent, no maternal awareness and no adverse effect on neonatal outcome reported. After delivery of baby, the concentration of halogenated agent can be increased and opioid can be given to deepen the plane of anesthesia and analgesia, respectively. If required, extra maintenances dose of muscle relaxant can be administered. Extubation should be done when patient is fully awake and is able to protect her airway. Peripheral nerve stimulator can be used to know the status of muscle paralysis.

Induction Agents

Thiopental: Sodium pentothal (4–5 mg/kg) is most preferred induction agent. It rapidly crosses the placenta but its adverse effect on fetus is not reported at this dose. It rapidly attains its level in umbilical venous blood within 1 min of injection and then is rapidly metabolized by fetal liver. Therefore, its concentration in the fetal brain is almost negligible. Neonatal depression is, however, found at very high doses of 8 mg/kg.[35]

Ketamine: Ketamine is a preferred induction agent for hemodynamically unstable patients. It is a sympathomimetic drug, which stimulates the cardiovascular system and acts through antagonism of N-methyl-D-aspartate (NMDA) receptor on the brain, which depresses neuronal activity. It also has

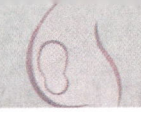

bronchodilator effect, therefore, preferred in patients with asthma. Because of its cardio-stimulatory effects, it is preferred in patients with hypovolemic shock. It is to be avoided in hypertensive patients as it increases arterial blood pressure by 10 to 25%. Its undesirable adverse effects are emergent delirium and hallucinations, which can be minimize with diazepam or midazolam as premedication. Patients can be induced with 1 mg/kg dose and no neonatal depression is reported. It rapidly crosses the placental barrier and low Apgar score and neonatal muscular hyper-tonicity are reported at higher dose. Study compared the ketamine 1 mg/kg and thiopental 4 mg/kg as induction found neonatal neurobehavioral score high in ketamine group.[36]

Propofol: Propofol can be used as IV induction agent. Role of propofol has not yet been approved in obstetric anesthesia. Placental transfer of propofol is same as thiopental and Apgar score is comparable to thiopental. Its unwanted effects, like pain on injection and propofol infusion syndrome, make it unpopular. It is contraindicated in patients with egg allergy.

Etomidate: It provides stable hemodynamic condition. Its induction dose is 0.3 mg/kg. It can be a preferred agent in patients with cardiac disease. It also causes pain on injection and associated with nausea and vomiting. It is contraindicated in epileptic patients due to activation of epileptogenic foci, which results into onset of seizures.[37] It also reduces fetal cortisol production but transiently.[38]

Midazolam: Midazolam can be used as induction agent but it is reserved only for those cases where other agents are contra-indicated. Higher concentration (0.2 mg/kg) of midazolam is associated with neonatal low Apgar score, prolonged respiratory depression, low general body tone, body temperature and arm recoil.[39]

Depolarizing muscle relaxant succinyl-choline (1–1.5 mg/kg) is most commonly used muscle relaxant for facilitation of endotracheal intubation. It has rapid onset of action and is rapidly metabolized by plasma pseudo-cholenesterase, therefore, it is considered as an ideal agent for difficult airway. If 'cannot intubate' condition arises, patient can be awakened and other alternative measures can be carried out. Neuromuscular blocking agents do not readily cross placental barrier. Only minimal amount is transferred to the fetus and no harmful effects are reported. Atracuronium, vecuronium, mivacuronium and rocuronium are intermediate-acting muscle relaxants and can be used for induction as well as for maintenance agent. Atracuronium may cause hypotension due to histamine-releasing action and is contraindicated in asthmatic patients. Rocuronium has rapid onset of action and longer duration of action and can be used where succinylcholine is contraindicated.

Nitrous oxide: Nitrous oxide is most commonly used inhalational agent for CS. It has very less effect on maternal blood pressure and uterine tone. It rapidly crosses placental barrier and rapid fetal tissue uptake reduces fetal arterial concentration. Oxygen with 70% N_2O produces neonatal depression and study showed oxygen with 50% nitrous oxide asso-ciated with maternal awareness.[40] Therefore, 50% N_2O need an anesthetic agent to prevent maternal awareness. In presence of 50% N_2O, the requirement of anesthetic agent is decreased and low concentration (0.5) MAC of halogenated agent produces adequate anesthesia with no recall or awareness and also does not produce neonatal depression.

Halogenated Agents

Requirement of anesthetic agents has become less due to decreased FRC and there is rapid induction of anesthesia. Hence, low doses isoflurane (0.75%), halothane (0.5%), sevoflurane (1.0%), desflurane (2–4%) and enflurane (1.0%) provide adequate level of anesthesia. At this concentration, no neonatal depression has been reported. Halogenated agents are highly lipophilic and have low molecular weight, therefore, rapidly cross placental barrier. Halothane and isoflurane has F/M ratio of 0.71–0.87 and 0.71, respectively.

FAILED INTUBATION (DIFFICULT AIRWAY)

The incidence of difficult intubation in the pregnant patient has been estimated to be 1 in 30 and incidence of failed intubation has observed 1 in 280 obstetric cases which is 8 times more than general population.[41] Most of these cases of difficult airway can be predicted preoperatively. According to Mckeen et al,[42] previously accepted risk factors, such as labor, pre-existing medical conditions and obstetrical disorders, did not predict any high risk of difficult tracheal intubation, while maternal age ≥35 years, weight 90 to 99 kg, and absence of active labor were found to predict increased risk.

Anesthesiologist must be able to deal with the anticipated or unanticipated difficult airway. This requires proper planning, evaluation and preparation. First and most important factor is proper assessment of airway. It should be performed in all kinds of surgery whether it is a routine or emergency, major or minor and whether it requires neuraxial or general anesthesia. Protruded incisors, retrognathia, restrictive neck movements either in flexion or extension, restricted mouth opening, short neck and high arched palate are predictors of difficult airway. Modified Mallampati classification by Samsoon and Young is first and most important assessment tool. Its class keeps on changing with advancing period of gestation. It may shifts to one or two class higher with stages of labor. Its class III and IV are supposed to be a case of difficult airway. To assess the Mallampati class, the patient should be asked to open her mouth as wide as possible either in supine or sitting position. All the oral and pharyngeal structures should be assessed and given score accordingly. Apart from Mallampati, assessment of thyromental distance (>6.5 cm), mouth opening (>3-finger breadth) and neck movement (flexion at lower cervical and extension at atlanto-occipital joint) should be done.

Appropriate position is needed for achieving successful airway. Increased body mass index and increased breast size require additional measures to be taken. Ramp position is useful in morbidly obese patient as it improves oxygenation and visualization of glottis during laryngoscopy. A role or stacked blankets should be kept under the shoulder so that head and neck falls away from the chest and two firm pillows under the head provide adequate lower cervical flexion and extension at atlanto-occipital joint. Confirm horizontal alignment of the external auditory meatus and the sternal notch. This aligns the oral, pharyngeal and laryngeal axis (Sniffing position) and facilitates insertion of laryngeal blade. 10–20° head up also displace the breast away from head.

Awake fiberoptic bronchoscopy is a preferred choice for endotracheal intubation in planned case of difficult airway. Optimum oral and nasal preparations are needed, if awake endotracheal intubation is planned. Nasal decongestion is done with adrenalized local anesthetic solution. Lidocain 4% with adrenaline or lidocaine 3%/phenylephrine 0.25% can be used to anesthetize the nasal mucosa. Intravenous glycopyrrolate should be administered to reduce the secretions. Intravenous dexamethasone 8 mg should be administered to prevent upper airway edema. Topicalization of oral and pharyngeal mucosa should be done with local anesthetic gargles. No sedative agent should be administered to the patient as it may cause respiratory depression and hypoxia and increase the fetal distress. Low dose opioid agent can be administered. Transtracheal injection of lidocaine is not recommended in parturient as

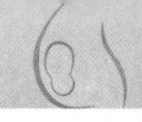

it increases the risk of aspiration. Superior laryngeal nerve block can be given. Bilateral glossopharyngeal nerve block through palato-glossal arches provides anesthesia to posterior one-third of tongue and pharyngeal wall.

In case of unanticipated difficult airway and if surgery is not an emergency, allow the patient to wake up and consider regional anesthesia or awake intubation. Cormack Lehane grade 3 is most common in parturient and it is associated with increased incidence of failed intubation. Repeated attempts of laryngoscopy should be avoided, it may cause injury to pharynx and larynx, edema and laryngospasm. The rise in circulatory catecholamines due to the stress response leads to decrease in uteroplacental blood flow thereby increasing the magnitude of fetal distress, which is already compromised due to maternal hypoxia. Call for help is must, if one is unable to achieve successful airway. If mask ventilation is possible, then ventilate the patient with 100% oxygen. General anesthesia without intubation can be an alternative technique but consider placing nasogastric tube first and maintain cricoid pressure, maternal oxygenation and adequate depth of anesthesia. In this technique, anesthesia can be maintained with 60% nitrous oxide in oxygen with low concentration of inhalational agent and if required it can be supplemented with IV fentanyl or low dose ketamine (0.1–0.25 mg/kg). A competent obstetrician can perform CS under local anesthesia mean while maternal airway management is in progress.

In case a 'cannot ventilate' condition occurs, then laryngeal mask airway or combitube should be considered for maintaining airway. If all the above methods have failed, surgical airway that is cricothyroidotomy or trans-tracheal jet ventilation or tracheostomy must be considered. Emergency cricothyroidotomy can be performed with 16G intravenous cannula, through which oxygen can be administered to maintain maternal oxygenation.

Remember that LMA is not meant for apneic patient or patient with full stomach. It is an emergency equipment of resuscitation. Use of LMA for GA in CS is recommended only in case of 'cannot ventilate or cannot intubate' situation, as risk of aspiration cannot be prevented by it.

CESAREAN SECTION FOR FETAL DISTRESS

Anesthesia techniques vary with the severity of fetal distress. If time constrains, general anesthesia is preferred choice over neuraxial. It provides faster onset of anesthesia, less hemodynamic changes, therefore, maintains good uteroplacental circulation. Fetal distress is a most common indication for emergency cesarean section. Fetal hypoxia means decrease in fetal oxygen tension that is umbilical venous PO_2 <15 mm Hg and fetal asphyxia means decrease in fetal oxygen tension along with increase in carbon dioxide tension (umbilical venous PCO_2 >40 mm Hg). Fetal cardiac output maintains the oxygen supply to the vital organs such as brain, heart, adrenal glands in case of fetal asphyxia. Fetal pH is decreased as blood supply to other organs is hampered and widespread anaerobic metabolism (produces lactic acidosis and metabolic acidosis) is occurred. In 1998, ACOG committee opine, "The fetal distress is imprecise and nonspecific term". Fetal distress may consist of severe fetal bradycardia, persistent late deceleration, severe repetitive variable deceleration or loss of beat-to-beat variability. A study conducted in 126 patients which compared GA with SA and EA in fetal distress and found that umbilical artery pH was consistently high in spinal and 1 minute Apgar score of 8–10 was found in 11% of babies in SA group and only 51% in GA.[41] The reason for the better outcome with regional techniques could be the lower stress response and lower maternal norepinephrine levels in mother under SA leading to less vasoconstriction.

There is still a controversy that which anesthesia technique is better. Both the anesthetic techniques (general as well as neuraxial) are good and provide effective anesthesia. Most of the anesthesiologist prefers to give SA over GA as single drug provides fast and adequate anesthesia. Other reason of preferring SA over GA is incidence of unanticipated difficult airway in parturients while providing general anesthesia can be avoided. Depressant action of various drugs on fetus can be avoided by not administering general anesthesia. Some anesthesiologists prefer GA for fetal distress as it takes less time to induce the parturient than SA. Time is an important issue, SA failure may occur and it may require administration of GA to the patient. Within the neuraxial technique, SA is preferred over epidural anesthesia, as placing the epidural catheter is time consumable procedure. However, labor epidural can be used to extend the anesthesia.

POSTPARTUM TUBAL LIGATION (PTL)

Postpartum period or postnatal period starts immediately after the delivery of baby and extends up to 6–8 weeks. During this period, maternal hormones and pregnant physiological state return to non-pregnant physiological state.

For initial few days, the physiological state of post-pregnancy is same to the pregnant state. Atrophy of uterus starts from 2nd day and continues till 6–8 weeks. The blood volume is increased to 15–35% due to autotransfusion and started declining to non-pregnant state within 2–3 weeks. Due to increased blood volume, cardiac output is also increased. Hematocrit may be low due to blood loss during vaginal and cesarean deliveries. White blood cell count may remain high (20,000–30,0000 per cumm), especially neutrophil count. Respiratory changes such as increased ventilatory drive, laryngeal and pharyngeal edema of pregnant state will remain there for few days. Laryngeal and pharyngeal edema may put the patient at an increased risk of upper airway infection.

Laryngitis, nasal congestion and voice changes are common presentation.

Spinal anesthesia is considered to be the safe and effective procedure and it has been most commonly used method for providing anesthesia for postpartum tubal ligation. Epidural anesthesia can be used, if epidural catheter has been placed earlier for labor analgesia or for cesarean section and remain *in situ* for providing postoperative analgesia. Epidural anesthesia has not been used solely for PTL because PTL is a short duration procedure. General anesthesia is reserved only for those cases where the spinal anesthesia is contraindicated such as coagulopathy, infection at the site and increased intracranial tension. If GA has been chosen for administering anesthesia for PTL, laryngoscopy should be gentle to avoid injury to the pharyngeal structures. If planning for early PTL, ideally 8 hours should be completed between the delivery and scheduled tubal ligation. This period is most preferred time of doing PTL because during this time uterus remains extra-pelvic and its fundus is at the umbilicus, therefore, easy to catch hold fallopian tube of both sides.

ASA Guidelines for Postpartum Tubal Ligation

- Oral intake of solid foods should be stopped 6 h prior to surgery.
- Aspiration prophylaxis should be administered.
- Time of procedure and type of anesthesia technique for PTL should be based on obstetric risk factor, anesthesia risk factors and patient preferences.
- Neuraxial techniques are preferred to general anesthesia for most postpartum tubal ligations.
- Gastric emptying will be delayed in patients who have received opioids during labor.
- There may be failure of induction through epidural catheter, if it has placed earlier for labor analgesia, due to longer postdelivery time interval.

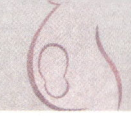

Pearls

- Proper evaluation of patient
- Aspiration prophylaxis
- Spinal anesthesia is safe and effective technique except certain specific situation
- Always keep difficult airway cart ready

Key Points

- Consent is an integral part of preanesthetic check-up. It should be informed and obtained in writing from the patient.
- Preanesthetic evaluation includes obtaining proper history and examination.
- Airway assessment should be performed with difficult airway indicators such as mouth opening, size of tongue, Mallampati classification, thyromental distance and neck mobility in all routine as well as emergency cases.
- Normal preoperative investigation includes complete blood picture with platelet count. Coagulation profile, liver function test and renal function test should be based on history and examination.
- Operation theatre should be well equipped with anesthesia machine, ASA standard monitors, resuscitation equipment, emergency drugs and defrillator.
- Patient should be maintained in left lateral tilt to avoid aortocaval compression which may lead to maternal hypotension and subsequent decrease in uteroplacental flow.
- Aspiration prophylaxis should be administered 30–40 minutes before induction of anesthesia.
- A wide bore intravenous cannula should be secured and crystalloid in a dose of 15–20 mL per kg of body weight should be infused before the neuraxial block as a preload.
- Neuraxial technique especially spinal anesthesia is most commonly used technique for cesarean section. It is considered as a simple, safe and effective technique. T4 dermatomal level of anesthesia is required for adequacy of block for cesarean section.
- Epidural anesthesia is reserved for high-risk medical conditions which require hemodynamic stability. Combined spinal epidural anesthesia can also be used to get advantages of both techniques.
- Adjuvant in local anesthetic agent maintains anesthesia for longer duration without hemodynamic instability and provides postoperative analgesia.
- General anesthesia is preferred technique in case of acute fetal distress, obstetric emergency (eclampsia, ruptured ectopic pregnancy with unstable hemodynamics or ruptured uterus), patient refusal for neuraxial anesthesia, failed neuraxial block and patient with seizure and coagulopathy disorder.
- Unpredictable difficult airway can be encountered in normal situation, therefore, always keep difficult airway cart ready while providing general anesthesia for cesarean section.
- Rapid sequence induction is the most commonly used technique as pregnant patients are prone for regurgitation and aspiration even with proper aspiration prophylaxis. This technique involves intravenous induction with rapid onset muscle relaxant along with cricoid pressure of 30 Newton to prevent aspiration until endotracheal tube is secured.
- In case of failed intubation, call for help is must and follow difficult airway algorithm to secure airway and try to maintain maternal oxygenation at every step.

SUMMARY

Obstetric anesthesia is a challenge to the anesthesiologists due to unpredictable difficult airway, blood loss, obesity and fetal distress. We had discussed in above section that neuraxial technique especially spinal anesthesia is a preferable, safe and widely acceptable technique over general anesthesia for cesarean section. It may be an individual decision based on the factors such as emergent nature of surgery, amount of fetal distress, expecting blood loss, comorbid condition and predictable difficult airway for inducing a pregnant patient. But both maternal and fetal wellbeing are the prime concerns to an anesthesiologist while choosing the technique.

REFERENCES

1. Lanigan C, Reynolds F. Risk information supplied by obstetric anaesthetists in Britain and Ireland to mothers awaiting elective caesarean section. Int J Obstet Anesth 1995;4(1):7–13.

2. Lin CJ, Huang CL, Hsu HW, Chen TL. Prophylaxis against acid aspiration in regional anesthesia for elective cesarean section: a comparison between oral single-dose ranitidine, famotidine and omeprazole assessed with fiberoptic gastric aspiration. Acta Anaesthesiol Sin 1996; 34(4):179–84.

3. Rout CC, Rocke DA, Gouws E. Intravenous ranitidine reduces the risk of acid aspiration of gastric contents at emergency cesarean section. Anesth Analg 1993;76(1):156–61.

4. Dewan DM, Floyd HM, Thistlewood JM, Bogard TD, Spielman FJ. Sodium citrate pretreatment in elective cesarean section patients. Anesth Analg 1985;64(1):34–7.

5. James CF, Gibbs CP. An evaluation of sodium citrate solutions. Anesth Analg 1983;62(2):241.

6. American College of Obstetricians and Gynecologist. Prophylactic antibiotics in labor and delivery. ACOG Practice Bulletin No. 47. Wasington, DC. ACOG, October 2003. Obstet Gynecol 2003;102: 875–82.

7. Dyer RA1, Farina Z, Joubert IA, Du Toit P, Meyer M, Torr G, Wells K, James MF. Crystalloid preload versus rapid crystalloid administration after induction of spinal anaesthesia (coload) for elective caesarean section. Anaesth Intensive Care 2004;32(3):351–7.

8. Lawrence C Ten. Anesthesia for cesarean delivery. In: David H Chestnut, Linda SP, Lawrence CT, Cynthia AW (Eds). Chestnut's Obstetric Anesthesia: Principles and Practice, 4th ed. Philadelphia: Mosby Elsevier 2009,p.519–73.

9. Cyna AM, Andrew M, Emmett RS, et al. Techniques for preventing hypotension during spinal anaesthesia for caesarean section. Cochrane Database Syst Rev 2006;(4):CD002251.

10. RipollésMelchor J, Espinosa A, Martínez Hurtado E, Casans Francés R, Navarro Pérez R, Abad Gurumeta A, Calvo Vecino J. Colloids versus crystalloids in the prevention of hypotension induced by spinal anesthesia in elective cesarean section. a systematic review and meta-analysis. Minerva Anestesiol 2014 Dec 11. [Epub ahead of print].

11. Moran C1, Ni Bhuinneain M, Geary M, Cunningham S, McKenna P, Gardiner J. Myocardial ischaemia in normal patients undergoing elective cesarean section: a peripartum assessment. Anaesthesia 2001;56(11):1051–8.

12. Shen CL, Ho YY, Hung YC, Chen PL. Arrhythmias during spinal anesthesia for Cesarean section. Can J Anaesth 2000;47(5):393–7.

13. Afolabi BB, Lesi FE. Regional versus general anaesthesia for caesarean section. Cochrane Database Syst Rev 2012;10:CD004350.

14. Staikou C1, Tsaroucha A, Vakas P, Salakos N, Haslakos D, Panoulis K, Petropoulos G. Maternal and umbilical cord oxygen content and acid-base balance in relation to general, epidural or subarachnoid anesthesia for term elective cesarean section. Clin Exp Obstet Gynecol 2013; 40(3):367–71.

15. Baraka A, Louis F, Dalleh R. Maternal awareness and neonatal outcome after ketamine induction of anaesthesia for Caesarean section. Can J Anaesth 1990;37(6):641–4.

16. Chatmongkolchart S, Prathep S. Supplemental oxygen for caesarean section during regional anaesthesia. Cochrane Database Syst Rev 2013;6: CD006161.

17. Ben-David D, Miller G, Gavril R, Guruvitch A. Low dose bupivacaine fentanyl spinal anaesthesia for caesarean delivery. Reg Anesth Pain Med 2000;25: 235–9.

18. Venkata HG, Pasupuleti S1, Pabba UG1, Porika S1, Talari G2. A randomized controlled prospective study comparing a low dose bupivacaine and fentanyl mixture to a conventional dose of hyperbaric bupivacaine for cesarean section. Saudi J Anaesth 2015;9(2):122–7.

19. Peterfreund RA, Datta S, Ostheimer GW. pH adjustment of local anesthetic solutions with sodium bicarbonate: laboratory evaluation of alkalinization and precipitation. Reg Anesth 1989;14(6):265–70.

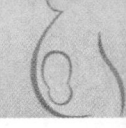

20. Choi DH, Ahn HJ, Kim MH. Bupivacaine sparing effect of fentanyl in spinal anesthesia for cesarean delivery. Reg Anesth Pain Med 2000;25:240–45.

21. NganKee WD, Khaw KS, Tan PE, Ng FF, Karmakar MK. Placental transfer and fetal metabolic effects of phenylephrine and ephedrine during spinal anesthesia for cesarean delivery. Anesthesiology 2009;111(3):506–12.

22. Krisanaprakornkit W. Spinal versus epidural anaesthesia for caesarean section: RHL commentary (last revised: 15 Dec. 2006). The WHO Reproductive Health Library; Geneva: World Health Organization. 2015 Review.

23. Ready LB, Cuplin S, Haschke RH, Nessly M. Spinal needle determinants of rate of transdural fluid leak. Anesth Analg 1989;69(4):457–60.

24. Mihic DN. Postspinal headaches, needle surfaces and longitudinal orientation of the dural fibers. Results of a survey. Reg Anaesth 1986;9(2):54–6.

25. Barrios-Alarcon J1, Aldrete JA, Paragas-Tapia D. Relief of post-lumbar puncture headache with epidural dextran 40: a preliminary report. Reg Anesth 1989;14(2):78–80.

26. Borgeat A, Ekatodramis G, Schenker CA. Postoperative nausea and vomiting in regional anesthesia: a review Anesthesiology 2003;98(2): 530–47.

27. Goll V, Akça O, Greif R, Freitag H, Arkiliç CF, Scheck T, Zoeggeler A, Kurz A, Krieger G, Lenhardt R, Sessler DI. Ondansetron is no more effective than supplemental intraoperative oxygen for prevention of postoperative nausea and vomiting. Anesth Analg 2001;92(1). 112–7.

28. Numazaki M, Fujii Y. Subhypnotic dose of propofol for the prevention of nausea and vomiting during spinal anaesthesia for caesarean section. Anaesth Intensive Care 2000;28(3): 262–5. Retraction in: Gibbs N. Anaesth Intensive Care 2013;41(2):275.

29. Hirmanpour A, Safavi M, Honarmand A, Hosseini AZ, Sepehrian M. The comparative study of intravenous ondansetron and sub-hypnotic propofol dose in control and treatment of intrathecal sufentanil-induced pruritus in elective caesarean surgery. J Res Pharm Pract 2015; 4(2):57–63.

30. Roy S, Levine AB, Herbison GJ, Jacobs SR. Intraoperative positioning during cesarean as a cause of sciatic neuropathy. Obstetrics & Gynecology 2002;99(4):652–3.

31. Rorarius M, Suominen P, Haanp ÄÄ M, Puura A, Baer G, Pajunen P, Tuimala R. Neurologic sequelae after caesarean. Acta Anaesthesiolo Scand 2001;45(1):34–41.

32. Maheshwari D1, Ismail S1. Preoperative anxiety in patients selecting either general or regional anesthesia for elective cesarean section. J Anaesthesiol Clin Pharmacol 2015;31(2):196–200.

33. Norris MC, Dewan DM. Preoxygenation for cesarean section: a comparison of two techniques. Anesthesiology 1985;62(6):827–9.

34. Cugell DW, Frank NR, Gaensler Ea, Badger TL. Pulmonary function in pregnancy I. Serial observations in normal women. Am Rev Tuberc 1953;67(5): 568–97.

35. Kosaka Y, Takahashi T, Mark LC. Intravenous thiobarbiturate anesthesia for cesarean section. Anesthesiology 1969;31(6):489–506.

36. Hodgkinson R, Marx GF, Kim SS, Miclat NM. Neonatal neurobehavioral tests following vaginal delivery under ketamine, thiopental, and extradural anesthesia. Anesth Analg 1977;56(4): 548–53.

37. Bergen JM, Smith DC. A review of etomidate for rapid sequence intubation in the emergency department. J Emerg Med 1997;15(2):221–30 Review.

38. Crozier TA, Flamm C, Speer CP, Rath W, Wuttke W, Kuhn W, Kettler D. Effects of etomidate on the adrenocortical and metabolic adaptation of the neonate. Br J Anaesth 1993;70(1):47–53.

39. Bland BA, Lawes EG, Duncan PW, Warnell I, Downing JW. Comparison of midazolam and thiopental for rapid sequence anesthetic induction for elective cesarean section. Anesth Analg 1987;66(11):1165–8.

40. Crawford JS. Awareness during operative obstetrics under general anaesthesia. Br J Anaesth 1971;43(2):179–82.

41. Boutonnet M, Faitot V, Keïta H. Airway management in obstetrics. Ann Fr Anesth Reanim 2011;30(9):651–64. doi: 10.1016j.annfar. 2011.03. 024. Epub 2011 Jun 25[Article in French].

42. McKeen DM, George RB, O'Connell CM, Allen VM, Yazer M, Wilson M, Phu TC. Difficult and failed intubation: Incident rates and maternal, obstetrical and anesthetic predictors. Can J Anaesth 2011;58(6):514–24.

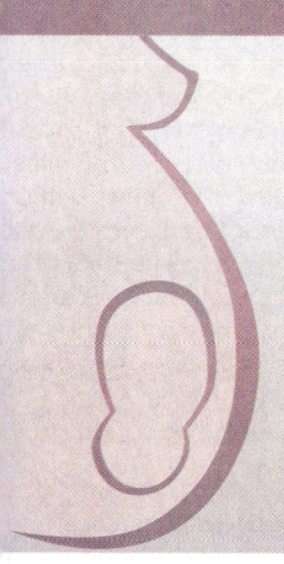

Maternal Obstetric Hemorrhage

Indrani Hemantkumar

INTRODUCTION

Maternal hemorrhage remains one of the major causes of both maternal mortality and morbidity all over the world.[1] Postpartum hemorrhage accounts for majority of these deaths. Deaths due to hemorrhage have dropped to sixth place following genital sepsis, pre-eclampsia, thromboembolism, amniotic fluid embolism and early pregnancy deaths. This may be because of the awareness and anticipation of the obstetrician and the well-defined multidisciplinary approach that aims to act quickly and effectively. Morbidity following a maternal hemorrhage can be equally dangerous, e.g. adult respiratory distress syndrome, coagulopathy, shock, loss of fertility, and pituitary necrosis (Sheehan syndrome). The blood loss assessment may be extremely difficult and challenging. Blood loss can take place over hours or days; may be concealed internally (e.g. placental abruption), or be hidden under drapes or on the floor. Blood collected via suction, the weighing of surgical swabs, and careful search for concealed blood loss on the floor or under the operating drapes must be included in the estimation of blood loss, especially in suspected major hemorrhage.[2-5]

DEFINITION

Obstetric hemorrhage is defined as blood loss from uterus or genital tract of >1500 mL or a decrease in hemoglobin of >4 gm/dL or acute loss requiring PRBC transfusion of more than 4 units.

Antepartum hemorrhage (APH) is one that occurs after 24th week of gestation and before delivery, e.g. placenta previa, placental abruption, bleeding from vaginal/cervical lesions or uterine rupture. The incidence of uterine rupture increases with previous cesarean section especially with a short time interval since the last cesarean section and with the induction of labor. Patients present with decreased uterine activity, abdominal pain continuing between contractions and vaginal bleeding. The uterine rupture may disrupt the placental circulation. Therefore, the first clinical sign may be deterioration in the cardiotocographic trace (CTG). Catastrophic uterine rupture is life-threatening to both mother and fetus and can cause severe hemorrhage with the need for hysterectomy.

Postpartum hemorrhage (PPH) is bleeding that occurs after delivery and can be either primary or secondary PPH.

- *Primary PPH* is bleeding that occurs within 24 hours of delivery, which is 500 mL following vaginal delivery and >1000 mL following a cesarean section. [6]
- *Secondary PPH* occurs from 24 hours to 6 weeks following delivery;[7,8] e.g. uterine atony, retained products of conception, genital tract trauma, uterine inversion, puerperal sepsis, etc.

PPH can be **minor** (500–1000 mL), **moderate** (1000–2000 mL) or **severe** (>2000 mL). [1]

CAUSES[7,8]

- Tone (uterine atony)
- Tissue (retained products)
- Trauma (vaginal and cervical trauma)
- Thrombosis (coagulation derangement)
- Others: Prolonged labor, multiple pregnancy, polyhydramnios, large baby, previous atony, etc.)

Tone[9-11]

Uterine atony and failure of contraction and retraction of myometrial muscle fibers can lead to rapid and severe hemorrhage and hypovolemic shock. Overdistension of the uterus is a major risk factor for atony. It can be due to multiple gestation, fetal macrosomia, polyhydramnios, or fetal abnormality (e.g. severe hydrocephalus); a uterine structural abnormality; or a failure to deliver the placenta or distension with blood before or after placental delivery. Poor myometrial contraction can result from fatigue due to prolonged labor or rapid forceful labor, especially if stimulated. It can also result from the inhibition of contractions by drugs such as halogenated anesthetic agents, nitrates, nonsteroidal anti-inflammatory drugs, magnesium sulfate, beta-sympathomimetics, and nifedipine. Other causes include placental implantation site in the lower uterine segment, bacterial toxins (e.g. chorioamnionitis, endomyometritis, septicemia), hypoxia due to hypoperfusion or Couvelaire uterus in abruptio placentae, and hypothermia due to massive resuscitation or prolonged uterine exteriorization. Recent data suggest that grand multiparity is not an independent risk factor for PPH.

Tissue

Complete detachment and expulsion of the placenta following uterine contraction and retraction permits continued retraction and optimal occlusion of blood vessels. Retention of a portion of the placenta is more common, if the placenta has developed with a succenturiate or accessory lobe.

The placenta is more likely to be retained at extreme preterm gestations (especially <24 weeks), and significant bleeding can occur. Failure of complete separation of the placenta due to invasion and adherence occurs in placenta accreta and its other variants. Significant bleeding from the area where normal attachment (and now detachment) has occurred may mark partial accreta. Complete accreta in which the entire surface of the placenta is abnormally attached, or more severe invasion (placenta increta or percreta), may not initially cause severe bleeding, but it may develop as more aggressive efforts are made to remove the placenta. This condition should be considered possible whenever the placenta is implanted over a previous uterine scar, especially if associated with placenta previa. Hence all such patients should be explained the risk of PPH and the need for blood transfusion or even hysterectomy. All patients with placenta previa should be informed and explained in their antenatal visit about the risk of severe PPH, including the possible need for transfusion and hysterectomy.

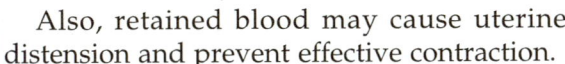

Also, retained blood may cause uterine distension and prevent effective contraction.

Ectopic pregnancy can cause torrential bleeding, if ruptured.

Trauma

Trauma to the genital tract can occur spontaneously or through manipulations to deliver the baby. Cesarean delivery results in twice the average blood loss of vaginal delivery. Incisions in the poorly contractile lower segment heal well but are more dependent on suturing, vasospasm, and clotting for hemostasis.

Uterine rupture is most common in patients with previous cesarean delivery scars. Any uterotomy or partial disruption as in fibroidectomy; uteroplasty for congenital abnormality; cornual or cervical ectopic resections and perforation of the uterus during dilatation, curettage, biopsy, hysteroscopy, laparoscopy, or intrauterine contraceptive device placement are considered at risk for rupture in a future pregnancy. Trauma is known to occur following very prolonged or vigorous labor seen as in absolute cephalopelvic disproportion and the uterus has been stimulated with oxytocin or prostaglandins. Using intrauterine pressure monitoring may lessen this risk. Trauma also may occur following extrauterine or intra-uterine manipulation of the fetus as in internal version and extraction of a second twin; however, uterine rupture may also occur secondary to external version. Finally, trauma may result secondary to attempt to remove a retained placenta manually or with instru-mentation. The uterus should always be controlled with a hand on the abdomen during any such procedure. An intraumbilical vein saline/oxytocin or saline/misoprostol injec-tion may reduce the need for more invasive removal techniques.

Cervical laceration is most commonly associated with forceps delivery, and the cervix should be inspected following all such deliveries. Vaginal side wall laceration is also most commonly associated with operative vaginal delivery, but it may occur sponta-neously, especially if a fetal hand presents with the head. Lacerations may occur during manipulations to resolve shoulder dystocia. The frequency of sidewall and cervical lacerations has decreased because of the reduction in the use of mid-pelvic forceps/mid-pelvic rotational procedures. Lower vaginal trauma occurs either spontaneously or because of episiotomy.

Thrombosis

In the immediate postpartum period, bleeding is well controlled due to the efficient contraction and retraction of the uterus. Fibrin deposition and formation of clots over the placental site and supplying vessels inhibit further bleeding in the hours and days following delivery, and abnormalities in these areas can lead to late PPH or exacerbate bleeding from other causes, especially, trauma. Thrombocytopenia can be primary as in as idiopathic thrombocytopenic purpura, or acquired secondary to HELLP syndrome (hemolysis, elevated liver enzymes, and low platelet count), abruptio placentae, dissemi-nated intravascular coagulation (DIC), or sepsis. Undiagnosed functional abnormalities of platelets can also occur.

There could be derangement in the clotting profile as in familial hypofibrinogenemia and von Willebrand disease. A proper history of bleeding in the past as in menorrhagia since menarche, family history of bleeding dis-orders, personal history of notable bruising without known injury, bleeding from the oral cavity or GI tract without obvious lesion, or epistaxis of longer than 10 minutes duration (possibly requiring packing or cautery) should be elicited to rule out a bleeding disorder. Acquired disorders are more dangerous and difficult to treat as in abruptio placentae, HELLP syndrome, intrauterine fetal demise, amniotic fluid embolism, sepsis, etc. Fibronogen levels which should be elevated in normal pregnancy are seen to drop in these conditions. Dilutional coagulopathy due to massive blood/crystalloid/colloid transfusion can occur.

PREVENTION[12–16]

The value of active management in the prevention of PPH cannot be overstated. They are: (1) uterotonic administration (preferably oxytocin) immediately upon delivery of the baby, (2) early cord clamping and cutting, and (3) gentle cord traction with uterine countertraction when the uterus is well contracted (i.e. Brandt-Andrews maneuver).

In addition, avoidance of prolonged labor, minimal trauma during assisted delivery, detection and treatment of anemia during pregnancy, identification of placenta previa in the antenatal period, and MRI for detection of accrete/percreta will help in prevention of massive bleeding.

Following delivery, administering a uterotonic drug that lasts at least 2–3 hours is acceptable. For example, 10 U of oxytocin in 500 mL of intravenous fluid by continuous drip, 200–250 mg of ergonovine intramuscularly, or 250 mg of 15-methyl prostaglandin F2α (carboprost) intramuscularly. The use of misoprostol and a long-acting oxytocin analogue (carbetocin) is being studied.

PATHOPHYSIOLOGY

Maternal blood volume (plasma volume more than total RBC volume) from 4 L to 6 L, leading to a fall in the hemoglobin concentration and hematocrit value. The increase in blood volume serves to fulfill the perfusion demands of the low-resistance uteroplacental unit and to provide a reserve for the blood loss that occurs at delivery.

At term, the estimated blood flow to the uterus is 500–800 mL/min, which constitutes 10–15% of cardiac output. Most of this flow traverses the low-resistance placental bed and also supplies the weave of myometrial fibers. During delivery, myometrial contraction and retraction occurs. Retraction is the unique characteristic of the uterine muscle to maintain its shortened length following each successive contraction. The blood vessels are compressed and kinked by this crisscross lattice work, and, normally, blood flow is quickly occluded forming 'living ligatures' or 'physiologic sutures' of the uterus.

Uterine atony, which is the most important cause of PPH, is a failure of the uterine myometrial fibers to contract and retract. Trauma to the genital tract at the time of delivery or otherwise (i.e. uterus, uterine cervix, vagina, labia, clitoris) results in significantly more bleeding than would occur in the non-pregnant state because of increased blood supply to these tissues.

PRESENTATION

The presentation of PPH can be dramatic or the bleeding may be slower and misleading and ultimately result in critical loss and shock. The common presentation of PPH is one of heavy vaginal bleeding quickly leading to signs and symptoms of hypovolemic shock. If the placenta remains in situ, then a significant unknown amount of blood can be retained in the uterus behind a partially separated placenta, the membranes, or both. An atonic uterus can collect blood. Hence, close observation and documentation of maternal vital signs and condition, vaginal blood loss, and uterine tone and size should be done frequently following delivery. The uterus should be periodically massaged to express any clots that have accumulated in the uterus or vagina. Bleeding from trauma may be concealed in the form of hematomas of the retroperitoneum, broad ligament or lower genital tract, or abdominal cavity.

The **clinical findings** in hypovolemia are given in Table 12.1.[17]

Table 12.1: Clinical findings in hypovolemia

Blood volume loss	Systolic blood pressure	Symptom and signs	Degree of shock
500–1000 mL (10–15%)	Normal	Palpitations, tachycardia, dizziness	Compensated
1000–1500 mL (15–25%)	Slight fall (80–100 mm Hg)	Weakness, tachycardia, sweating	Mild
1500–2000 mL (25–35%)	Moderate fall (70–80 mm Hg)	Restlessness, pallor, oliguria	Moderate
2000–3000 mL (35–50%)	Marked fall (50–70 mm Hg)	Collapse, air hunger, anuria	Severe

Rapid recognition and diagnosis of PPH is essential to successful management. The amount of lost blood volume by visualizing clots as well as the masking of the hemodynamics with the birthing position (semi-recumbent and leg elevated) may delay recognition and treatment of PPH. The major factor in the adverse outcomes associated with severe hemorrhage is a delay in initiating appropriate management.

Management of Anticipated Maternal Hemorrhage[10,19]

- Two large bore IV cannulas
- Rapid infusion devices or pressure bags
- Blood warmers and warming blanket
- Blood crossmatched and available
- Consider preoperative invasive monitoring
- Cell savage, if available
- Interventional radiology standby

Management of Unanticipated Maternal Hemorrhage[20]

- Allocate roles to team members and practice fire drills, if department guidelines exist.
- ABC, high flow oxygen.
- Left lateral position, if antepartum, and head down, if postpartum.
- IV access: Two large bore cannulas. Start infusion of warmed crystalloids until crossmatched blood available.

- O negative blood should be available in the labor unit or should be quickly available from blood bank, if required.
- Send blood for grouping and crossmatching (at least 6 units), FFP (4–6 units).
- Send for Hb, coagulation profile, urea, electrolytes and ABG, even if patient is moderately symptomatic. Point of care test (POCT), e.g. TEG and thromboelastometry give quick results.
- Call for help and establish a multidisciplinary approach to patient management (obstetrician, anesthesiologist, blood bank, radiologist alert, intensivist alert, lab technicians for tests, porters to bring blood, etc.
- Aim to replace losses with blood and products ASAP and warming all fluids. Ratio of blood to FFP is 1:1 with early replacement of platelets, if <50,000/cu.mm, cryoprecipitate, if fibrinogen <1 g/dL.
- O negative blood should be given in the presence of worsening cardiovascular instability.
- Tranexamic acid—1 g over 10 min and SOS 1 g more over 1hour (CRASH 2 and WOMAN trial).
- If further blood loss, surgical/interventional radiology considered which is tailored to individual patients.
- If blood loss has stopped, continue crystalloid and blood products until normovolemia.
- Monitor Hb with POCT (Hemacue or ABG).

- Transfer to intensive care area for monitoring.

   Treatment goals used by the UK military provide useful guidelines for patients with MOH:
- Hct >0.3.
- Plt >100 × 10^9 litre—1.
- Fibrinogen >2 g litre—1.
- Ionized Ca >1.
- Temp. >36°C.

Non-Surgical Intervention for Uterine Atony[21,22]

- Bimanual compression of uterus (rubbing of fundus to stimulate contractions)
- Ensure bladder is empty (Foley catheter)
- Syntocinon 5 units by slow IV injection. SOS repeat the dose.
- Ergometrine 0.5 mg by slow IV/IM injection (contraindicated in heart disease and hypertension)
- Syntocinon infusion (40 units over 4 hours)
- Carboprost 0.25 mg by IM injection and repeated at intervals not less than 15 min to a maximum of 8 doses (contraindicated in women with asthma—causes bronchospasm, flushing and hypertension)
- Direct intramyometrial injection of carboprast 0.5 mg (hemabate or prostaglandin F2α). Can be repeated up to 5 doses. However, it is not licensed for intrauterine injection.
- Misoprostol 1000 mg rectally.

   Patients should be quickly transferred to the operation theatre sooner rather than later, if above measures fail.

SURGICAL TREATMENT AND OTHER INTERVENTIONS

The most common cause is atony. However, other reasons should be excluded.

Trauma of the genital tract: The entire genital tract (perineum, vagina and cervix) is assessed either in the labor ward or in the operation room for bleeding sources and pressure should be applied to bleeding areas and repair attempted. If the patient is shocked and the amount of vaginal bleeding is normal, intra-abdominal sources such as ruptured uterus, broad ligament hematoma, uterine inversion, subcapsular liver rupture, ruptured spleen, and ruptured aneurysm should be considered.

   Tissue (retained products of conception)—usually due to retained placenta, cotyledon or membranes: The placenta is assessed for missing tissues. If placenta is adherent, oxytocic dose is repeated, bladder is emptied and patient transferred to theatre for manual removal of placenta.

Thrombin (abnormalities of coagulation): Rarely the primary cause of PPH and usually the consequence of massive hemorrhage and treated with blood and blood products as mentioned above.

Intrauterine balloon tamponade:[23] It is first tried for atonic uterus. Depending on the clinical circumstances, if above fails, following conservative surgical interventions should be attempted.

Other Surgical Interventions[24–26]

- Hemostatic brace suturing (B-Lynch or modified compression sutures)
- Bilateral ligation of uterine arteries
- Bilateral ligation of internal iliac arteries
- Selective arterial embolization or balloon occlusion radiologically
- Compression/clamping aorta to buy time
- Uterine replacement, if uterine inversion
- Hysterectomy (discussed with patient especially in placenta percreta) sooner than later.

Intervention Radiological Techniques

Intervention radiological techniques are especially useful in anticipated bleedings as in placenta accreta because balloon may be placed in the internal iliac artery before the C-section. Should a bleed occur, the balloons

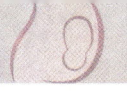

may be inflated. Selective internal iliac artery or uterine artery embolization can be performed. Complications of this procedure include hematoma, false aneurysms and lower limb ischemia.

Intraoperative Cell Salvage[27]

Intraoperative cell salvage is a process in which shed blood is collected, filtered and washed to produce autologous red cells for transfusion to the patient. However, there are concerns reinfusion of fetal cells which can cause hemolytic disease in future pregnancies and a potential to cause amniotic fluid embolus. Separate suction should be utilized for amniotic fluid. A leukocyte depletion filter should be used during retransfusion.

Use of Recombinant Factor VII (rVIIa)[28]

Even though the effectiveness of recombinant factor VIIa is not proven in PPH, it can be used in a life-threatening situation as an adjuvant to standard pharmacological and surgical treatment after consulting a hematologist. A dose of 90 mcg/kg repeated, if needed within 30 min should be given. Recombinant factor VIIa is not effective in the presence of hypofibrinogenemia and low platelets. In such a scenario, cryoprecipitate and platelets should be administered ahead of recombinant factor VIIa.

ANESTHETIC CONSIDERATIONS IN THE PRESENCE OF PPH[29,30]

- GA with rapid sequence intubation is advocated, if patient is actively bleeding or if there is coagulopathy.
- Spinal/epidural anesthesia contraindicated but if there is an existing epidural, one can use it if bleeding is controlled.
- Induction agent dosages should be reduced/titrated to the response of the patient. Inj. ketamine/etomidate with midazolam useful

in the presence of hypotension and should be used after volume resuscitation.

- In the presence of ongoing bleeding, maternal early warning system (MEWS), blood bank and hematologist should be alerted.
- Trendelenburg position is given.
- Monitoring is stepped up by taking an arterial line, CVP line and urinary catheter.
- Baseline investigations: Hb, PCV, ABG, coagulation profile, S. creatinine and S. electrolytes are sent.
- If coagulation monitors, like Hemacue or thromboelastography, are available, Hb and coagulation should be monitored in regular intervals.
- Call for help. Crystalloids/colloids and blood/blood products given through warming and rapid infuser system or pressure bags. PRBC, FFP, cryoprecipitate and platelets in accordance to Hb and coagulation results administered in the ration 4:2:1 (Blood:FFP:Platelets).
- 100% oxygen given.
- Calcium citrate injections administered in presence of massive transfusion and documented hypocalcemia.
- Fluid warmers and convection warmers should be used to maintain normothermia.
- Use of hemostatic agents, like aprotonin, tranexamic acid, etc., can be considered.
- Recombinant factor VIIa is used in life-threatening situations, if fibrinogen and platelets are at least near normal.
- Various surgical/radiological possibilities to arrest bleeding should be discussed with the surgical colleagues.
- Patients shifted to ICU for continuous monitoring as after the bleeding has stopped, they can develop thrombosis after 1 or 2 days. Hence thromboprophylaxis considered in these patients. In presence of thrombocytopenia, pneumatic compression is given to avoid thrombosis.

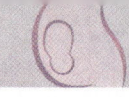

Pearls

- Maternal obstetric hemorrhage can be unanticipated and every obstetric unit should have systems in place to tackle it.
- Assessment of blood loss can be notoriously difficult as the blood loss can be concealed.
- Most common cause of PPH is tone (uterine atony), tissue (retained products), trauma (vaginal and cervical trauma), thrombosis (coagulation derangement), others: Prolonged labor, multiple pregnancy, polyhydramnios, large baby, previous atony, etc.).
- Uterotonic agents should be the first-line treatment for postpartum hemorrhage due to uterine atony.
- Anticipated hemorrhages should be managed by being prepared with 2 large bore IV cannulas, rapid infusion devices or pressure bags, blood warmers and warming blanket, blood crossmatched and available, preoperative invasive monitoring, cell savage if available and interventional radiology standby.
- Unanticipated torrential hemorrhages should be alerted to the seniors in the department. Patient should be initially resuscitated immediately. However, if there is hemodynamic instability, O negative blood should be infused before the group specific blood arrives to maintain tissue oxygenation.
- PRBC:FFP:Platelet transfusion ratio is 4:2:1.
- Normothermia maintained.
- Coagulation profile, hemoglobin, ABG, and S. electrolyte should be performed at various intervals.
- General anesthesia is the choice in the presence of active bleeding and coagulopathy.
- Postoperative care is essential in these patients as they are prone to thrombosis, ARDS, etc.

SUMMARY

Major obstetric hemorrhage management is managed by multidisciplinary approach. Each hospital should have their protocol in place and regular 'bleeding drill' should be conducted. Early timely resuscitation is very important and help should be sought to control the bleeding with uterotonics initially and later with blood/blood products. If the bleeding was anticipated, appropriate planning and precautionary steps should be taken.

Severe bleeding is the single most significant cause of maternal death worldwide. Sequelae following maternal hemorrhage include adult respiratory distress syndrome, coagulopathy, shock, loss of fertility, and pituitary necrosis (Sheehan syndrome). Although many risk factors have been identified, it often occurs without any warning. Also, the bleeding may be concealed making it difficult to assess the gravity of the bleeding until the patient suddenly slips into shock. All tertiary units should have proper facilities, personnel and equipment to manage this life-threatening emergency properly. Management may vary between patients, depending on etiology and available treatment options, and a multidisciplinary approach is required.

REFERENCES

1. Rajashree Chavan, Latoo MY. Recent advances in the treatment of major obstetric haemorrhage. BJMP 2013;6(1):a604.
2. Dildy GA, Paine AR, George NC, Velasco C. Estimating blood loss: can teaching significantly improve visual estimation? Obstet Gynecol 2004; 104:601–6.
3. Stafford I, Dildy GA, Clark SL, Belfort MA. Visually estimated and calculated blood loss in vaginal and cesarean delivery. Am J Obstet Gynecol 2008;199:e511–7.
4. Glover P. Blood losses at delivery: how accurate is your estimation? Aust J Midwifery 2003;1 6:21–4.
5. Toledo P, McCarthy RJ, Hewlett BJ, Fitzgerald PC, Wong CA. The accuracy of blood estimation after simulated vaginal delivery. Anesth Amalga 2007;105: 1736–40.
6. Mousa HA, Alfirevic Z. Treatment for primary postpartum haemorrhage. Cochrane database Syst Rev 2007;(1): CD003249. DOI:10.1002/14651858. CD003249.pub2.

7. Alexandra J, Thomas PW, Sanghera J. Treatments for secondary haemorrhage. Cochrane database Syst Rev 2002;(1): CD002867. DOI:10.1002/14651858. CD002867.

8. Cunningham FG, Leveno KJ, Bloom SL, Hauth JC, Gilstrap L 3rd, Wenstrom KD. Obstetric hemorrhage. In: Williams Obstetrics, 22nd ed. New York: McGraw-Hill; 2005, p. 809–54.

9. Lutomski J, Byrne B, Devane D, Greene R. Increasing trends in atonic postpartum haemorrhage in Ireland: a 11 year population-based cohort study. BJOG 2012;119(3):306–14.

10. John R Smith. Postpartum Hemorrhage In: Ronald M Ramus (Chief Ed) et al. emedicine.medscape.com/article/275038; September 23, 2014.

11. Sheiner E, Sarid L, Levy A, Seidman DS, Hallak M. Obstetric risk factors and outcome of pregnancies complicated with early postpartum hemorrhage: a population-based study. J Matern Fetal Neonatal Med 2005;18(3):149–54.

12. Khan GQ, John IS, Wani S, Doherty T, Sibai BM. Controlled cord traction versus minimal intervention techniques in delivery of the placenta: a randomised controlled trial. Am J Obstet Gynecol 1997;177(4):770–4.

13. McDonald S, Abbott JM, Higgins SP. Prophylactic ergometrine-oxytocin versus oxytocin for the third stage of labour. Cochrane Database Syst Rev 2004;(1):CD000201.

14. Elbourne DR, Prendiville WJ, Carroli G, Wood J, McDonald S. Prophylactic use of oxytocin in the third stage of labour. Cochrane Database Syst Rev 2001;CD001808.

15. Dansereau J, Joshi AK, Helewa ME, et al. Double-blind comparison of carbetocin versus oxytocin in prevention of uterine atony after cesarean section. Am J Obstet Gynecol 1999;180(3 Pt 1): 670–6.

16. Oladapo OT, Fawole B, Blum J, Abalos E. Advance distribution of misoprostol for preventing and treating excessive blood loss after birth. Cochrane Database of Systematic Reviews, Feb. 15, 2012.

17. American College of Obstetricians and Gynecologists. ACOG educational bulletin. Hemorrhagic shock. Number 235, April 1997 (replaces no. 82, December 1984). American College of Obstetricians and Gynecologists. Int J Gynaecol Obstet 1997;57(2):219–26.

18. Prevention and management of postpartum haemorrhage, RCOG Green-top Guideline No. 52, March 2011.

19. De Groot AN. Prevention of postpartum haemorrhage. Baillieres Clin Obstet Gynaecol 1995;9:619–31.

20. Stainsby D, MacLennan S, Hamilton PJ. Management of massive blood loss: a template guideline. Br J Anaesth 2000;85(3):487–91.

21. Boucher M, Horbay GL, Griffin P, Deschamps Y, Desjardins C, Schutz M, et al. Double blind, randomized comparison of the effect of carbetocin and oxytocin on intraoperative blood loss and uterine tone of patients undergoing caesarean sections. J Perinatol 1998;18: 202–7.

22. Gulmezoglu AM, Forna F, Villar J, Hofmeyr GJ. Prostaglandins for prevention of postpartum haemorrhage. Cochrane Database Syst Rev 2007;(3):CD000494.

23. Johanson R, Kumar M, Obhrai M, Young P. Management of massive postpartum haemorrhage: use of a hydrostatic balloon catheter to avoid laparotomy BJOG 2001;108(4):420–2.

24. Lingam K, Hood V, Carty MJ. Angiographic embolisation in the management of pelvic haemorrhage. BJOG 2000;107(9):1176–8.

25. Stanco LM, Schrimmer DB, Paul RH, Mishell DR Jr. Emergency peripartum hysterectomy and associated risk factors. Am J Obstet Gynecol 1993;168(3 Pt 1):879–83.

26. O'Leary JA. Uterine artery ligation in the control of postcesarean hemorrhage. J Reprod Med 1995; 40(3):189–93.

27. Catling SJ, Williams S, Fielding AM. Cell salvage in obstetrics: an evalution of the ability of cell salvage combined with leucocyte depletion filtration to remove amniotic fluid from operative blood loss at caesarean section. Int J Obstet Anesth 1999;8:79–84.

28. Birchall J, Stanworth S, Duffy M, Doree C, Hyde C. Evidence for the use of recombinant factor VIIa in the prevention and treatment of bleeding in patients without haemophilia. Transfus Med Rev 2008;22:177–87.

29. Levy D. Obstetric Haemorrhage In: Johnson I. Harrop-Griffiths W, Gemmell L, eds. AAGBI core topics in anaesthesia. Chichester:Wiley-Blackwell Ltd, 2012; 105–23.

30. Parekh N, Hussaini SWU, Russell IF. Caesarean section for placenta praevia: a retrospective study of aneesthetic management. Br J Anaesth 2000;84: 725–30.

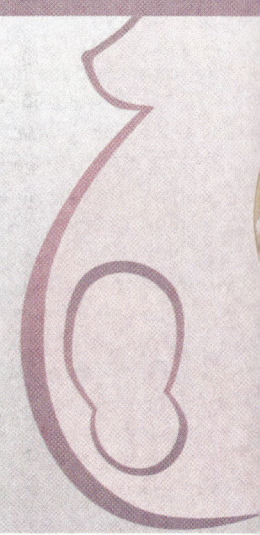

CHAPTER 13

Cardiovascular Disease and Pregnancy

Sona Dave, Minal Harde

Pregnancy imposes unique physiological strains on the cardiovascular system which are magnified in presence of heart diseases. Maintaining maternal cardiovascular stability with adequate placental perfusion can be challenging. Many mothers are asymptomatic and the physiological changes of pregnancy may precipitate decompensation. The risk and the preferred anesthetic techniques differ amongst the various cardiac conditions. Goal of anesthetic management is to maintain hemodynamic parameters within a narrow therapeutic range. The risk in mother and fetus doubles increasing the peripartum morbidity and mortality. Thus multidisciplinary planning should be at the helm of peripartum management.[1]

Cardiac disease in pregnancy accounts for 0.1–4% in the developed nations of which 70–80% are patients with congenital heart disease who survive to adulthood because of better surgical techniques and newer and better drugs. As women present at a much advanced age in recent times ischemic heart disease also may complicate pregnancies.[1] There is usually deterioration by 1 grade (NYHA class) during pregnancy in patients with pre-existing cardiac disease (Table 13.1).[1]

While assessing a pregnant patient certain warning signs may point to a cardiac pathology in an otherwise unsuspected case.

- A rising pulse rate may be a harbinger of cardiac decompensation. The radial pulse is difficult to detect when the heart rate is fast or irregular. Hence, auscultating the heart with a stethoscope is more prudent and accurate.
- The blood pressure (BP) should be recorded with the woman sitting comfortably with a manual sphygmomanometer with an appropriate-sized cuff. The arm should be at an angle and supported to ensure that the cuff is at the level of the left atrium.

Table 13.1: New York Heart Association (NYHA)— functional classification	
NYHA Class	Symptoms
I	No symptoms and no limitations on ordinary physical activity
II	Ordinary activity may cause mild symptoms and slight limitation
III	Marked limitation in activity. Less than ordinary activity will cause symptoms
IV	Severe limitations and symptoms at rest

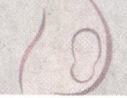

- Crackles may sometimes develop in late pregnancy due to the splinting effect of the enlarged uterus resulting in poor lung expansion. These crackles disappear on asking the woman to take several deep breaths and then cough several times. Crackles posteriorly in the lung bases may be pathognomonic of incipient cardiac failure.[1]

The risk and the preferred anaesthetic techniques differ amongst the various cardiac conditions which are enumerated in Table 13.2.

The FDA classifies drug risk during pregnancy based on available data (Table 13.3).

The various cardiac conditions complicating pregnancy and their management are discussed below.

CONGENITAL HEART DISEASE

Grown up with congenital heart disease (GUCH) is now becoming the most common cardiac disease in pregnant patients as due to improved medical and surgical management as many congenital heart disease (CHD) patients reach childbearing age.[2] Maternal and fetal mortality varies depending upon the lesion associated. If complete repair and normal cardiovascular function is achieved by

Table 13.2: The choice of anesthesia for cesarean section complicated by cardiac diseases

Risk	Likely complication/ treatment	Preferred anesthetic technique
Arrhythmias	May require DC cardioversion	General anesthesia
Cyanotic CHD, aortic stenosis	Any fall in SVR will be fatal	General anesthesia
Impaired cardiac contractility	Negative inotropic of general anesthetics	Guarded neuraxial
Tracheal intubation, coughing	Acute TTT crisis	Neuraxial
Cardiac mechanical valve	Anticoagulations are required due to risk of thromboembolism	General anesthesia
Cardiac procedure to be performed postpartum	Elective postoperative ventilation on invasion	General anesthesia

Table 13.3: Effect of various cardiac drugs on pregnancy

Drug	Class	Indication	Risk
Amiodarone	D	Atrial fibrillation	Transient fetal hypo-/hyperthyroidism
Propranolol	C	Tachydysrhythmias	IUGR. Hypoglycemia/bradycardia in newborns
Labetalol	C	Hypertension	May be associated with IUGR
Esmolol	C	Hypertension/tachydysrhythmias	If given during a period of uteroplacental insufficiency may cause fetal distress
Nicardipine/ nifedipine	C	Stable angina/hypertension	May decrease uteroplacental blood flow
Verapamil	C	Atrial tachycardia	Prolong PR interval in fetus
Hydralazine	C	Hypertension	Maternal hypotension and tachycardia, higher incidence of stillbirths
Nitroglycerine	C	Angina/hypertension	Maternal hypotension tachycardia
Adenosine	C	Supraventricular tachycardia	

successful surgery during childhood, then patients often require no special management except antibiotic prophylaxis as per the current recommendations. Some patients present during pregnancy with uncorrected lesion or partially corrected lesion, which may decompensate during the course of pregnancy and labor and their management is a challenge.[2–4]

Major categories of CHD are:
- Left-to-right shunts which include atrial septal defect (ASD), patent ductus arteriosus (PDA), ventricular septal defect (VSD).
- Right-to-left shunts include tetralogy of Fallot (TOF), Eisenmenger's syndrome.
- Congenital valvular and vascular lesions—aortic stenosis, pulmonary stenosis and coarctation of aorta.

In these entire lesions, the anesthetic goal should include antibiotic prophylaxis, avoid factors which can cause reversal of shunts such as hypoxia and hypercarbia.

Left-to-Right Shunts

Either small ASD, VSD or PDA with modest left-to-right shunt without pulmonary hypertension is often well tolerated during pregnancy. However, mortality is high with coexisting pulmonary hypertension. Physiological changes during pregnancy may increase left-to-right shunt and worsen the degree of pulmonary hypertension. There may be increased risk of pre-eclampsia and small

for gestational age babies in case of unrepaired lesions.[2–4]

There is increased incidence of supraventricular arrhythmias (atrial fibrillation and flutter) due to:
- Chamber enlargement
- Pulmonary hypertension (PH)

Paradoxical embolus is common during pregnancy as:
- Respiratory efforts may increase due to physiological changes in pregnancy
- Straining during parturition

Complications associated with ASD
- Incidence of supraventricular arrhythmia is high
- Increased incidence of thromboembolism
- Increased incidence of paradoxical embolus

Neonatal complications
- Heart disease in offspring
- Preterm delivery
- Small for gestation age

Anesthesia Management

The major goal in peripartum management is maintenance of systemic vascular resistance (SVR) and pulmonary vascular resistance (PVR) ratio as alteration in them may lead to ventricular failure, shunt reversal and hypoxia.[5] Continuous monitoring (standard monitoring plus transesophageal echocardiography [TEE], if available) and supplemental oxygen therapy is essential.[6] Accidental intravenous infusion of air bubbles should be avoided.

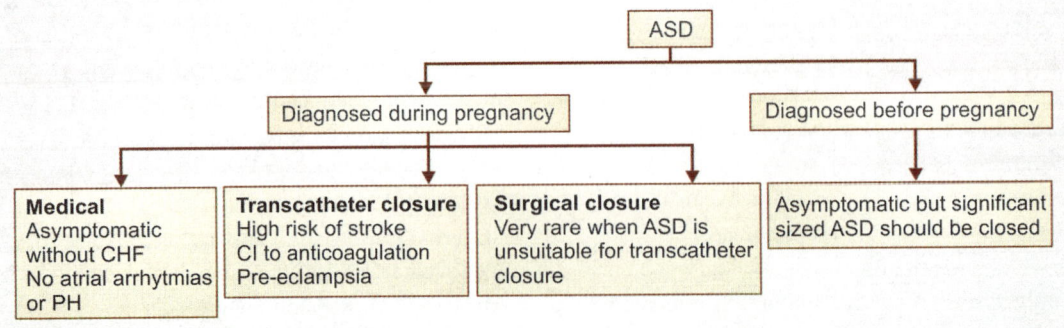

Fig. 13.1. Management of ASD in a woman of childbearing age

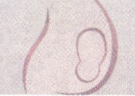

Early lumbar epidural analgesia for labor and vaginal delivery is desirable to avoid pain and resulting increase in SVR.[5] For cesarean section, slow-graded segmental epidural anesthesia is preferred. During epidural space localization, loss of resistance to saline is preferable than air as identification of the epidural space with air might result in systemic air embolization especially in pregnancy due to high epidural venous pressure and engorged veins. General anesthesia is also well tolerated and combined opioid and inhalation technique is preferred.[5–7] Oxytocin is used to induce uterine contractions and reduce bleeding following delivery of the baby. This should be given as slow intravenous infusion and not as a bolus.

Presence of isolated ventricular septal defects (VSD) possesses a low risk during pregnancy. However, when complicated by pulmonary hypertension and/or Eisenmengerization, there is a high risk of cardiac complications. If the VSD has been repaired prior to the development of pulmonary hypertension, risk is minimal.

General precautions during transcatheter closure of ASD during pregnancy
- Should be performed during second trimester
- Long venous sheath to reduce radiation dose to pelvic area
- Intracardiac echocardiography for balloon sizing and deployment of device reduces radiation dose

Pearls
- Avoid accidental injection of air
- Treat arrhythmia promptly
- Infective endocarditis prophylaxis

Right-to-Left Shunts

Eisenmenger's syndrome: Uncorrected left-to-right shunt (ASD, VSD or PDA) may result in right ventricular hypertrophy, elevated pulmonary artery pressure and eventually right ventricular dysfunction. The conglo-meration of these signs and symptoms are known as Eisenmenger's syndrome. After irreversible pulmonary hypertension occurs, correction of primary lesion does not help. Patients with Eisenmenger's syndrome who become pregnant should be consulted to terminate pregnancy as there are chances of sudden profound hypoxemia and death. Maternal mortality is as high as 30–50% in these patients.[2,7]

Management includes early hospitalization, continuous oxygen administration, pulmonary vasodilators and prophylactic anticoagulation. Patient may, however, not respond to above treatment and pregnancy may be fatal.[21]

Anesthetic Management

Supplemental oxygen must be provided to combat the hypoxia and prevent further increase in PA pressures. Continuous monitoring including central venous and intra-arterial catheter facilitates rapid detection of sudden changes in hemodynamics and cardiac filling pressures. However, a pulmonary artery catheter is relatively contraindicated as it is difficult to position and carries the risk of pulmonary artery rupture. Transesophageal echocardiography (TEE) is preferred.

For labor analgesia, as anticoagulation may contraindicate regional techniques, intravenous remifentanil infusion or patient-controlled analgesia (PCA) may be the modalities of choice.[8,9] If not contraindicated epidural or intrathecal opioid or cautious segmental epidural analgesia provided the SVR is maintained, can be considered.[8] For emergency cesarean section, general anesthesia is the anesthesia of choice. However, few authors mention use of slow onset epidural anesthesia for elective cesarean.[9] It is essential to maintain preload, SVR and oxygen saturation. To maintain adequate venous return, avoid aortocaval compression and judicious intravenous crystalloids and small doses of phenylephrine are considered.

Regardless of the anesthetic technique, many life-threatening complications may occur in the postpartum period mainly hypoxemia, cardiac dysrhythmias, and thromboembolic events. Hence continued use of invasive monitoring, oxygen, inhaled nitric oxide and extreme vigilance is recommended in the peripartum period.[7,9]

Pearls

- Maintain in SVR: PVR ratio
- Prevent hypoxia, hypercapnia, acidosis

Tetralogy of Fallot (TOF)

It is the most common right-to-left shunt lesion in women of childbearing age. Four components of TOF include VSD, overriding of aorta, infundibular or right ventricular outflow tract obstruction, and right ventricular hypertrophy. Presence of cyanosis, history of syncope, polycythemia (hematocrit >60), decreased arterial oxygen saturation (<80%), right ventricular hypertension, and congestive heart failure indicates poor prognosis.[2,10]

Goals of management should include:

- Avoid decrease in SVR
- Maintain adequate intravascular volume and venous return
- Avoid myocardial depressants
- Infective endocarditis prophylaxis

For labor analgesia and vaginal delivery in these patients, systemic or intrathecal opioids or pudendal block may be considered. Segmental epidural analgesia is not recommended because of chances of decrease in SVR. For forceps-assisted deliveries, low dose ketamine may be considered. Anesthesia of choice for cesarean section is general anesthesia with invasive monitoring and TEE.

Patients with corrected TOF, even if asymptomatic, 2D echocardiography is must along with 12-lead electrocardiogram (ECG) as they may have residual lesions and atrial

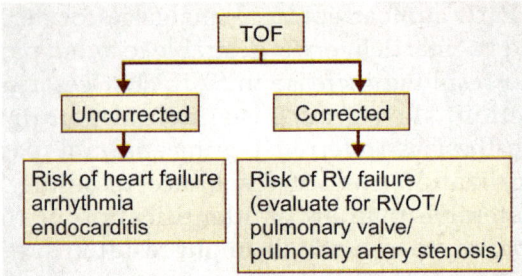

Fig. 13.2. Management of TOF in a woman of child-bearing age

and ventricular arrhythmias due to surgical injury to the cardiac conduction system.[11]

Pearls

- Regional anesthesia may lead to worsening of right-to-left shunt and should be avoided.
- In corrected TOFs, RV and RVOT should be assessed.

PRIMARY PULMONARY HYPERTENSION

It is a rare disease entity affecting young women of childbearing age with very high mortality reaching nearly 30%.[12] There is reduction in vascular nitric oxide and prostacyclin synthesis. At the same time, there is increase in endothelin and thromboxane production. The pulmonary artery pressure (PAP) is raised above 25 mm Hg at rest without any obvious cause. Pregnancy should be avoided as far as possible. However, use of oral contraceptives is unadvisable as they are known to accelerate the progression of the disease.[13]

Management

Any factors which increase the pulmonary vascular resistance (PVR) should be avoided such as hypoxia, hypercarbia and acidosis. Avoidance of myocardial depression and aortocaval compression and maintenance of SVR, intravascular volume and venous return should be the goal.

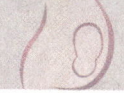

Anticoagulation is a must in any patient with primary pulmonary hypertension. As warfarin is known to be teratogenic, subcutaneous enoxaparin (1 mg/kg twice daily) is recommended.[13] Oxygen to counter the hypoxia and diuretics for right heart failure should be administered. IV epoprostenol should be administered by continuous infusion as it has a very short half-life of less than 6 minutes and can cause rebound increase in pressures, if abruptly discontinued. Endothelin receptor antagonists are contraindicated. Calcium channel blockers are not favored because of their negative inotropic effects.[12]

Timing of Delivery

The delivery should ideally be carried out between 32 to 34 weeks.[14] Vaginal delivery using low dose epidural analgesia would be the safest mode. If elective cesarean section is planned, single shot spinal anesthesia should be avoided as the RV may not be able to respond to decreased venous return. In fact it is prudent to avoid regional anesthesia in any form. Vasopressors are avoided as they increase the pulmonary artery pressure. Stress associated with laryngoscopy and intubation may also increase the PVR.[6]

Careful titration of oxytocin is required as it may decrease the SVR. Carboprost should be avoided because of its pulmonary side effects and methergin should be avoided as it causes vasoconstriction.

Fluid management in these patients is challenging as neither hypovolemia nor hypervolemia are tolerated. Fluid should be administered monitoring the central venous pressure or echocardiography. Right ventricular diastolic dysfunction is best treated with diuretics or hemofiltration.[12]

Inotropic agents may be required for systolic failure of the RV. Dobutamine at doses less than 10 µg/kg/min decreases the pulmonary vascular resistance but at higher doses

may have a detrimental effect on vasculature. Dopamine is avoided for its propensity of causing tachyarrhythmias. Phosphodiesterase inhibitors, like milrinone, have been known to reduce the pulmonary vascular resistance. Nebulized milrinone has the advantage of direct effect on pulmonary vasculature with less incidence of systemic hypotension.[12]

Vasopressors, like norepinephrine, may be used to maintain the systemic vascular resistance above the pulmonary vascular resistance. However, their effect is offset by the rise in pulmonary vascular pressure which may result in RV failure. Also the effect of α-adrenergic agents on the α-receptors of the uterus may result in reduced uterine blood flow.[12]

Patients should be monitored in high dependency units for 72 hours postpartum as the fluid shifts associated with delivery may decompensate the right ventricle.

Pearls

- Factors which increase pulmonary artery pressures must be avoided.
- Pulmonary vasodilators and oxygen form the mainstay of therapy.
- Anticoagulation is must.
- Regional anesthesia should be avoided as decrease in systemic vascular resistance may result in RV ischemia.
- Inotropic agents which do not increase the PVR should be used.

HYPERTROPHIC OBSTRUCTIVE CARDIOMYOPATHY (HOCM)

It is a genetically transmitted cardiac disease characterized by left ventricular hypertrophy. There is reduced left ventricular size and compliance. Chest pain, dyspnea and palpitations which may be confused with normal symptoms of pregnancy are the hallmark of HOCM. Any reduction in the preload or the afterload can result in increased outflow gradient and decreased left ventricular filling.

Thus regional anesthesia is relatively contraindicated in these patients. Invasive monitoring is indicated and any hypotension should be promptly treated with fluids and phenylephrine. Since it is a pure α-agonist, it does not have a positive inotropic effect and at the same time it slows the heart which may be advantageous for the perfusion of the hypertrophied ventricle. The morbidity directly correlates with the preconception NYHA status of the patient.[15]

Tachyarrhythmias including atrial fibrillation should be aggressively treated.[2]

Beta blockers should be continued throughout the pregnancy. In patients with history of syncope, an automatic implantable cardiac defibrillator (AICD) should be implanted preconception.

Pearls

- Chest pain, dyspnea and palpitations are the hallmark of HOCM.
- Phenylephrine and beta blockers are the drugs of choice.
- Adequate intravascular volume, maintain SVR and avoiding increase in myocardial contractility and pulse rate are the goals in anesthesia management.

ISCHEMIC HEART DISEASE

It is uncommon in pregnancy with an incidence of 1 in 10000 pregnancies. Myocardial infarction can commonly occur in third trimester or in the puerperium of the first or second pregnancies. The mortality may be very high up to 45%, if myocardial infarct occurs within 2 weeks postpartum. The presenting symptoms are usually ischemic chest pain, with ECG abnormalities and elevated cardiac troponin I levels (>0.15 ng/mL). Creatinine kinase levels may increase during normal labor and is not a sensitive indicator. In 78% of the women, there is no predisposing cause. However, increasing maternal age, smoking amongst young women and prevalence of type 2 diabetes mellitus may be some of the contributory causes.

Management

Management consists of early coronary angiography as spontaneous coronary dissection is the most common cause. 84% of the lesions involve left anterior descending artery. Coronary stenting or coronary artery bypass grafting may be the treatment options. Thrombolysis using tissue plasminogen activator (TPA) 100 mg over 90 min may be used. However, its use in early postpartum period is contraindicated due to the risk of hemorrhage.

Intramuscular or intravenous ergometrine may be associated with myocardial infarction due to coronary artery spasm. It would be best to avoid ergometrine in patients at risk of ischemic heart disease and to use it intramuscularly or small incremental intravenous doses, if required in high-risk patients. Ergometrine acts rapidly with 2 minutes of intravenous administration. Glyceryl trinitrate 10–400 mg/min injected immediately intravenously or sublingually 300 mg may be used to prevent infarct, if coronary artery spasm is suspected. If this is not effective, immediate coronary angiography and intracoronary injection of GTN or aspiration of thrombus may be undertaken.

Another rare cause of myocardial infarction is the use of nifedipine for the treatment of preterm labor where the cause may be either hypotension or reflex tachycardia associated with it.[15]

Differential diagnoses are pre-eclampsia, acute pulmonary embolism, sickle crisis hemorrhage and aortic dissection. Diagnosis can be confirmed by ischemic chest pain, with ECG abnormalities and elevated cardiac troponin I levels (>0.15 ng/mL).

Pearls

- Ergometrine to be avoided, if there is risk of myocardial ischemia
- Early thrombolysis
- Coronary stenting or coronary artery bypass grafting may be the treatment options

---

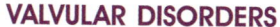
VALVULAR DISORDERS

Valvular heart diseases are most frequently encountered in pregnant women in developing nations. Many of these women are asymptomatic and the physiological changes of pregnancy may precipitate failure. Rheumatic mitral stenosis is the most commonly encountered valvular lesion during pregnancy. Complications during pregnancy include failure, atrial dysrhythmias, systemic or pulmonary embolism, and infective endocarditis. Regurgitant lesions are well tolerated during pregnancy due to physiological changes of pregnancy, however, stenotic lesions are poorly tolerated due to the risk of failure and pulmonary edema.[16]

Goal of anesthetic management is to maintain hemodynamic parameters within a narrow therapeutic range. Patients with symptomatic disease warrant invasive monitoring.

The incidence of complications is greater in:
1. Patients with prior history of arrhytmias, heart failure, transient ischemic attacks or stroke
2. If the baseline NYHA class is III or more or presence of cyanosis.
3. Ejection fraction less than 40%
4. Pulmonary artery pressure 50% of systemic pressure
5. Patients with aortic or mitral regurgitation who have NYHA class III or IV symptoms.

Mitral Stenosis (MS)

The normal area of the mitral valve is 4–6 cm^2. The symptoms of MS begin to appear when the valve area is reduced to less than 2 cm^2. As a result of MS, the filling of the left ventricle from the left atrium is hindered. This results in decreased stroke volume and cardiac output. A state of fixed cardiac output ensues and it is difficult for the heart to meet the increased cardiac output demanded by the pregnant state.[17]

The increased heart rate in pregnancy limits the time for diastolic filling with the resulting increased left atrial pressure and the propensity for pulmonary edema. Thus there is a downhill course and the patient's NYHA status usually worsens by one grade. The situation becomes further grim with the onset of atrial fibrillation and there is 80% incidence in systemic emboli in these patients.

There is a sudden increase in preload due to autotransfusion immediately after delivery and there is high incidence of pulmonary edema and death which can occur in the immediate peripartum and postpartum period and require close monitoring.

Medical Management

Bed rest, oxygen therapy and diuretics form the basis of therapy. Beta blockers can be used to reduce the heart rate. They reduce the incidence of maternal cardiac failure without adverse effects on the fetus. Recent evidence does not show any beneficial role of digoxin in treatment of cardiac failure. If there is atrial fibrillation, then aggressive treatment with digoxin, beta blockers and anticoagulation is required. Anticoagulation has proven to be beneficial even in the absence of atrial fibrillation.

Increased stenosis	Progressive LA dilatation	Increased LA pressures	Back pressure on pulmonary vasculature	Pulmonary congestion and pulmonary edema

The standard guidelines for anticoagulation during pregnancy are:

- Up to 12 weeks antepartum SC/IV heparin (aPTT 1.5–2.5 times the normal)
- Between 12 and 36 weeks warfarin (INR 2.5–3.0)
- After 36 weeks SC/IV heparin

Unfractionated heparin has been replaced by low molecular weight heparin. When anticoagulation is necessary, especially in women with mechanical valves, warfarin or low-molecular-weight heparin should be replaced by unfractionated heparin 36 h before induction of labor. Unfractionated heparin should be discontinued 4–6 h before delivery and restarted 4–6 h after delivery. Antibiotic prophylaxis for bacterial endocarditis is reserved for those patients who have previous history of endocarditis or in presence of infection.

Surgical Management

Mitral commissurotomy is preferred, if mitral stenosis is diagnosed prior to pregnancy.

Percutaneous valvuloplasty is the treatment of choice during the second trimester in pregnant women. After valvulopasty, the valve area increases to 1.5 cm² with a 100% success rate. Fetal loss is high in open commissurotomy though maternal outcome is same for both the procedures. In severe cases where there is a calcified valve or thrombus, valve replacement may be indicated. In open valve replacement, there are high chances of losing the fetus 16–33%. Maternal mortality may be also as high as 1.5–5%.[18,19]

Anesthesia Management

For vaginal delivery, labor analgesia is a must as it attenuates pain and associated sympathetic response which might precipitate failure. Segmental lumbar epidural analgesia is gold standard.

For cesarean section, plain epidural or combined spinal epidural (CSE) technique is preferred as it produces controlled hemodynamics. Spinal anesthesia is contraindicated as sympathetic blockade produced by single shot can lead to cardiovascular collapse in severe MS.[14] However, general anesthesia is the method of choice in cases of decompensated heart failure, obstetric emergency or when patient is on anticoagulation. Avoiding tachycardia, hypotension and judicious fluid management along with ICU care in postoperative period is the key to management.

Mitral Insufficiency/Regurgitation (MR)

Mitral valve regurgitation is the second commonest valvular lesion in pregnancy. Though most patients with MR tolerate pregnancy well some present with atrial fibrillation, bacterial endocarditis, systemic embolization, and pulmonary edema during late pregnancy. However, if associated with coexisting MS, morbidity and mortality increases significantly.[18] Congenital mitral valve prolapse (MVP) is well-tolerated during pregnancy and therapeutic interventions are thus rarely necessary.[18,20]

In MR, regurgitation through an incompetent mitral valve results in chronic volume overload of the left atrium and dilatation with resultant pulmonary venous congestion. Physiologic decrease in SVR improves forward flow. However, increases in SVR due to sympathetic stimulation during labor pain, uterine contractions, or surgical stimulation, may lead to acute left ventricular failure.

Anesthesia Management

Adequate analgesia for labor will decrease peripheral vasoconstriction and thus attenuate the increase in left ventricular afterload and forward flow. Segmental lumbar epidural analgesia is the preferred technique. Controlled sympathetic blockade which decrease SVR and is beneficial. However, to augment preload, adequate intravenous fluid infusion to maintain left ventricular filling volume is must.

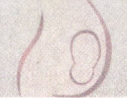

For cesarean section, plain epidural or combined spinal epidural (CSE) technique can be considered. Graded epidural supplementation produces minimal sympathetic blockade and hemodynamic changes with the advantage of better pain relief in the postoperative period.

Pearls in management of MS and MR	
MS	**MR**
Prevent tachycardia	Prevent bradycardia
Avoid fluid overload	Avoid increase in SVR
Avoid decrease in SVR and increase in PVR	Avoid myocardial depression
Maintain sinus rhythm	Maintain sinus rhythm

Aortic Stenosis and Regurgitation (AS, AR)

Rheumatic mitral stenosis is the most commonly encountered valvular lesion during pregnancy, but aortic valvular involvement has greater functional significance. Mild to moderate aortic stenosis during pregnancy can rapidly deteriorate the hemodynamics and precipitate congestive heart failure, carrying a high risk of maternal and fetal mortality.

Bicuspid aortic valve is the most common congenital cardiac malformation occurring in 1–2% of the population.[18] It can present either as a regurgitant or stenotic pathology. Calcification of the bicuspid aortic valve occurs at an early age due to degeneration caused by mechanical strains on the valve.[21] However, it is a rare entity in childbearing age. Regurgitant valvular lesions are well tolerated during pregnancy, whereas stenotic lesions have a greater potential for decompensation and left ventricular failure.[22,23] The incidence of complications, like preterm birth (44%), intrauterine growth retardation (IUGR) (22%), and lower birth weight (LBW), is more in these patients.[19,20]

Anesthesia goals in aortic stenosis include maintenance of intravascular volume and preload, avoiding aortocaval compression, myocardial ischemia and prevent and treat arrhythmias promptly. Regional and general anesthesia (GA) has been used successfully. High dose opioid technique and volatile agents for general anesthesia induction are mentioned but both are depressant for the fetus. However, during emergency LSCS, when patient is on anticoagulation and in decompensated heart failure, GA should be chosen.

Single shot spinal anesthesia may cause marked sympathetic blockade leading to cardiovascular collapse and is contraindicated in severe AS.[14] Due to autotransfusion and relief of vena caval compression, cardiac output and stroke volume increases by almost 80% in the immediate postpartum period.[24] Hence, furosemide should be considered for induced controlled diuresis to offset the effects of autotransfusion. Postpartum hemorrhage (PPH) due to uterine atony is a major concern, and is managed with infusion of uterotonic drugs in slow titrated doses. Cardiac failure can occur after rapid infusion of IV oxytocin (>5 U over 5 min) due to hypotension, tachycardia and fluid retention, so oxytocin should be used slowly (an infusion pump is preferred over drip) with extreme vigilance.[25]

The final decision of GA versus regional anesthesia for valvular diseases in pregnancy is still unconvincing and anesthetic plan should be individualized for each patient. Perioperative use of invasive monitoring should be considered and high-dependency postpartum care should be available.

Pearl
Single shot spinal anesthesia is contraindicated in severe aortic stenosis

Pearls in management of AS and AR	
AS	**AR**
Avoid decrease in SVR	Avoid marked increase in SVR
Avoid bradycardia	Avoid bradycardia
Maintain ventricular filling and preload	Avoid myocardial depression

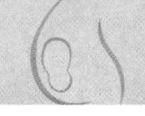

PERIPARTUM CARDIOMYOPATHY (PPCM)

Peripartum cardiomyopathy may present in late pregnancy or in the puerperial period up to five months postpartum. There should be a high index of suspicion in a woman during pregnancy or in the postpartum period who complains of increasing breathlessness especially on lying flat or at night. This entity may be confused with pre-eclampsia as 25% of these women may be hypertensive.[26] The incidence ranges from 1:1500 to 1:4000 live births. It may impose substantial risk to the life of the mother with mortality reaching 18–56%.[1]

The exact etiology is not known. However, viral and autoimmune causes have been attributed in certain cases. Predisposing factors include advanced maternal age, multiparity, multiple gestations, presence of pre-eclampsia, prolonged use of tocolytics, diabetes, obesity and Afro-Caribbean descent have been implicated.[1,27,28] An electrocardiogram (ECG), echocardiogram (Echo) and X-ray chest is volunteered as early as possible in all these patients.[26] After excluding pre-eclampsia and other cardiac conditions, PPCM is diagnosed.

Prolonged tocolysis using terbutaline has been mentioned as one of the causative factors but whether β-agonist therapy is a causative agent or it is manifesting a clinically silent heart disease is not clear.[15]

Close differential diagnoses of PPCM include myocardial infarction, severe pre-eclampsia, sepsis, pulmonary thromboembolism and amniotic fluid embolism.[15]

The PPCM criteria were first described by Demakis in the year 1971:[27]

- Absence of any heart disease before the last month of pregnancy
- Etiology unknown
- Heart failure developing towards end of pregnancy or in the puerperal period up to five months.

To complement this, the echocardiographic evidence has been added:[27]

- Ejection fraction (EF) reduced to 45% or less.
- Left ventricular end diastolic dimensions >2.7 cm/m^2
- Fractional shortening (FS) <30%

ECG criteria may include:

- There may be sinus tachycardia or dysrhythmias. The rhythm may be normal.
- Other changes which may include left ventricular hypertrophy, inverted T waves, non-specific ST changes and presence of Q waves.

Cardiomegaly is usually seen on X-ray chest. Thus diagnosis lays mainly on echocardiographic findings which should be done in all suspected patients urgently.

In cases where diagnosis is unclear, an endomyocardial biopsy can be done which reveals myocarditis in 76% of the patients.[15]

Treatment includes supportive management and urgent delivery of the fetus which may alleviate the symptoms. Salt restriction and diuretics to decrease the pulmonary congestion and fluid overload may be necessary. Vasodilators are used to decrease the afterload in patients with systolic dysfunction. Use of angiotensin-converting enzyme inhibitors is contraindicated in pregnancy because of risk of teratogenicity, neonatal anuric renal failure and even neonatal death. Hydralazine may be added to amlodipine or nitrate. Angiotensin-converting enzyme inhibitors are to be used in the postpartum period even in lactating mothers. Carvedilol, a beta blocker, improves survival in PPCM. Immunosuppressive therapy and use of pooled polyclonal human antibodies are the latest treatments available.

Digoxin is used to treat atrial arrhythmias. It also has positive inotropic effect. Amiodarone is avoided as it may result in fetal hypothyroidism and premature delivery. Fetal bradycardia, hypotension and heart blocks may be some of the side effects of verapamil. Anticoagulation is necessary in patients with poor cardiac function (EF <35%) as there is a risk of thromboembolism in these patients. Unfractionated or low molecular weight heparin may be used.[1,15]

Anesthetic management: The best option is vaginal delivery with low dose epidural analgesia. Blood pressure and fluid status need vigilant monitoring. General anesthesia with invasive monitoring should be provided for cesarean sections.

Pearls
- Echocardiography with EF <45% is diagnostic.
- Diuretics to decrease pulmonary congestion and vasodilators like hydralazine, amlodipine and nitrates are the treatment of choice.

ARRHYTHMIAS IN PREGNANCY

Arrhythmias are common in pregnancy but arrhythmias causing hemodynamic instability or requiring invasive management are rare. They may be due to exacerbations of pre-existing arrhythmias in pregnancy or may manifest for the first time.[29] Patients with pre-existing arrhythmias, congenital heart disease and those with structural heart disease are at highest risk for developing arrhythmia during pregnancy.[29,30] Supraventricular tachycardias are the most common arrhythmias occurring during pregnancy. Regarding safety of antiarrhythmic drugs (AADs) or guidelines for management of arrhythmias in pregnant women, little data on the efficacy and very few randomized studies are available.[29]

Etiology and Mechanism of Arrhythmia

Cardiac arrhythmias are caused by disorders of impulse formation, impulse conduction, or both. Cardiac arrhythmia, if left untreated, may lead to reduction in cardiac output, or precipitation of life-threatening serious arrhythmia. Exact cause in a pregnant woman is unknown, however, because of a combination of hemodynamic, hormonal, and autonomic factors, arrhythmogenesis may occur. Due to the increase in effective circulating blood volume during pregnancy, preload increases stretching cardiac chambers and atrial and ventricular myocytes thereby activating stretch activated channels. These result in membrane depolarization, shortened refractory period, slowed conduction and a spatial dispersion through activation of stretch-activated ion channels.[31–33] Thus above CVS changes, increased adrenergic activity and autonomic stimuli together are proarrhythmic.[32,33]

Clinical Presentation

Patient may be asymptomatic and may be diagnosed during evaluation of a murmur. Palpitations, dizziness, syncope are the most common presenting symptoms followed by breathlessness or chest pain. In patients with pre-existing arrhythmia, episodes are increased in frequency and intensity during pregnancy.[29]

A detailed history, clinical examination and a thorough preoperative evaluation are crucial. Laboratory investigations including complete blood count, blood glucose, electrolytes (Na, K, Ca, and Mg), coagulation profile, and thyroid function tests are essential. To detect structural heart disease, an electrocardiograph (ECG) and 2D echocardiography should be done. In high-risk patients, Holter monitoring can be done but stress test should be avoided as there is risk of fetal bradycardia.[31]

While interpreting of ECG, physiological changes during pregnancy should be kept in mind. There is increase in resting heart rate and decreased PR, QRS and QT intervals with left axis deviation. Cardiac conduction abnormalities are common due to stretching of the chamber walls mainly the left atrium (LA). Also supraventricular tachycardias and ventricular extrasystoles, T wave inversion and Q waves are also seen commonly.[31, 34]

Paroxysmal supraventricular tachycardias (PSVT) are the most common arrhythmias occurring during pregnancy followed by ventricular premature beats (VPBs), ventricular tachycardia (VT), and ventricular fibrillation (VF), however, is rare.[29,30] Atrial tachycardia, fibrillation/flutter and bradyarrhythmias are rare in pregnancy and usually associated with structural heart disease.

Common Arrhythmias and Their Management (Fig. 13.3)

Supraventricular Tachycardia

During acute episode, management starts with vagal maneuvers (Valsalva, carotid sinus massage) followed by adenosine.[29] Fetal heart rate monitoring is recommended. Intravenous beta-blockers can be used as a next step. Verapamil should be avoided due to its long half-life and risk of maternal hypotension. If the above treatment is unsuccessful or the patient is hemodynamically unstable, then electrical cardioversion is the treatment of choice.[29,34]

To control recurrent and sustained symptomatic arrhythmias, digoxin can be considered. Amiodarone causes intrauterine growth retardation (IUGR), premature delivery and thyroid abnormalities and should not be used except in emergencies.[35] For recurrent symptomatic episodes resistant to drug therapy, radiofrequency ablation is the treatment of choice.[29] It is preferably done in the second or third trimester under fluoroscopy by abdominal shielding or pulsed fluoroscopy. Magnetic navigation system is advocated, if available to minimize screening.[36.]

Atrial Fibrillation/Flutter

Management is mainly to control the rate using digoxin, beta-blockers and calcium channel blockers.[37] Electrical cardioversion can be performed, if mother is hemodynamically unstable or within the first 48 hours to avoid the need for anticoagulation. Cardioversion considered safe for fetus as minimal electrical energy is delivered to the fetus and high fetal fibrillation thresholds.

Ventricular Arrhythmias

Ventricular tachycardias are usually secondary to structural heart disease or may be the first presentation of a peripartum cardiomyopathy or myocardial infarction.[29,30,34] If the patient is hemodynamically stable, mainstay of management is correction of electrolyte abnormalities and withdrawal of precipitating factor. If the patient takes a diuretic regularly, assume hypomagnesemia is present and correct it with IV magnesium. This helps to stabilize myocardial cell membranes.

Other treatment options are IV lignocaine bolus of 100 mg followed by a maintenance infusion of 4 mg/min for 30 min, 2 mg/min for 2 hours, then 1 mg/min which will chemically cardiovert the rhythm back to sinus rhythm in 30–40% of cases. If lignocaine fails,

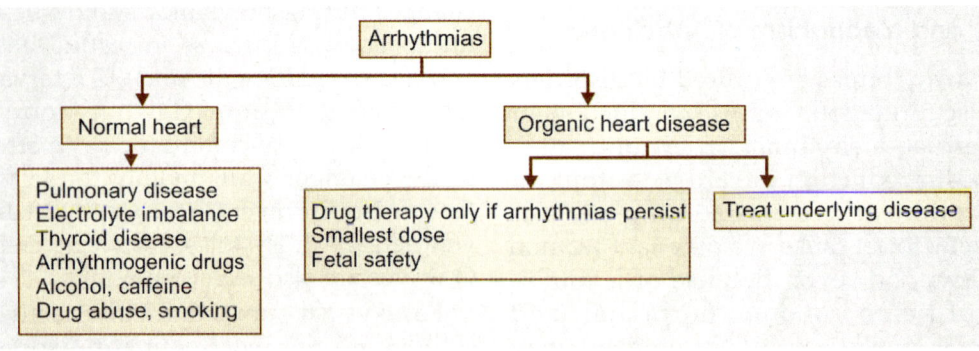

Fig. 13.3. Arrhythmias

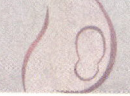

sotolol 100 mg IV over 5 min or procainamide 100 mg IV over 5 min infusion can be considered.

An implantable defibrillator (ICD) may be necessary in select cases and it should be implanted using an abdominal shield or ultrasound guidance to minimize radiation exposure to the fetus.[29,30,36,37] Pregnancy can be safely continued with an ICD *in situ* but it should be switched off during cesarean section due to the use of electrocautery causing discharge.

Arrhythmias recur in the postpartum period and patients should be on their prophylatic beta-blockers.[31]

Bradyarrhythmias

For symptomatic bradycardia, ideal management is implantable pacemakers with the ability to respond to changing hemodynamic demands. If the patient is symptomatic, preoperative pacing should be considered and atropine and/or isoprenaline (infusion 1–10 µg/min) can be used.

Anesthetic Considerations

Parturient with history of arrhythmia especially AF controlled on medications should be continued on their current anti-arrhythmic drugs perioperatively. Doses should be adjusted with expert cardiologist opinion to achieve ventricular rate between 90 and 110 bpm. Patients with pre-existing heart disease, if develops new onset arrhythmias, should be treated promptly. If associated with hemodynamic instability, immediate DC cardioversion should be instituted.

In the perioperative period, recognize and treat the reversible cause. Administer 100% O_2 and normalize CO_2 (intubate, ventilate). Deepen the plane of anesthesia but switch off volatile agents and administer adequate analgesia. Correction of reversible factors, mainly electrolyte and acid-base imbalances, should be done rapidly.

Antiarrhythmic Drugs during Pregnancy

Large data based on randomized controlled trials of antiarrhythmic drug for safety in pregnant women is not available. Therefore, the potential risk must be taken into account when treating arrhythmia. On the other hand, it is important to avoid hemodynamic instability and significant risk to mother and fetus. No antiarrhythmic is classified as A due to the lack of available trials on the other hand none is absolutely contraindicated. Most are classified as C, lignocaine and sotalol are classified as B and only amiodarone and atenolol are classified as D (Table 13.3).[29,30,34,37]

> **Pearls**
> - Treat arrhythmia promptly
> - Continue antiarrhythmics perioperatively

DISEASES OF AORTA

Coarctation of Aorta

It is characterized by narrowing of the aorta at or near the insertion of ductus arteriosus. Hypertension in the upper half of the body is the presenting sign. Left ventricular failure, aortic rupture or dissections may be the complications associated with uncorrected or partially corrected coarctation of aorta in a pregnant lady. As a result of decreased uterine perfusion, distal to the narrowed segment fetal mortality may be as high as 20%. The lower limb systolic blood pressure should be maintained above 100 mm Hg to ensure adequate uterine perfusion. General anesthesia is preferred for cesarean sections. Since it is a fixed output state regional anesthesia with the fall in SVR is a relative contraindication. For this, it may be necessary to cannulate the postductal artery for continuous blood pressure monitoring. Ephedrine and dopamine are the vasopressors of choice with their positive chronotropic effects being advantageous.

Thus the anesthetic goals include invasive hemodynamic monitoring, maintenance of a slightly elevated SVR and heart rate. It is advisable to maintain an adequate intravascular volume and venous return.[2]

Pearls

- The lower limb systolic BP to be maintained above 100 mm Hg.
- General anesthesia is preferred.
- Maintenance of a slightly elevated SVR and heart rate.

INFECTIVE ENDOCARDITIS: ANTIBIOTIC PROPHYLAXIS

Patients at high risk of infective endocarditis should be administered intravenous amoxicillin and gentamicin irrespective of the mode of delivery (vaginal/cesarean).[38] These include:

- Patients with prosthetic cardiac valves or in those where prosthetic material is used for valve repair.
- Unrepaired cyanotic heart disease including palliative shunts.
- Repaired congenital heart disease with residual defects.
- In case of repaired congenital heart disease where prosthesis is used prophylaxis should be given for first six months after repair.
- Where there is history of previous endocarditis.
- Post-transplant patients who develop valvulopathies.

Mortality

Based on the specific lesions, the mortality and outcome varies accordingly (Table 13.4). The danger to the mother's life does not end with a safe delivery. Postpartum surveillance is required for at least 15 days post-delivery. Conditions, such as peripartum cardiomyopathy, may occur for up to 5 months postpartum.

For successful management of the pregnant patient with heart disease, exquisite cooperation among the obstetrician, the cardiologist and the anesthesiologist involved in peripartum care is essential. A comprehensive understanding of physiology of pregnancy and pathophysiology of underlying cardiac disease is of primary importance in obstetric and anesthetic management of this high-risk group of parturients to improve maternal and fetal outcomes.

SUMMARY

- Avoid aortocaval compression.
- Infective endocarditis prophylaxis in indicated patients.
- Prevent hypoxia, hypercapnia, acidosis.
- Maintain SVR:PVR ratio.
- Avoid accidental injection of air.
- Labor analgesia with low dose epidural infusion and assisted shortened second stage is advisable management in most obstetric patients with heart disease.
- Regional anesthesia vs GA to be decided depending on risk benefit ratio and the cardiac lesion.

Table 13.4: Various cardiac lesions and associated mortality

Low risk (mortality 0.1–1%)	Intermediate risk (mortality 1–5%)	High risk (mortality 5–30%)
• Most repaired lesions • Uncomplicated left to right shunts • Mitral valve prolapse • Bicuspid aortic valve • Pulmonary stenosis • Regurgitant lesions	• Mechanical valves • Unrepaired cyanotic lesions • Switch procedures • Single ventricles • Stenotic lesions (mild/moderate aortic, mitral and severe pulmonary)	• Severe pulmonary hypertension • Severe ventricular dysfunctions • Patient symptomatic preconception (NYHA class III or IV) • Aortic stenosis • Marfan's disease with aortic involvement

- Controlled graded epidural should be preferred technique over single shot spinal.
- Goal of anesthetic management is to maintain hemodynamic parameters within a narrow therapeutic range.
- Treat arrhythmia promptly.
- Oxytocin should be used with caution.

REFERENCES

1. Blackburn D, Bracco D. Heart Disease in Pregnancy—the Anesthesiologist's Perspective Anesthesiology Rounds, Vol 9, Issue 3.
2. Maitra G, Sengupta S, Rudra A, Debnath S. Pregnancy and non-valvular heart disease—anesthetic considerations. Ann Card Anaesth 2010;13:102–9.
3. Ruys TP, Cornette J, RoosHesselink JW. Pregnancy and delivery in cardiac disease. J Cardiol 2013;61;107–12,
4. Fernandes SM, Arendt KW, Landzberg MJ, Economy KE, Khairy P. Pregnant women with congenital heart disease: cardiac, anesthetic and obstetrical implications. Expert Rev Cardiovasc Ther 2010;8(3):439–48.
5. Krzysztof M, Kuc Arnoski TMD, Ana aha aha for the parturient with cardiovascular disease. Southern African Journal of Anesthesia and Analgesia 2003;9:2,18–25.
6. Harnett M, Mushlin PS, Camann WR. Cardiovascular disease. In: Chestnut DH. Obstetric Anesthesia: Principles and Practice. Philadelphia: Elsevier Mosby; 2004, p. 707–33.
7. Kansaria JJ, Salvi VS. Eisenmenger syndrome in pregnancy. J Postgrad Med 2000;46:101–3.
8. Owen MD, Poss MJ, Dean LS, Harper MA. Prolonged intravenous remifentanil infusion for labor analgesia. Anesth Analg 2002;94:918–9.
9. Kuczkowski KM. Labor analgesia for the parturient with cardiac disease: What does an obstetrician need to know? Acta Obstet Gynecol Scand 2004;83:223–33.
10. Ghai B, Mohan V, Khetarpal M, Malhotra N. Epidural anesthesia for cesarean section in a patient with Eisenmenger's syndrome. Int J Obstet Anesth 2002;11:44–7.
11. Veldtman GR, Connolly HM, Grogan M, Ammash NM, Warnes CA. Outcomes of pregnancy in women with tetralogy of Fallot. J Am Coll Cardiol 2004;44:174–80.
12. Bassily-Marcus AM, Yuan C, Oropello J, Manasia A, Kohli-Seth R, Benjamin E. Pulmonary hypertension in pregnancy: Critical care management. Pulm Med 2012;2012:709407.
13. Rosengarten D, Kramer MR. Pulmonary hypertension and pregnancy: Management and outcome. Harefuah 2013;152(9):547–51,562,563.
14. Shaikh SI, Lakshmi RR, Hegade G. Perioperative anesthetic management for cesarean section in patients with cardiac disease. Anesth Pain & Intensive Care 2014;18(4):377–85.
15. Ray P, Murphy GJ, Shutt LE. Recognition and management of maternal cardiac disease in pregnancy. British Journal of Anesthesia 2004:93 (3):428–39.
16. Warnes CA. Pregnancy and heart disease. In: Libby P, Bonow RO, Mann DL, Zipes DP, (Eds). Braunwald's Heart Disease: A Textbook of Cardiovascular Medicine, 8th ed. Philadelphia: Saunders; 2007, pp 1967–82.
17. Kannan K, Vijayanand G. Mitral stenosis and pregnancy: Current concepts in anesthetic practice. Indian J Anaesth 2010;54(5):439–44
18. Nanna M, Stergiopoulos K. Pregnancy complicated by valvular heart disease: An update. J Am Heart Assoc 2014; 3:e000712.
19. Drenthen W, Boersma E, Balci A, Moons P, RoosHesselink JW, Mulder BJ. Predictors of pregnancy complications in women with congenital heart disease. Eur Heart J 2010; 31:2124–32.
20. Malhotra M, Sharma JB, Tripathii R, Arora P, Arora R. Maternal and fetal outcome in valvular heart disease. Int J Gynaecol Obstet 2004;84:11–6.
21. Fedak PW, Verma S, David TE, Leask RL, Weisel RD, Butany J. Clinical and pathophysiological implications of a bicuspid aortic valve. Circulation 2002;106:900–4.
22. Naidoo DP, Moodley J. Management of the critically ill cardiac patient. Best Pract Res Clin Obstet Gynaecol 2001;15:523–44.
23. Tumelero RT, Duda NT, Tognon AP, Sartori J, Giorgo S. Percutaneous balloon aortic valvuloplasty in a preg adolescent. Arq Bras Cardiol 2003;82:98–101.
24. Ibrahim H, Parkin J. Aortic stenosis and pregnancy: A case report and review of peripartum anesthetic management. Kuwait Med J 2008; 40:64–6.
25. Thomas JS, Koh SH, Cooper GM. Hemodynamic effects of oxytocin given as i.v. bolus or infusion

in women undergoing Caesarean section. British J Anaesth 2007;98:116–9.

26. Cardiac disease in Pregnancy. Good practice No. 13. Royal college of Obstetricians and Gynaecologists June 2011.

27. Tiwari AK, Agrawal J, Tayal S, Chadha M, Singla A, et al. Anesthetic management of peripartum cardiomyopathy using "epidural volume extension" technique: A case series. Annals of Cardiac Anesthesia 2012;15(1):44–6.

28. Indira K, Sanjeev K, Sunanda G. Sequential combined spinal epidural anesthesia for caesarean section in peripartum cardiomyopathy. Indian J Anaesth 2007;51:137.

29. Enriquez AD, Economy KE, Tedrow UB. Contemporary management of arrhythmias during pregnancy. Circ Arrhythm Electrophysiol 2014;7:961–7.

30. Knotts RJ, Garan H. Cardiac arrhythmias in pregnancy. Semin Perinatol 2014;38:285–8.

31. Silversides CK, Harris L, Haberer K, et al. Recurrence rates of arrhythmias during pregnancy in women with previous tachyarrhythmia and impact on fetal and neonatal outcomes. Am J Cardiol 2006;97:1206.

32. Ninio DM, Saint DA. The role of stretch-activated channels in atrial fibrillation and the impact of intracellular acidosis. Prog Biophys Mol Biol 2008;97:401.

33. Drenthen W, Boersma E, Balci A, et al. Predictors of pregnancy complications in women with congenital heart disease. Eur Heart J 2010;31:2124.

34. Joglar JA, Page RL. Management of arrhythmia syndromes during pregnancy. Curr Opin Cardiol 2014;29:36–44.

35. Bartalena L, Bogazzi F, Braverman LE, Martino E. Effects of amiodarone administration during pregnancy on neonatal thyroid function and subsequent neurodevelopment. J Endocrinol Invest 2001;24:116–30.

36. Ferguson JD, Helms A, Mangrum JM, DiMarco JP. Ablation of incessant left atrial tachycardia without fluoroscopy in a pregnant woman. J Cardiovasc Electrophysiol 2011;22(3):346–9.

37. Blomstrom-Lundqvist C, Scheinman MM, et al. "ACC/AHA/ESC guidelines for the management of patients with supraventricular arrhythmias–execution summary". JACC 2003;42:1493–1531.

38. Ravi J, Sukhwinder KB, Sukhminder JSB, Ratika J. Pregnancy in cardiac disease: clinical, obstetric and anesthetic concerns. Sri Lanka Journal of Obstetrics and Gynaecology 2011;33:174–82.

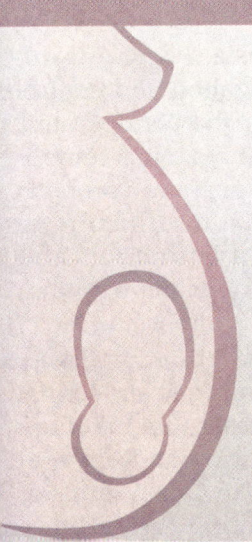

Endocrine Disorders and Pregnancy

Gayathri Bhat, Kausalya Chakravarthy

14.1 GENERAL CONSIDERATIONS

Pregnancy causes profound anatomical and physiological changes in the body. These adaptations enable the pregnant woman to accommodate and cater to the needs of the growing fetus. Endocrine adaptations to the pregnant state begin soon after conception. The subtle changes in pituitary, adrenal and pancreas almost completely revert back to the non-pregnant state after delivery while thyroid dysfunction (hypothyroidism and hyperthyroidism) may have long-term implications. The metabolic changes induced by the placental hormones affect the glucose and lipid metabolism of the pregnant woman predisposing to a diabetogenic state which may persist or recur in the next pregnancies.

The circulating concentrations of the hypothalamic stimulatory hormones, like gonadotropin-releasing hormone (GnRH), corticotropin-releasing hormone (CRH), growth hormone-releasing hormone (GHRH), thyrotropin-releasing hormone (TRH), and prolactin-releasing factors, rise during pregnancy due to placental production of identical or variant hormones. The anterior lobe of the pituitary gland enlarges up to threefold during gestation because of hyperplasia and hypertrophy. There is an increase in serum adrenocorticotropic hormone (ACTH) concentrations[1] causing a state of relative hypercortisolism.[2]

The major changes in thyroid function during pregnancy are an increase in serum thyroxine-binding globulin (TBG) concentrations and stimulation of the thyrotropin (TSH) receptor by human chorionic gonadotropin (hCG).[3] While a modest elevation in serum TSH may be noted at term due to increase in renal iodine clearance and placental degradation of thyroid hormone.[3,4] During pregnancy, TSH retains its normal circadian rhythm (nocturnal surge), indicating an intact pituitary-thyroid axis. There is a decline in the PTH levels in the first half of pregnancy, reaches a nadir in the second trimester, and rises thereafter.

METABOLIC ADAPTATIONS

Placental hormones affect both glucose and lipid metabolism to ensure adequate supply of glucose and amino acids to the growing fetus, while providing extra free fatty acids, ketones, and glycerol as sources of maternal fuel.[5,6] There is a hyperplasia of the insulin-secreting pancreatic beta cells, increased insulin secretion, and a progressive increase in insulin resistance.[5] Maternal glucose homeostasis shows transient maternal hyperglycemia after meals due to increasing insulin resistance and transient hypoglycemia between meals and at night to facilitate the placental transfer of glucose.[5] The insulin resistance in pregnancy is important in understanding the pathology of gestational diabetes mellitus. Serum total cholesterol and triglyceride concentrations increase markedly during pregnancy. Maternal obesity or a pre-pregnancy BMI is a risk factor for development of obstetric syndromes (gestational diabetes mellitus, pre-eclampsia, preterm birth).

The deviation from the normal physiological adaptations is reflected as endocrinal disorder encountered in pregnancy. The most common endocrinal disorders in pregnancy are hypo-/hyperthyroidism, pheochromocytoma and diabetes.

Anesthetic Implications of Endocrinal Disorders in Pregnancy

The presence of endocrinological disorders complicating pregnancy demands eternal vigilance on the part of anesthesiologist to tackle the perioperative problems. A thorough preanesthetic evaluation, proper planning of anesthesia technique and perioperative care can decrease the perioperative morbidity in these patients. Cardiac evaluation should be done in uncontrolled diabetic patients, pregnant patients with pheochromocytoma and thyrotoxicosis.

Hypothyroidism lowers the metabolic rate and can prolong the effect of anesthesia causing delayed recovery. Uncontrolled hyperthyroidism can precipitate thyroid storm a dire emergency. Pheochromocytoma though rare can present in pregnancy as uncontrolled hypertension/pre-eclampsia. Proper evaluation, preoperative optimization and control of pressures are crucial for the perioperative management of pheochromocytoma complicating pregnancy. Diabetes can pose a problem to the anesthesiologist due to difficulty in securing airway, renal dysfunction and autonomic neuropathy. Perioperative optimization of glycemic control is important.

The intrinsic difficulty of obstetric airway is compounded by the presence of endocrinal disorders. General anesthesia (GA) is more challenging in these patients. Regional anesthesia is much safer than GA in terms of airway management, blunting the catecholamine surge and postoperative pain relief.[7]

Management of pregnant patients with co-morbid endocrinal pathologies needs a multidisciplinary approach with the involvement of obstetrician, endocrinologist, obstetric anesthesiologist and intensivist, cardiologist and fetal medicine experts.

REFERENCES

1. Mastorakos G, Ilias I. Maternal hypothalamic-pituitary-adrenal axis in pregnancy and the postpartum period. Postpartum-related disorders. Ann N Y Acad Sci 2000;900:95.
2. Frim DM, Emanuel RL, Robinson BG, Smas CM, Adler GK, Majzoub JA. Characterization and gestational regulation of corticotropin-releasing hormone messenger RNA in human placenta. J Clin Invest 1988;82(1):287.
3. Glinoer D. What happens to the normal thyroid during pregnancy? Thyroid 1999;9(7):631.
4. Brent GA. Maternal thyroid function: interpretation of thyroid function tests in pregnancy. Clin Obstet Gynecol 1997;40(1):3.
5. Butte NF. Carbohydrate and lipid metabolism in pregnancy: normal compared with gestational diabetes mellitus. Am J Clin Nutr 2000;71(5 Suppl):1256S.
6. Homko CJ, Sivan E, Reece EA, Boden G. Fuel metabolism during pregnancy. Semin Reprod Endocrinol 1999;17(2):119.
7. Bajwa SJS, Bajwa SK, Ghuman GS. Pregnancy with comorbidities: Anesthetic aspects during operative intervention. Anesth Essays Res 2013;7(3):294–301.

14.2 DIABETES MELLITUS (Pathophysiology, Clinical Presentation, Interaction with Pregnancy and Anesthetic Management)

INTRODUCTION

Diabetes mellitus results from either an absolute deficiency in insulin secretion (type 1) or a combination of resistance to insulin in target tissues and inadequate insulin secretion (type 2). Pregnancy is a state of chronic low grade inflammation, associated with increased circulating levels of C-reactive protein (CRP) Interleukin-6 (IL-6). Both these factors enhance insulin resistance. A pregnancy complicated by diabetes mellitus (DM) requires a multidisciplinary co-operation amongst obstetricians, endocrinologists, anesthesiologists, nurse educators and dieticians to facilitate a healthy outcome of mother and child.

PREVALENCE OF DIABETES IN PREGNANCY

The global prevalence of diabetes was estimated to be 9% among adults aged 18+ years.[1] In India, the disease affects more than 62 million Indians, which is more than 7.1% of India's adult population. It is estimated to increase to more than 100 million by 2030.[2] Using the screening and diagnostic criteria proposed by the International Association of Diabetes and Pregnancy Study Groups (IADPSG) in 2010, the global prevalence of hyperglycemia in pregnancy has been estimated at 17%.[3] The prevalence of gestational diabetes mellitus (GDM) in India was

found to be 16.2% in urban areas and 9.9% in rural areas.[4]

Terminology of Diabetes in Pregnancy

Diabetes in pregnancy can be either pregestational (PGDM) or gestational diabetes mellitus (GDM):

- *Pregestational diabetes mellitus (PGDM):* The term pregestational diabetes refers to pre-existing type 1 or type 2 diabetes mellitus diagnosed prior to a woman's pregnancy.
- *Gestational diabetes mellitus (GDM)* is defined as "any degree of glucose intolerance with onset or first recognition during pregnancy".

Pathophysiology of Diabetes Mellitus in Pregnancy

Insulin is a peptide hormone secreted by the beta cells of the islets of Langerhans in the pancreas. Insulin binds to specific cell-surface receptors in insulin-responsive target tissues (e.g. liver, skeletal muscle, fat). Normal hepatic glucose metabolism represents a balance between the effects of insulin and several 'counter regulatory' hormones (e.g. glucagon, cortisol, epinephrine, growth hormone). Insulin deficiency (absolute or relative due to increased resistance) associated with DM results in abnormal metabolism of carbohydrates, lipids, and amino acids.

During pregnancy, there is an increase in the insulin resistance. The insulin resistance during GDM is post-cellular defect evidenced by a decrease in phosphorylation of tyrosine residues in insulin receptors and insulin receptor substrate-1.[6] The main causes of insulin resistance are the increasing levels of cortisol, estrogen and progesterone. The increase in HPL and TNF-α and the decrease in adiponectin during pregnancy also contribute to the development of insulin

---

Classification of Diabetes Mellitus[5]

I. Type 1 diabetes (β-cell destruction, usually leading to absolute insulin deficiency)
  A. Immune mediated
  B. Idiopathic
II. Type 2 diabetes (may range from predominantly insulin resistance with relative insulin deficiency to a predominantly secretory defect with insulin resistance)
III. Other specific types
IV. Gestational diabetes mellitus

resistance. Most pregnant women counteract the insulin resistance with enhanced insulin production both in the basal state and in response to meals thus maintaining normal blood glucose levels. This increase in insulin production is not seen in those with β-cell insufficiency and they tend to show hyper- glycemia and hypo- or normoinsulinemia. Thus the insulin resistance together with beta cell insufficiency contribute to the develop- ment of impaired glucose tolerance and gestational diabetes mellitus.

Human Placental Lactogen

Human placental lactogen (HPL) is a single polypeptide chain held together by disulphide bonds. It is secreted in both the maternal and fetal circulations after the sixth week of preg- nancy. Structurally, HPL is similar to human growth hormone (HGH), but has only 3% of HGH activity and a short half-life of only 15 minutes. HPL is a potent antagonist to insulin. It causes lipolysis and increases the maternal circulating free fatty acids, thus sparing the glucose and amino acids for the fetus.[6,7]

Consequences of Maternal Hyperglycemia

Maternal hyperglycemia poses a risk for both mother and neonate. It was well established by the HAPO study (hyperglycemia and adverse pregnancy outcome) which is a multi- national epidemiological study, including 25,000 pregnant women (Table 14.2.1).[8]

Fetal Effects of Maternal Hyperglycemia

Glucose transport across the placenta takes place on the basis of concentration gradient from higher maternal concentration to lower fetal concentration. The first gradient drives the glucose from maternal blood to the placenta. The placenta consumes glucose depending upon the fetal glucose levels. With low fetal glucose levels, placental glucose consumption decreases making more glucose available to the fetus. Maternal diabetes and maternal hyperglycemia alter the fetal glucose levels, prompting fetal adaptations to hyperglycemia that may have long-term consequences on organ develop- ment of the offspring (Table 14.2.2).[8–10]

Table 14.2.1: Consequences of maternal hyperglycemia

Effects on mother	Effects on fetus
1. Pre-eclampsia	1. Macrosomia and large for gestational age infant
2. Hydramnios	2. Fetal organomegaly (hepatomegaly, cardiomegaly)
3. Maternal and infant birth trauma	3. Perinatal mortality
4. Operative delivery	4. Neonatal respiratory problems and metabolic complications (hypoglycemia, hyperbilirubinemia, hypocalcemia, erythremia)

Table 14.2.2: Fetal effects of maternal hyperglycemia

Immediate effects	Long-term effects
Macrosomia	Increased risk of diabetes in the offspring
Congenital malformation	Obesity
Fetal hypoxia	Neuropsychological deficits (poor intellectual performance
Hypoglycemia in neonates	and deficits in memory recognition)
Hypocalcemia and hypomagnesemia	Poor psychomotor development
Polycythemia and hyperbilirubinemia	Minimal brain dysfunction in children with neonatal hypogly-
Cardiomyopathy	cemia who were born to diabetic mothers
Respiratory distress syndrome	Poor auditory–verbal function

Table 14.2.3: Risk factors for gestational diabetes mellitus (GDM)

High-risk factors	Low-risk factors
History of impaired glucose tolerance or GDM	No history of glucose intolerance or adverse pregnancy outcomes due to GDM
Family history of DM/belonging to a race with high prevalence of DM	No first degree relative with diabetes/non-hispanic white
Prepregnancy BMI >30 kg/m^2/weight $\geq$110% of IBW/excessive gestational weight gain	Normal BMI (<25 kg/m^2)
Maternal age >25 years of age	Younger age (<25 years of age)
Other high-risk factors	
Previous delivery of a baby >9 pounds (4.1 kg)	
Previous unexplained perinatal loss or birth of a malformed infant	
Maternal birth weight >9 pounds (4.1 kg) or <6 pounds (2.7 kg)	
Glycosuria at the first prenatal visit	
Concurrent metabolic syndrome, PCOS, current use of glucocorticoids, hypertension	

Impaired fasting glucose—IFG: FBG—100 mg/dL to 125 mg/dL (5.6 to 6.9 mmol/L)
Impaired fasting glucose tolerance—IGT; 2hr OGTT—140 to 199 mg/dL (7.8 to 11.0 mmol/L)
HbA1c of 5.7 to 6.4%-cut-off of >5.8% (38 to 47 mmol/mol)

GESTATIONAL DIABETES MELLITUS

Risk Factors for Gestational Diabetes Mellitus (GDM)

There are certain risk factors which predispose the pregnant women to develop GDM. They are further identified as high-risk and low-risk factors.[13–15] Presence of multiple factors increases the risk of developing overt GDM (Table 14.2.3).[16–18]

Diagnostic Criteria for Gestational Diabetes Mellitus

Recommendations for Screening Women at Increased Risk of Overt Diabetes

1. International Association of Diabetes and Pregnancy Study Groups (IADPSG) criteria (endorsed by the ADA) recommend that patients at increased risk for type 2 diabetes and those at high risk of GDM be screened for diabetes using standard diagnostic criteria at their first antenatal visit.[21,22]
2. Pregnant women present with overt signs or symptoms of hyperglycemia such as polyuria, polydipsia, or glycosuria.

3. Confirmed fasting glucose levels of $\geq$7.0 mmol/L ($\geq$126 mg/dL) or random glucose levels $\geq$11.1 mmol/L ($\geq$200 mg/dL) are diagnostic of overt rather than gestational diabetes.
4. The ADA and IADPSG recommended that high-risk women with diabetes diagnosed on the basis of standard diagnostic criteria receive a diagnosis of overt rather than gestational diabetes.
5. As per ADA guidelines, women diagnosed with diabetes in the first trimester should receive a diagnosis of overt (rather than gestational) diabetes.

Recommendations for Screening Pregnant Women for Low Risk of GDM

As only less than 10% of women belong to low-risk group, it is recommended that all pregnant women be screened for GDM. The ADA guidelines recommend either one- or two-step screening methods (Table 14.2.4).[21]

Step-by-step Diagnostic Approach

At 24 to 28 weeks' gestation, all women not known to have diabetes (including high-risk

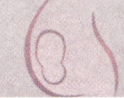

Table 14.2.4: Screening for gestational diabetes mellitus (GDM)

Pregnant women at 24 to 28 weeks not previously diagnosed with DM		
One-step strategy	Two-step strategy	

• 75 gm OGTT
• Overnight fast of at least 8 hrs
• The plasma glucose values suggestive of GDM are
  • Fasting ≥92 mg/dL (≥5.1 mmol/L)
  • 1 hour ≥180 mg/dL (≥10.0 mmol/L)
  • 2 hours ≥153 mg/dL (≥8.5 mmol/L)
	STEP 1
	• 50 gm non-fasting Sample
	• If plasma glucose after 1 hr >140—proceed to Step 2 ⟶
		STEP 2
		300 mg OGTT
		• Fasting ≥95 mg/dL (≥5.3 mmol/L)
		• 1 hour ≥180 mg/dL (≥10.0 mmol/L)
		• 2 hours ≥155 mg/dL (≥8.6 mmol/L)
		• 3 hours ≥140 mg/dL (≥7.8 mmol/L)

women, if the initial testing was normal) should undergo screening with a glucose tolerance test. It can be:

1. A one-step method using the 75 gm oral glucose tolerance test, or
2. Two-step method: 1-hour 50 gm non-fasting test, followed by a 3-hour 100 gm test, if the initial test is positive.

The IADPSG recommends a one-step test, while the National Institute of Health and the American Congress of Obstetricians and Gynecologists (ACOG) recommend a two-step test. The ADA endorses both the approaches.[21–24]

One-step method: 75 gm OGTT:

• Used to screen all pregnant women at 24 to 28 weeks gestation not previously diagnosed with overt diabetes
• The OGTT is done after an overnight fast of at least 8 hours.
• The plasma glucose values suggestive of GDM are:
  • Fasting ≥92 mg/dL (≥5.1 mmol/L)
  • 1 hour ≥180 mg/dL (≥10.0 mmol/L)
  • 2 hours ≥153 mg/dL (≥8.5 mmol/L)

Two-step approach:

• Includes a 1-hour 50 gm OGTT, which does not have to be fasting.

• Glucose thresholds of 130 or 140 mg/dL (7.2 or 7.8 mmol/L) are considered abnormal.
• If glucose levels are ≥140 mg/dL (7.8 mmol/L), then a 3-hour 100 gm OGTT is performed.
• This test is performed when the patient is fasting.
• Two or more plasma glucose levels at or above the following thresholds establish diagnosis.

Other Screening Guidelines

WHO Recommendations[25]

Table 14.2.5: WHO recommendations: 75 g, OGTT after an 8- to 14-hours fast

The diagnosis of gestational diabetes mellitus at any time during pregnancy should be based on any one of the following values:
• Fasting plasma glucose = 5.1–6.9 mmol/L (92–125 mg/dL)
• 1-hour post-75 gm oral glucose load ≥10.0 mmol/L (180 mg/dL)*
• 2-hours post-75 gm oral glucose load 8.5–11.0 mmol/L (153–199 mg/dL)

*There are no established criteria for the diagnosis of diabetes based on the 1-hour post-load value

National Institute for Health and Care Excellence (NICE) Guidelines[26,27]

NICE guidelines for screening for diabetes in pregnancy are depicted in Table 14.2.6.

Table 14.2.6: NICE guidelines for screening for diabetes in pregnancy[27,28]

The NICE guidelines recommended:
- Screening with WHO OGTT criteria at 24 to 28 weeks' gestation
- Except in women with previous GDM, who are screened at 16 to 18 weeks and again at 28 weeks if the first OGTT was normal
- First-trimester screening of high-risk women was suggested

High risks are:
- BMI >30 kg/m^2
- Previous macrosomic baby weighing >4.5 kg
- Previous GDM
- Family history of DM (first-degree relative with DM)
- Family origin in an area with high prevalence of DM
  - South Asian (specifically women whose country of family origin is India, Pakistan, or Bangladesh)
  - Black Caribbean
  - Middle Eastern

Role of HbA1c in Diagnosing GDM

HbA1c is a measure of glycosylated RBC hemoglobin. It reflects ambient glucose levels over the preceding 2 to 3 months.[26–28] Elevated preconceptional HbA1c levels are associated with fetal abnormality. HbA1c levels should be measured in all pregnant women with pre existing diabetes at the booking appointment and in the second and third trimesters of pregnancy as the level of risk for the pregnancy increases with an HbA1c level above 48 mmol/mol (6.5%).[29] HbA1c levels can be measured in all women with gestational diabetes at the time of diagnosis to identify those who may have pre-existing type 2 diabetes, but routine use of HbA1c levels in GDM in the second and third trimesters of pregnancy is not warranted.[28–31]

Antenatal Care of Pregnant Patients with Diabetes

Pregnant women diagnosed as GDM need regular antenatal checkups, risk assessment and treatment. A trial of diet control and exercise should be offered to women with fasting glucose <7 mmol/L (126 mg/dL).[33] Traditionally, short- and intermittent-acting insulin is used for control of diabetes in pregnancy. Most insulins belong to category B drugs.

Role of Oral Antidiabetic Agents in Diabetes in Pregnancy

The use of oral antidiabetic agents (ADA) in diabetes in pregnancy is controversial and has not been approved by FDA. Nevertheless ADA is being used with good results in pregnant diabetic patients. Rowan and colleagues[34] compared metformin and insulin in women with GDM. There was no difference in the neonatal complications between the 2 subject groups. They concluded that hypo-glycemia was less severe in the infants of mothers on metformin and metformin is safe to use in pregnancy. Recent NICE guidelines[28] have included oral ADA for glycemic control in pregnancy. NICE 2015 recommends metformin, if sugars are not controlled with diet and exercise alone. If metformin is contraindicated or unacceptable to the woman with a fasting glucose <7 mmol/L (126 mg/dL), insulin should be started for a better glycemic control. In pregnant women with fasting glucose >7 mmol/L at diagnosis, insulin with or without metformin should be started. For a patient with fasting glucose of 6.0 and 6.9 mmol/L with complications such as macrosomia or hydramnios, NICE 2015 recommends insulin, with or without metformin. Glibenclamide may be considered for women with gestational diabetes, in whom blood glucose targets are not achieved with metformin but who decline insulin therapy or who cannot tolerate metformin.[28]

Role of Long-acting Insulin in Diabetes in Pregnancy

Short- or intermediate-acting insulins have been used safely in pregnancy. Rapid-acting insulin analogues have superior pharmacological profiles, and more patient compliance and better glycemic control.[35,36] Insulin can be administered either as subcutaneous multiple daily injections (MDI) or as continuous subcutaneous insulin infusion pump (CSII). There was no difference either in the pregnancy outcomes or glycemic control using CSII over MDI in pregnant diabetic women.[37,38] There is limited data on using long-acting insulin analogues insulin detemir and insulin glargine in pregnancy. The regular and NPH insulins and lispro are FDA category B whereas aspart, glargine and glulisine are category C insulins. Though no harm has been documented by their use, the long-acting

insulins still need approval for use in pregnancy.[39] Informed consent should be obtained and documented before their use.

Monitoring Pregnant Women with Diabetes
(Table 14.2.7)

Monitoring Blood Glucose

Pregnant women should regularly monitor their blood glucose levels. The frequency of monitoring depends on the type of diabetes and the treatment received.

Monitoring also includes ketone testing and diabetic ketoacidosis, retinal assessment for diabetic retinopathy in type 1 diabetes, renal assessment for raising serum creatinine and nephrotic range proteinuria. Investigations should include 24 hours urine for proteinuria, liver function tests and LDH, for early detection of pre-eclampsia.[40] Fetal congenital malformations should be ruled out and fetal growth and amniotic fluid volume be assessed by ultrasound.

Timing of Delivery and Birth

Patients with well controlled DM may be allowed to progress to their expected date of delivery, as long as antenatal testing remains reassuring.[41] The ACOG states that in preGDM, optimal timing of delivery relies on

Table 14.2.7: Monitoring pregnant women with diabetes		
Type of diabetes	Monitoring required	ACOG goals for self-monitoring blood glucose
Type 1, type 2 or GDM on multiple insulin regimes	• Fasting • Pre-meal • 1-hour post-meal • Bedtime	• Fasting glucose ≤95 mg/dL (5.3 mmol/L) • Preprandial glucose concentrations no higher than 100 mg/dL (5.6 mmol/L) • One-hour postprandial glucose concentrations no higher than 140 mg/dL (7.8 mmol/L) • Two-hour postprandial glucose concentrations no higher than 120 mg/dL (6.7 mmol/L) • Mean capillary glucose 100 mg/dL (5.6 mmol/L) • During the night, glucose levels should not decrease to less than 60 mg/dL (3.3 mmol/L)
Type 2 or GDM • On diet/exercise • Oral therapy • Single dose of insulin	• Fasting • 1-hour post-meal	

Indications for continuous glucose monitoring: (1) Severe hypoglycemia (with or without impaired awareness); (2) Unstable blood glucose levels (to minimize variability) or (3) To gain information about variability in blood glucose levels.

balancing the risk of IUFD with the risks of preterm birth.[42] Decision of delivery before 37 weeks should be taken in type 1 or type 2 diabetics, if there are metabolic, maternal or fetal complications. Diabetes is not a contraindication for steroid cover in case of preterm labor. The rise in blood sugar levels induced by steroids should be corrected with additional dose of insulin, if needed.

Target Blood Glucose during Labor and Vaginal Birth

Managing glycemic control during labor is prudent to prevent maternal hyperglycemia. Avoiding intrapartum maternal hyperglycemia may prevent fetal hyperglycemia and reduce the likelihood of neonatal hypoglycemia.[43] During labor, sugars can be controlled with an intravenous infusion of 6–8 units of conventional regular insulin or analogue like lispro or aspart in 500 mL dextrose normal saline (DNS) titrated to maintain hourly readings of blood glucose between 72 and 144 mg/dl (4–8 mmol/L).[43] Patients who are using an insulin pump may continue their basal infusion during labor. During active labor, insulin use may be greatly reduced and sometimes may not be needed at all. In mothers who are GDM on lifestyle modification, monitoring blood sugars once in every 4–6 h is sufficient.[43, 44]

ANESTHESIA/ANALGESIA FOR PREGNANT WOMEN WITH DIABETES

Analgesia for Labor and Vaginal Delivery

The diabetic mother carries high chances of interventions during vaginal delivery in terms of prolonged labor, shoulder dystocia, risk of PPH due to uterine overdistention by the big baby. Adequate analgesia during the labor is best provided with labor epidural analgesia. Labor epidural has the added advantage of decreasing the maternal catecholamine levels. It also improves the uteroplacental perfusion.[45] The other modes of analgesia can be parenteral opioids either as a continuous IV infusion or patient-controlled IV infusion. Inhalation with entonox has been described but may not be ideal in diabetic parturient with high risk of aspiration. The epidural catheter can be used for providing surgical anesthesia as in case of operative delivery or assisted vaginal delivery or for procedures like retained placenta.

Anesthesia for Cesarean Section

The perioperative management of pregnant patient with diabetes starts with the preanesthetic evaluation for glycemic control and other existing comorbidities like preeclampsia. Elective cesarean should be preferred in the morning hours. Patient should be given the night dose of intermediate-acting insulin and the morning dose of insulin has to be withheld. An 8-hr fasting is required to decrease the risk of aspiration.

Regional anesthesia is preferred either as a subarachnoid block or an epidural or combined spinal epidural anesthesia. The decreased local anesthetic requirement of pregnancy can be exaggerated by the increased sensitivity of diabetics to local anesthetic drugs. Aim should be to avoid hypotension with low dose local anesthetics for cesarean section. Regional anesthesia can decrease the catecholamine surge and also can be extended for postoperative pain relief.[45,46]

General anesthesia, if opted for, needs more vigilance. Acid aspiration prophylaxis is mandatory. The obstetric difficult airway situation can be amplified by the limited atlanto-occipital joint extension and the associated high BMI. Rapid sequence induction with cricoids pressure should be opted. Laryngosympathetic response should be suppressed by drugs like dexmedetomidine started as an infusion at the time of premedication, especially in patients with associated pre-eclampsia. The association of preeclampsia with end organ damage, like diabetic nephropathy and autonomic neuropathy, can add to the perioperative risk of pulmonary edema due to low colloid osmotic pressure.[45–47]

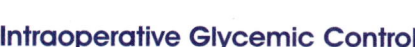

Intraoperative Glycemic Control

All the patients posted for cesarean delivery should have the fasting blood sugar done on the day of surgery. Intraoperative glycemic control depends on the perioperative control of sugars. Patients with GDM on diet control and type 2 diabetics with well-controlled sugars can be managed with non-dextrose solutions and monitoring of capillary blood glucose. Intraoperative insulin infusion is required in patients with uncontrolled sugars. The insulin requirement falls after placental delivery and should be monitored.

Postpartum Care

1. Glycemic control: Following delivery, HPL decreases returning the insulin sensitivity to pre-pregnancy state. If the patient is started on intraoperative insulin infusion, the rate of infusion should be decreased or stopped depending on the capillary glucose levels. Well-controlled diabetic patients on low dose of insulin may not require insulin supplementation after delivery.
2. Women on oral agents or diet before pregnancy, insulin should be used only if the patient has documented postpartum hyperglycemia.
3. Care should be taken to prevent wound infection.
4. Postpartum thromboprophylaxis should be given either as mechanical (stockings or SCD—sequential compression device) or with pharmacological agents like LMWH or a combination of both.
5. Postoperative analgesia can be provided either by epidural infusion of local anesthetic and opioid. Parenteral opioids and NSAIDs can be used in patients who do not have an epidural.

Neonatal Care

Neonates of diabetic mothers need extra care due to high risk of respiratory distress, hypoglycemia and hypocalcemia. Blood tests for polycythemia, hyperbilirubinemia, hypocalcemia and hypomagnesemia should be done where indicated. Breastfeeding should be commenced as early as possible. Though insulin and metformin get secreted in small amounts in breast milk, they are unlikely to cause hypoglycemia.[48] In general, infants born to diabetic mothers should have glucose testing done immediately and 2–4 hours after birth. Oral feeds or IV dextrose should be given, if blood glucose level <2 μmol/L (<36 mg/dL).

SUMMARY

- The insulin resistance together with beta cell insufficiency contribute to the development of impaired glucose tolerance and gestational diabetes mellitus.
- Maternal hyperglycemia prompts fetal adaptations to fetal hyperglycemia that may have long-term consequences on organ development of the offspring.
- Screening is done at 24 to 28 weeks' gestation in pregnant women not known to have diabetes. It can be a one-step method using the 75 gm oral glucose tolerance test or two-step method.
- WHO recommendations: 75 gm OGTT after an 8- to 14-hour fast.
- HbA1c levels should be measured in all pregnant women with pre-existing diabetes at the booking appointment and in the second and third trimesters of pregnancy.
- Routine use of HbA1c levels in GDM in the second and third trimesters of pregnancy is not warranted.
- Recent NICE guidelines[28] have included oral antidiabetic agents for glycemic control in pregnancy. NICE 2015 recommends metformin for GDM, if sugars are not controlled with diet and exercise alone.
- During labor, sugars should be controlled to maintain hourly readings between 72 and 144 mg/dL (4–8 mmol/L).
- Labor epidural has the added advantage of decreasing the maternal catecholamine levels and improves the uteroplacental perfusion.

- Regional anesthesia is preferred to general anesthesia as the later has increased risk of aspiration and airway difficulty.
- Postpartum thromboprophylaxis should be started in high-risk diabetic mothers.
- Neonates of diabetic mothers need extra care due to high risk of respiratory distress, hypoglycemia and hypocalcemia.
- A pregnancy complicated by diabetes mellitus (DM) requires a multidisciplinary approach to facilitate a healthy outcome of mother and child.

REFERENCES

1. Global status report on noncommunicable diseases 2014. Geneva, World Health Organization, 2012. WHO fact sheet

2. Abishek R, Jayashree TM, Felix AJW, Ethirajan N, Senthil Murugan TK. Study on frequency and duration of peripheral neuropathy among known case of type 1 diabetes mellitus ≥30 years in chidambaram urban population. Asian J Pharm Res 2014;4(3)141–5.

3. International Association of Diabetes and Pregnancy Study Groups Consensus Panel, Metzger BE, Gabbe SG, et al International association of diabetes and pregnancy study groups recommendations on the diagnosis and classification of hyperglycemia in pregnancy. Diabetes Care 2010;33:676.

4. Arivudainambi Kayal, Ranjit Mohan Anjana, Viswanathan Mohan. Gestational diabetes—an update from India. Diabetes Voice 2013;58(2).

5. American Diabetes Association Diagnosis and classification of diabetes mellitus. Diabetes Care 2010;33(Suppl 1):S62–S69.

6. M C Al-Noaemi, M HF Shalayel. Pathophysiology of Gestational Diabetes Mellitus: The Past, the Present and the Future, ISBN: 978-953-307-581-5, In Tech, Available from: http://www.intechopen.com/books/gestationaldiabetes/pathophysiology-of-gestational-diabetes-mellitus-the-past-the-present-and-the-future

7. Kautzky–Willer, Alexandra. Pathogenesis of Gestational DM [internet] 2015 Jan 13; Diapedia 41040851394 rev.no.19.

8. Metzger BE, Lowe LP, Dyer AR, et al. HAPO Study Cooperative Research Group. Hyperglycemia and adverse pregnancy outcomes. N Engl J Med 2008;358:1991–2002.

9. Lager S, Powell TL. Regulation of nutrient transport across the placenta. Journal of Pregnancy, Volume 2012 (2012), Article ID 179827, 14 pages.

10. Hay WW. Placental-fetal glucose exchange and fetal glucose metabolism. Trans Am Clin Climatol Assoc 2006;117:321–40.

11. Oma d D Persaud. Maternal diabetes and the consequences for her offspring. Journal on Developmental Disabilities, vol. 13 no. 1, 2007.

12. Lila-Sabrina Fetita, Eugéne Sobngwi, Patricia Serradas, Fabien Calvo, Jean-François Gautier. REVIEW: Consequences of Fetal Exposure to Maternal Diabetes in Offspring The Journal of Clinical Endocrinology & Metabolism 91(10):3718–24.

13. Setji TL, Brown AJ, Feinglos MN. Gestational diabetes mellitus. Clinical Diabetes 2005;23:17–24.

14. Hiller TA, Pedula KL Schmidt MM. Childhood obesity and metabolic imprinting: the ongoing effects of maternal hyperglycemia. Diabetes Care 2007;30:2287.

15. Landon MB , Varner MM , Willet WC, Carey VJ. A prospective study of gestational diabetes mellitus JAMA 1997;278:1078

16. Kim C, Liu T, Valdez R, Beckles GL. Does frank diabetes in first-degree relatives of a pregnant woman affect the likelihood of her developing gestational diabetes mellitus or nongestational diabetes? Am J Obstet Gynecol 2009;201:576.

17. Hedderson MM, Williams MA, Holt VL. Body mass index and weight gain prior to pregnancy and risk of gestational diabetes mellitus. Am J Obstet Gynecol 2008;198:409.

18. Heddeson MM, Gunderson E, Ferrara. A gestational weight gain and risk of gestational diabetes mellitus. Obstet Gynecol 2010;115:597.

19. Gibson KS, Waters TP, Catalano PM. Maternal weight gain in women who develop gestational diabetes mellitus. Obstet Gynecol 2012;119:560.

20. Carreno CA, Clifton RG, Hauth JC. Ecessive early gestational weight gain and risk of gestational diabetes mellitus in nulliparous women. Obstet Gynecol 2012;119:1227.

21. American Diabetes Association. Standards of medical care in diabetes–2015. Diabetes Care 2015;38:S1–S93.

22. Metzger BE, Gabbe SG, Persson B, et al. International Association of Diabetes and Pregnancy Study Groups Consensus Panel. International association of diabetes and pregnancy study groups recommendations on the diagnosis and classification of hyperglycemia in pregnancy. Diabetes Care 2010;33:676–82.

23. Committee on Practice Bulletins–Obstetrics. Practice Bulletin No. 137: gestational diabetes mellitus. Obstet Gynecol 2013;122(2 Pt 1):406–16.

24. Vandorsten JP, Dodson WC, Espeland MA, et al. NIH consensus development conference: diagnosing gestational diabetes mellitus. NIH Consens State Sci Statements 2013;29:1–31.

25. Berggren EK, Boggess KA, Stuebe Alison M, Funk MJ. National Diabetes Data Group versus Carpenter-Coustan Criteria to Diagnose Gestational Diabetes. Am J Obstet Gynecol 2011;205(3): 253.1–253.7.

26. World Health Organization, International Diabetes Federation. Definition and diagnosis of diabetes mellitus and intermediate hyperglycemia: report of a WHO/IDF consultation, 2006.

27. National Collaborating Centre for Women's and Children's Health. Diabetes in pregnancy: management of diabetes and its complications from preconception to the postnatal period. July 2008.

28. Diabetes in pregnancy: Management of diabetes and its complications from preconception to the postnatal period NICE guideline Published: 25 February 2015 nice.org.uk/guidance/ng3

29. Homko CJ, Khandelwal M. Glucose monitoring and insulin therapy during pregnancy. Obstet Gynecol Clin North Am 1996;23:47–74.

30. Agarwal MM, Dhatt GS, Punnose J, et al Gestational diabetes: a reappraisal of HBA1c as a screening test. Acta Obstet Gynecol Scand 2005;84:1159–63.

31. Agarwal MM, Hughes PF, Punnose J, et al. Gestational diabetes screening of a multiethnic, high-risk population using glycated proteins. Diabetes Res Clin Pract 2001;51:67–73.

32. Gavard JA, Artal R. Effect of exercise on pregnancy outcome. Clin Obstet Gynecol 2008;51: 467–80.

33. Rowan JA, Hague WM, Gao W, et al. Metformin versus insulin for the treatment of gestational diabetes. N Engl J Med 2008;358:2003–15.

34. Durnwald CP. Insulin analogues in the treatment of gestational diabetes mellitus. Clin Obstet Gynecol 2013;56(4):816–26.

35. Deepaklal MC, Joseph K, Rekha K, Nandita T. Insulin aspart in patients with gestational diabetes mellitus and pregestational diabetes mellitus. Indian J Endocr Metab 2015;19:658–62.

36. Farrar D, Tuffnell Dj, West J. Continuous subcutaneous insulin infusion versus multiple daily injections of insulin for pregnant women with diabetes. Cochrane Database Syst Rev 2007;18(3).

37. Mukhopadhyay A, Farrell T, Fraser RB. Continuous subcutaneous insulin infusion vs intensive conventional insulin therapy in pregnant diabetic women: a systematic review and metaanalysis of randomized, controlled trials. Am J Obstet Gynecol 2007;197(5):447–56.

38. Ansar S, Mian S, Roth S, Hebdon GM, Aldasouqi S, et al. (2013). Safety of Insulin Glargine in Pregnancy. J Diabetes Metab 4: 240. doi:10.4172/ 2155-6156.1000240

39. Yogev Y, Langer O, Brustman L, Rosenn B. Preeclampsia and gestational diabetes mellitus: does a correlation exist early in pregnancy? J Matern Fetal Neonatal Med 2004;15(1):39.

40. Peled Y, Perri T, Chen R, Pardo J, Bar J, Hod M. Gestational diabetes mellitus—implications of different treatment protocols. J Pediatr Endocrinol Metab 2004;17:847–52.

41. American College of Obstetricians and Gynecologists Committee on Practice Bulletins— Obstetrics. ACOG Practice Bulletin. Clinical management guidelines for obstetrician-gynecologists. No. 30, Sept. 2001 (replaces Technical Bulletin Number 200, December 1994). Gestational diabetes. Obstet Gynecol 2001;98:525–38.

42. Hen Y Sela, Itamar Raz, Uriel Elchala. Managing labor and delivery of the diabetic mother. Expert Rev Obstet Gynecol 2009;4(5):547–54.

43. Pramila Kalra, Manjunath Anakal. Peripartum management of diabetes. Indian J Endocrinol Metab 2013;17(Suppl 1):S72–S76. doi: 10.4103/ 2230-8210.119510

44. Glosten B. Anesthesia for obstetrics. In: Miller RD (Ed). Churchill-Davidson's A Practice of Anesthesia. 5 th ed. Vol. 2. London: Arnold. 2003; pp. 2024–68.

45. Richard N Wissler. Endocrine Disorders. In: Chestnut's Obstetric Anesthesia: Principles and Practice, 4th ed, Philadelphia: Elsevier 2009; pp. 913–22.

46. Nibedita Pani, Mishra SB, Rath SK. Diabetic parturient—anaesthetic implications. Indian J Anaesth 2010;54(5):387 93.

47. Gabbe SG, Graves CR. Management of diabetes mellitus complicating pregnancy. Obstet Gynecol 2003;102:857–68.

48. Glatstein MM, Djokanovic N, Bournissen FG, Finkelstein Y, Koren G. Use of hypoglycemic drugs during lactation. Can Fam Physician. 2009; 55(4):371–73.

14.3 THYROID DISORDERS (Pathophysiology, Clinical Presentation, Interaction with Pregnancy and Anesthetic Management)

INTRODUCTION

Thyroid disorders are not uncommon in pregnancy. Both hypothyroidism and hyper-thyroidism can be detected first time in pregnancy. The screening, evaluation of the disorder and treatment of the pregnant patient should be much more meticulous than in the non-pregnant population. A better under-standing of the physiological changes in pregnancy helps in evaluating the thyroid function tests in pregnancy.

PHYSIOLOGY OF THYROID GLAND

The follicular cells of the thyroid gland sequester iodine and synthesize thyroglobulin, an iodinated precursor protein. Thyroglobulin is secreted into the lumen of the microscopic thyroid follicles before it undergoes reuptake, proteolysis, and transfer to lysosomes, where it undergoes degradation. This process results in the systemic release of the thyroid hormones: thyroxine (T4) and 3,5,32-triiodo-thyronine (T3).

Thyroid hormone synthesis and release are controlled primarily by thyroid-stimulating hormone (TSH)—a tropic hormone from the pituitary and the supply of iodine. There is a negative feedback loop that regulates TSH secretion and thyrotropin-releasing hormone production in the hypothalamus. Thyroid hormones are highly bound to protein in the blood.

In euthyroid non-pregnant humans, the normal total serum concentrations of T4 and T3 are 50 to150 nmol/L and 1.4 to 3.2 nmol/L, respectively. A proportion of T4 and T3 are bound to three major plasma proteins which are (1) thyroxine-binding globulin (70 to 80%), (2) thyroxine-binding prealbumin or trans-thyretin (10 to 20%), and (3) albumin (10 to 15%). Thyroid hormones are temporarily inert while bound to plasma proteins.

The unbound or free fractions of T4 and T3 are 0.03 and 0.3% of total circulating T4 and T3, respectively. The serum concentration of unbound or free T4 is typically the major determinant of thyroid hormone activity in target tissues. Thyroid hormone action does not change with fluctuations in the total concentration of T4 as long as the concen-tration of free T4 remains constant.

Effect of Thyroid on Various Systems

Thyroid hormone is an endocrine regulator in many target organs (e.g. liver, kidneys, skeletal and cardiac muscles, brain, pituitary, and placenta).

The physiologic effects include:
1. Somatic and nervous system develop-ment
2. Calorigenesis
3. Augmented skeletal and cardiac muscle performance
4. Intermediary metabolism
5. Feedback control

In target tissues, the molecular actions of T4 begin with the enzymatic deiodination of T4 to T3 by iodothyronine deiodinase. Only 20% of the daily T3 production is secreted by the thyroid gland; the rest is formed by peripheral deiodination. In the classic model of thyroid hormone action, T3 enters the nuclei of target cells, binds to specific thyroid hormone receptors, and alters genomic transcription of specific proteins. Research has now characterized other mechanisms of thyroid hormone action, including mito-chondrial transcription and cytoplasmic or cell-surface non-transcriptional effects. The thyroid hormone receptor belongs to a family of structurally related, intracellular ligand binding proteins.

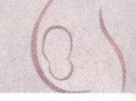

Anatomical and Physiological Adaptations of Thyroid during Pregnancy

The thyroid gland enlarges by 50 to 70% during pregnancy because of follicular hyperplasia and increased blood supply. The major changes in thyroid function during pregnancy are due to stimulation of the thyrotropin (TSH) receptor by human chorionic gonadotropin (hCG) (Table 14.3.1). hCG has weak thyroid-stimulating activity due to structural similarity between the beta-subunits of hCG and TSH. There has been inverse relationship between the level of hCG and TSH during pregnancy. During early pregnancy (10–12 weeks), serum hCG concentrations peak and serum TSH concentrations are appropriately reduced. This decrease in TSH is accompanied by an increase in serum free T4 and T3 levels manifesting as a physiological subclinical hyperthyroidism. As the pregnancy progresses, hCG secretion decreases, serum free T4 and T3 and serum TSH concentrations return to within the normal range.

Maternal TBG, T4 and T3 Levels

Increased estrogen levels in pregnancy increases the production and decreases the clearance of TBG (thyroxine-binding globulin). This results in a twofold increase in serum TBG concentrations and leads to an increase in both serum total triiodothyronine (T3) and thyroxine (T4) concentrations. The overall production rate of thyroid hormones returns to prepregnancy state by 20 weeks of gestation.

Increased maternal T4 increases the iodine requirement in pregnancy. Added to this the increased renal clearance of iodide in pregnancy due to increased GFR and decreased dietary intake can cause maternal iodine deficiency. Severe maternal iodine deficiency can cause decreased maternal thyroxine production, decreased placental transfer of thyroxine, resulting in impaired neurologic development in the fetus. 250 µg of iodine daily during pregnancy and lactation is the recommendation by the World Health Organization (WHO).

Thyroid Function Tests in Pregnancy—Laboratory Values

The guidelines of the American Thyroid Association (ATA) for the diagnosis and management of thyroid disease during pregnancy and postpartum recommend trimester-specific reference ranges for TSH and trimester/method-specific reference ranges for serum free T4. Direct free T4 measurements may be unreliable during pregnancy. Serum total T4 measurements are more reliable and can be measured to assess thyroid function during pregnancy. During pregnancy, the increase in TBG may cause 1.5-fold higher total T4 and T3 levels than in non-pregnant women.

THYROID DISORDERS IN PREGNANCY

Hyperthyroidism Complicating Pregnancy

The prevalence of hyperthyroidism in the general population is 0.2 to 1.9%. The incidence in pregnancy ranges from 0.1 to 0.4% of pregnant women. Most common causes of hyperthyroidism in pregnancy are Graves' (0.1 to 1% of all pregnancies) and hCG-mediated hyperthyroidism (1 to 3%). The other causes are rare in pregnant population.

Table 14.3.1: Physiological changes in pregnancy in thyroid

1. Increase in the size of the gland
2. Decreased TSH levels depending on the gestational age
   - First trimester: 0.24–2.99
   - Second trimester: 0.46–2.95
   - Third trimester: 0.43–2.78
3. Increased production and decreased clearance of TBG (estrogen effect)
4. Increased total serum T4 and total serum T3 (1.5 × normal)
5. Normal serum free T4 and free T3
6. Increased renal iodide clearance (due to increased GFR)

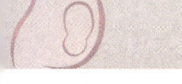

Etiology of Hyperthyroidism

Abnormal thyroid stimulation

- Graves' disease
- Gestational trophoblastic neoplasia
- TSH-secreting pituitary tumor

Intrinsic thyroid autonomy

- Toxic adenoma
- Toxic multinodular goiter

Inflammatory disease

- Subacute thyroiditis

Extrinsic hormone source

- Ectopic thyroid tissue
- Thyroid hormone ingestion

Hyperthyroid States Peculiar to Pregnancy

Gestational transient thyrotoxicosis (GTT): It occurs in the first trimester with peak hCG concentrations (10 to 12 weeks). Diagnosed by the laboratory findings of raised total serum T4 and T3 concentrations and decreased TSH levels. Free T4 and T3 are usually within the normal range. Mostly asymptomatic, the clinical features and laboratory finding subside as the pregnancy progresses.

Hyperthyroidism with hyperemesis gravidarum: Serum hCG and estradiol concentrations are found to be more in pregnant patients with hyperemesis gravidarum. The thyroid-stimulating activity was also found to be more in women with hyperemesis. hCG-mediated hyperthyroidism subsides as hCG production falls with progression of pregnancy.

Trophoblastic hyperthyroidism: Gestational trophoblastic diseases, hydatidiform mole and choriocarcinoma are associated with high and abnormal isoforms serum hCG. They manifest hCG-stimulated hyperthyroidism. Patients present with nausea and vomiting. Patients with advanced gestational age may have clinical findings of hyperthyroidism and a diffuse goiter, but typically no ophthalmopathy.

Brémont et al. described *'Familial gestational hyperthyroidism'* caused by a mutant thyrotropin receptor hypersensitive to physiological hCG.

Postpartum hyperthyroidism: Pregnant patients with Graves' disease may have an exacerbation in the postpartum period. Postpartum thyroiditis also can cause features of hyperthyroidism after delivery.

Pathophysiology

Graves' disease is an autoimmune thyroid disease. The immune modulated state of pregnancy lowers the incidence of auto-immune disorders in the pregnant patients. Prevalence of Graves' disease in pregnancy is 0.2%, which is lower than in the general population. Pathophysiology of Graves' disease involves the presence of autoanti-bodies or thyroid receptor antibodies (TRAbs) directed against the TSH receptor in the thyroid gland. These antibodies may either augment or inhibit TSH action.

Clinical Presentation

Hyperthyroidism presents as a physiologic state dominated by an increased metabolic rate. A hyperthyroid symptom scale has been developed on the basis of the following 10 clinical factors: nervousness, sweating, heat intolerance, hyperactivity, tremor, weakness, hyperdynamic precordium, diarrhea, appetite, and level of incapacitation. These symptoms may be confused with the non-specific symptoms of pregnancy. Specific signs, like goiter or ophthalmopathy, suggest Graves' hyperthyroidism. hCG-mediated hyperthy-roidism may occur transiently in the early weeks of pregnancy, is less severe than Graves' disease and not associated with goitre.

Subclinical hyperthyroidism is an abnor-mally suppressed TSH with a normal FT4 level. Incidence is 1.5% of pregnant women. It is more common in patients with hyperemesis gravidarum and is not associated with any adverse pregnancy outcomes.

Thyroid nodules occur in 4 to 7% of adults. Pregnancy is associated with increase in the number and size of thyroid nodules. Pregnancy probably does not affect the development or progression of thyroid carcinoma, but this conclusion remains controversial.

Laboratory Findings

1. TSH levels <0.1 mU/L (suppressed) or <0.01 mU/L (undetectable).
2. High serums free T4 and/or free T3 or total T4 and/or total T3.

   (In Graves' disease, T3 toxicity only T3 is elevated whereas both T4 and T3 are elevated in hCG-mediated hyperthyroidism).
3. Thyrotropin (TSH) receptor antibodies (TRAb), using a second-generation thyrotropin-binding inhibitory immunoglobulin (TBII) assay should be done, if Graves' disease is suspected (universal screening for thyroid autoantibodies in pregnancy is not recommended).
4. US thyroid with Doppler flow to distinguish Graves' disease (high blood flow) from painless or postpartum thyroiditis (low blood flow).
5. Fine-needle aspiration or percutaneous needle biopsy useful in nodules.

   Radionuclide imaging to distinguish Graves' disease from thyroiditis is contraindicated in pregnant women and should be delayed till postpartum.

Management of Hyperthyroidism in Pregnancy

Pregnant patients with hyperthyroidism can be asymptomatic where no treatment is essential. These patients need to be monitored with TSH, free T4 and/or total T4 or total T3 every four to six weeks.

A. No treatment is necessary in (Low TSH. Total T4 or T3 <1.5 times the upper limit of the non-pregnant normal):

1. Patients with hCG-mediated hyperthyroidism

2. Pregnant women with subclinical hyperthyroidism (low TSH, normal free T4)
3. Pregnant patients with asymptomatic hyperthyroidism (low TSH, normal free T4/T3) due to Graves' disease toxic adenoma, or toxic multinodular goiter may be followed with no treatment

B. Symptomatic patients with hyperthyroidism (Low TSH. Total T4 and/or total T3 >1.5 times the upper limit of the non-pregnant normal): The treatment options can be medical or surgical. Radio-iodine is contraindicated in pregnancy.

1. Medical Management

Thiamides: Propylthiouracil (PTU), methimazole (MMI) and carbimazole (CBZ), which is completely metabolized to MMI, are the antithyroid medications available. These drugs interfere with the incorporation of iodine into thyroglobulin and with subsequent coupling reactions in the thyroid gland. Propylthiouracil also inhibits iodothyronine deiodinase in peripheral tissues. Medical management can be summarized as in Table 14.3.2.

The goal is to control maternal hyperthyroidism and at the same time minimize fetal hypothyroidism. Euthyroid state has to be maintained and confirmed with thyroid function tests performed two to four weeks after switching to MMI and every four weeks throughout pregnancy.

2. Surgery for Hyperthyroidism in Pregnancy

Thyroidectomy is indicated during pregnancy for the patients with non-compliance to thioamides. Surgery should be opted in the second trimester to minimize the risk of spontaneous abortion and premature delivery. Higher rates of surgical complications are encountered in pregnant than non-pregnant women.

Preoperative optimization includes beta-blockers (atenolol or propranolol) for 7–10 days and potassium iodine solution

Table 14.3.2: Antithyroid and adjuvants in medical management of hyperthyroidism

S.no.	Drug	Gestational age	Dose	Side effects
1.	Propylthiouracil	1st trimester	50–100 mg times	Sudden onset and a rapidly progressive liver disease Leukopenia
2.	Methimazole	From 2nd trimester	5 to 20 mg twice daily	Congenital anomalies if used in 1st trimester/rash/leukopenia
3.	Carbimazole	From 2nd trimester	Atenolol 25–50 mg/day	Rash/leukopenia
4.	Beta blockers for symptomatic control	Should be tapered by 2–6 weeks	Propranolol 20 mg × 6–8 hourly	Neonatal growth restriction, hypoglycemia, respiratory depression and bradycardia

(35 to 50 mg iodine per drop, 1 to 3 drops daily). Iodine lowers serum thyroid hormone concentrations acutely and, in addition, decreases thyroid gland vascularity.

Thyroid storm: Thyroid strom also known as thyroid crisis is a life-threatening exacerbation or decompensation of a pre-existing hyper thyroid state. It is a clinical diagnosis based on signs and symptoms. Pregnancy itself is a precipitant of thyroid storm (Table 14.3.3).

Perioperative complications of thyroid surgery

1. Unilateral or bilateral vocal cord paralysis secondary to laryngeal nerve injury
2. Wound hematoma
3. Pneumothorax
4. Hypoparathyroidism
5. Thyroid storm
6. Hypocalcemia

Table 14.3.3: Thyroid—signs and symptoms and their management

Signs and symptoms	Precipitating events	Management
Hyperthermia	Surgery	1. Propylthiouracil 300–600 mg followed by 150–300 mg every 6 hours oral/NG tube/rectally (or)
Tachycardia	Labor and delivery	
Tachypnea	Trauma	
Abdominal pain	Iodinated contrast agents	2. Methimazole (20–25 mg 6 hourly)
Mental and emotional disturbances	Treatment with iodine-131	3. Saturated solution of KI 2–5 drops every 8 hours (or)
Diarrhea diaphoresis and dehydration	Emotional stress	4. NaI 0.5–1 g IV 8th hourly
Congestive cardiac failure	Pulmonary embolism	5. β-Blockers to decrease CV effects
Arrhythmias and atrial fibrillation	Stroke	6. Cold fluids, antipyretics cooling blanket
		7. Dexamethasone 2 mg/hydrocortisone 100 mg every 6 hours
Cardiovascular collapse	Infection	8. Correction of electrolyte imbalance
Laboratory findings		9. Phenobarbitone for restlessness
Leukocytosis	Diabetic ketoacidosis	10. Plasma exchange
Elevated LFT	Hypoglycemia	
Low TSH, high free T4 and/or T3	Congestive heart failure	
Hypercalcemia	Bowel infarction in the perioperative period	

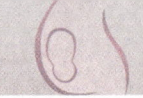

Table 14.3.4: Cause and effect of thyroid on fetus	
Effect of hyperthyroidism on pregnancy	Effect on fetus
1. Maternal hypertension/pre-eclampsia 2. Preterm labor 3. Anemia 4. Iodine deficiency 5. Thyroid storm	1. Early pregnancy loss 2. Fetal growth restriction 3. Low birth weight 4. Cardiac failure and hydrops 5. Stillbirth 6. Fetal goiter 7. Neonatal thyrotoxicosis

Obstetric Concerns of Hyperthyroidism Complicating Pregnancy

Pregnant patients with treated hyperthyroidism have perinatal outcomes similar to those for euthyroid parturients. Poorly controlled hyperthyroidism during pregnancy increases the risks to both mother and the fetus (Table 14.3.4).

Fetal monitoring: In women with Graves' disease, the placental transfer of antithyroid medications or thyroid-stimulating antibodies may result in fetal hyperthyroidism. All fetuses must be monitored for fetal tachycardia (>160 beats/minute) suggestive of fetal hyperthyroidism. Ultrasound can be used to detect fetal growth restriction, fetal goitre, advanced bone age, and craniosynostosis. Umbilical vein sampling after 20 weeks of gestation carries high risk of fetal loss and should be restricted only to the cases of ultrasound suspicion of fetal hyperthyroidism. The development of fetal goiter can interfere with vaginal delivery or lead to airway obstruction in the newborn and is best managed by *ex utero* intrapartum treatment (EXIT) procedure.

Anesthetic Management of Hyperthyroidism Complicating Pregnancy

The anesthetic management in patients is affected by:
1. The hyperdynamic cardiovascular system and the possibility of cardiomyopathy,
2. Partial airway obstruction secondary to an enlarged thyroid gland,
3. Respiratory muscle weakness, and
4. Electrolyte abnormalities.

Planned elective LSCS for obstetric indication should be only after control of the hyperthyroid state. Pregnant women with uncontrolled hyperthyroidism can be encountered for emergency cesarean delivery or vaginal delivery in labor.

When planning the mode of anesthesia, regional anesthesia seems safer than general anesthesia technique. Central neuraxial blockade both subarachnoid block and epidural are found to be safe in hyperthyroidism complicating pregnancy. Direct acting vasopressors, like phenylephrine, should be preferred over ephedrine or mephenteramine. Glycopyrrolate should be preferred over atropine for spinal-induced bradycardia.

Labor epidural can be safely administered and is advantageous by decreasing the sympathetic stimulation. Both obstetrician and the anesthesiologist should be aware of the fact that thyroid storm can be precipitated in uncontrolled hyperthyroid mothers during labor and childbirth. Precautions should be taken to prevent and tackle the problem, if arises.

General anesthesia when required is associated with intrinsic obstetric difficult airway compounded with the difficulty associated with hyperthyroidism. It is prudent to avoid medications associated with tachycardia. Anticholinergic drugs (i.e. atropine) may precipitate tachycardia and alter heat-regulating mechanisms and are better avoided.

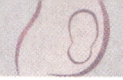

Premedication with barbiturate, benzodiaze-pine, and/or a narcotic are not routinely advised in pregnancy due to risks of maternal aspiration and neonatal depression. In emergency cases, the use of an intravenous β-blocker, ipodate, cortisol, or dexamethasone and PTU can be resorted to, with meticulous invasive hemodynamic monitoring. Thiopen-tone sodium has the theatrical advantage of decreasing the peripheral conversion of T4 to T3 but propofol gives the required depth of anesthesia. Drugs that stimulate the SNS, like ketamine, pancuronium, atropine, and epine-phrine, should be avoided. Rapid sequence induction (RSI) has been used safely with succinylcholine or rocuronium. Non-depolari-zing agents with limited hemodynamic effects and minimal or no histamine release are preferred (vecuronium, rocuronium). Inhala-tion agents may be used for maintenance of anesthesia, and for decreasing the awareness during general anesthesia. The increased BMR increases the minimum alveolar concentration (MAC) and may cause hepatotoxicity. Eye protection with eye pads is important in all, more so for patients with proptosis. Glyco-pyrrolate should be used for reversal instead of atropine in combination with an acetylcho-linesterase inhibitor. Every precaution should be taken to prevent and treat thyroid storm and malignant hyperthermia.

Goals of Anesthesia

Regional techniques preferred (SAB/epidural/CSE)

Phenylephrine preferred for spinal hypotension

Anticipate airway difficulty

Glycopyrrolate preferred over atropine

Avoid sympathetic stimulation

Maintain adequate depth

Anticipate/avoid and keep things ready to tackle thyroid storm

---

Hypothyroidism in Pregnancy

Definition and Epidemiology

Hypothyroidism is defined as an abnormal decrease in the serum concentration of unbound or free thyroid hormones. The prevalence of hypothyroidism in the general population is 0.1 to 2%, which is similar to that of hyperthyroidism. Hypothyroidism is more common in women and the elderly.

Pathophysiology

Hypothyroidism complicates between 1 and 3, in 1000 pregnancies. Hypothyroidism can be divided into primary and secondary. Primary is inadequate thyroid hormone production despite pituitary gland stimulation and insufficient stimulation of the thyroid by the pituitary or hypothalamus is secondary or central hypothyroidism. **Tertiary hypo-thyroidism** is the disorder where the hypo-thalamus is damaged or conditions where the delivery of TRH to the pituitary is prevented by the interference of hypothalamic–pituitary portal blood flow.

Etiology of Hypothyroidism

Etiology of hypothyroidism in pregnancy is given in Table 14.3.5.

Clinical Presentation

Table 14.3.6 shows clinical presentation of hypothyroidism in pregnancy.

Diagnosis of Hypothyroidism In Pregnancy

Thyroid function tests should be interpreted with knowledge of the changes in thyroid physiology during normal pregnancy. During pregnancy, there is a decrease in TSH, increase in TBG, and increased serum total T4 and T3 (1.5-fold higher than in nonpregnant women).

Serum TSH is more sensitive than free T4 for detecting hypothyroidism. Evaluation of free T4 is recommended if the TSH is abnormal. Based on this, the pregnant patient may be diagnosed as having, overt (elevated TSH and low free T4) or subclinical (elevated TSH, free T4 in normal reference range) hypothyroidism.

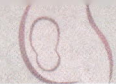

Table 14.3.5: Etiology of hypothyroidism in pregnancy

Primary	Secondary
Autoimmune	*Pituitary dysfunction*
• Hashimoto's thyroiditis	• Irradiation
• Atrophic hypothyroidism	• Surgery
Iatrogenic	• Neoplasm
• Radioiodine therapy for hyperthyroidism	• Sheehan's syndrome
• Subtotal thyroidectomy	• Idiopathic
Pharmacologic	
• Iodine deficiency or excess	
• Lithium	
• Amiodarone	
• Antithyroid drugs	
Congenital	*Hypothalamic dysfunction*
• Dyshormonogenesis	• Irradiation
• Thyroid gland dysgenesis or agenesis	• Granulomatous disease
	• Neoplasm

Table 14.3.6: Clinical presentation of hypothyroidism in pregnancy

	Symptoms	Signs
Fatigue and weakness	Edema	Ascites
Hoarseness	Weight gain	Bradycardia
Cold intolerance	Myalgia and paresthesia	Coarse skin
Constipation	Menorrhagia	Carotenemia
Clots and menorrhagia	Arthralgia	Delayed tendon reflexes
Cognitive dysfunction	Pubertal delay	Galactorrhea
Dyspnea on exertion	Mental retardation (infantile onset)	Puffy facies, Large tongue
Decreased hearing		Periorbital edema
Dry skin		Pleural and pericardial effusions
Depression		Slow movement and slow speech

1. *Overt hypothyroidism*: The upper limit of normal for TSH in the first trimester of pregnancy is approximately 2.5 mU/L ,(3.0 mU/L in the second and third trimesters) rather than 4.5 to 5.0 mU/L used in non-pregnant population.
2. *Subclinical hypothyroidism:* Normal free T4 with elevated TSH.
3. *Isolated maternal hypothyroxinemia:* Low free T4 levels (free T4 concentration in the lower 5th or 10th percentile of the reference range), in conjunction with a normal TSH.

Screening: Universal screening during the first trimester of pregnancy in asymptomatic pregnant women for thyroid dysfunction is no longer supported by American Thyroid Association (ATA), the Endocrine Society, and the American College of Obstetricians and Gynecologists.

Criteria for screening pregnant women for hypothyroidism

1. If the pregnant woman is from an area of known moderate to severe iodine insufficiency.
2. Signs and symptoms of hypothyroidism.
3. Positive family or personal history of thyroid disease.
4. Positive personal history of TPO antibodies.
5. Type 1 diabetes.
6. History of preterm delivery or miscarriage.
7. History of head or neck radiation.
8. Morbid obesity (bone mineral density [BMD] $\geq$40 kg/m^2.
9. Age >30 years.
10. History of infertility.

Obstetric Outcome in Hypothyroidism Complicating Pregnancy

The risk of complications during pregnancy and adverse neonatal outcomes are is lower in women with subclinical, rather than overt hypothyroidism (Table 14.3.7).

Management of Hypothyroidism in Pregnancy

American Thyroid Association (ATA) recommends treatment with thyroid supple-mentation in:

1. All pregnant patients with laboratory evidence of overt hypothyroidism
2. Pregnant patients with subclinical hypo-thyroidism with positive thyroid peroxidase (TPO) antibodies
3. Treatment of pregnant women with isolated hypothyroxinemia (low free T4, normal TSH) or subclinical hypothyroidism with TPO negative is not recommended.

Management: The treatment of choice is levothyroxine sodium. The goal of therapy is to achieve thyroid hormone levels to within the reference range. It is important to treat dietary iodine deficiency and add iodine supplementation of 200 µg/day.

In patients with overt hypothyroidism (moderate to severe), treatment should be initiated with a dose of 1.6 µg/kg body weight per day, while patients with TSH <10 mU/L may become euthyroid with lower doses of 1 µg/kg daily. Thyroid-stimulating hormones should be measured after 6 weeks and levo-thyroxine doses adjusted in 25 or 50 g increments. A low normal TSH is the goal throughout the pregnancy in the trimester-specific reference range, for the first (0.1 to 2.5 mU/L), second (0.2 to 3 mU/L), and third (0.3 to 3 mU/L) trimesters.

For maintenance, the patients can be advised to take a 'double dose' of levothy-roxine on two days out of seven (e.g. Monday and Thursday). TSH should be monitored every 6–8 weeks.

Postpartum care: Postpartum TSH should be checked in 6–8 weeks and levothyroxine should be returned to the pre-pregnant dose. Though excreted in breast milk, the levels of levothyroxine are too low to alter thyroid function in the infant.

Postpartum thyroiditis (PPT) is a condition where there is a rebound in thyroid autoimmunity after delivery, leading to lymphocytic infiltration of the thyroid gland and transient changes in thyroid function. Women with high TPO antibody titers in early

Table 14.3.7: Maternal complications and neonatal outcome	
Maternal complications	Neonatal outcome
1. Pre-eclampsia and gestational hypertension	1. Preterm delivery, including very preterm delivery (before 32 weeks)
2. Placental abruption	2. Low birth weight (due to pre-eclampsia)
3. Non-reassuring fetal heart rate tracing	3. Perinatal morbidity and mortality
4. Increased rate of cesarean section[13]	4. Neuropsychological and cognitive impairment
5. Postpartum hemorrhage	

pregnancy and those with type 1 diabetes are most commonly affected. 20–50% of women identified with PPT will develop permanent hypothyroidism within 2–10 years.

Anesthetic Management of Hypothyroidism Complicating Pregnancy

Pregnant patients with hypothyroidism can present for both elective and emergency surgeries. The anesthetic implications depend upon the extent of control of the disease. In euthyroid patients, both regional and general anesthesia can be safely administered. In uncontrolled hypothyroidism for emergency surgery, the anesthetic implications can be as given in Table 14.3.8.

Regional anesthesia is recommended, if there are no contraindications. Ephedrine is preferred over phenylephrine for spinal hypotension. Epidural analgesia preferred for labor pain relief instead of parenteral opioids.

In emergencies, with uncontrolled hypothyroidism and unconfirmed fasting status, if general anesthesia is indicated, airway should be secured with RSI and ETT intubation. These patients are extremely sensitive to narcotics and sedatives and tend to hypoventilate, if allowed to breathe spontaneously. Delayed emergence should be anticipated requiring postoperative ventilatory support. Regional techniques or a small dose of opioids and/or ketorolac with adequate monitoring is best suited for the postoperative analgesia.

Myxedema Coma in Pregnancy

Myxedema coma presents as a medical emergency. It is rare in pregnancy. It can be precipitated by sepsis, hypothermia, congestive heart failure, gastrointestinal bleeding, trauma, anesthesia and surgery. Hypothermia is the cardinal feature of myxedema coma. The definitive treatment is thyroid hormone replacement administered as intravenous initial bolus of I-thyroxine (T4) 200 to 500 µg followed by 50–100 µg daily. IV triiodothyronine (T3) 10–25 µg every 8 hours can be used, if available. Combinations of T4 and T3 can also be used. Intravenous hydrocortisone 100 to 300 mg/day is prescribed to treat possible adrenal insufficiency (AI). Treatment of the precipitating cause along with other supportive therapy is critical for rapid recovery.

April 2015 ACOG Recommendations

1. Do not do universal screening for thyroid disease in pregnancy.
2. TSH screening test is firstline screening to assess thyroid status in pregnancy.

Table 14.3.8: Anesthetic challenges	
Hypodynamic CVS, reduced CO, decreased blood volume, abnormal baroreceptor function	Increased sensitivity to anesthetic drugs
Decreased hepatic metabolism and decreased renal excretion	Delayed recovery
Decreased ventilatory responsiveness to hypoxia and hypercarbia	
Hypothermia, electrolyte imbalances (hyponatremia), hypoglycemia	
Myxedematous changes, swollen oral cavity, edematous vocal cords or goitrous enlargement/OSAS	Airway compromise
Decreased gastric emptying	Increased risk of regurgitation and aspiration
Anemia and platelet and coagulation factor (especially VIII) dysfunction	Risk of spinal hematoma in Central neuraxial block
Decreased neuromuscular excitability	Abnormal response to NM monitoring

3. TSH and FT4 should be measured to diagnose thyroid disease in pregnancy.

4. Treat overt hypothyroid disease in pregnancy with adequate thyroid hormone to minimize risk of adverse outcomes.

5. TSH should be monitored in pregnant women who have overt hypothyroidism and the dosage of thyroid replacement adjusted accordingly.

6. Pregnant women with overt hyperthyroidism should be treated with thioamide to minimize risk adverse outcomes.

7. FT4 should be monitored in pregnant women with hyperthyroidism and thioamide dose adjusted accordingly.

SUMMARY

• The physiological changes in pregnancy include increase in serum total T3 and T4 levels and decrease in TSH along with increase in TBG.

• Graves' disease should be differentiated from hCG-mediated hyperthyroidism.

• Thyroid storm can be precipitated by child birth. It should be anticipated in uncontrolled hyperthyroidism and tackled efficiently.

• The diagnosis of hypothyroidism in pregnancy is based on TSH levels above 2.5 or 3.0 U/L. Subclinical hypothyroidism is defined as an elevated serum TSH concentration and a normal free T4 concentrations specific to trimesters.

• The screening of asymptomatic pregnant women for thyroid dysfunction during the first trimester of pregnancy is no longer recommended.

• Patients with overt hypothyroidism should be started replacement doses of thyroxine approximately 1 µg/kg daily. T4 dose requirements may increase during pregnancy in women with pre-existing hypothyroidism.

• Uncontrolled hypothyroidism is associated with increased maternal and fetal morbidity.

• Myxedema coma, though rare, is a dire medical emergency with high mortality

• Anesthetic complications in hyperthyroidism is basically due to increased metabolic rate. Thyroid storm is the dreaded perioperative complication.

• Regional anesthesia is preferred in both hyperthyroidism and in hypothyroid patients.

• Epidural analgesia, if not contraindicated for other reasons, should be the preferred mode of labor pain relief.

REFERENCES

1. David H, Chestnut, Wong, Cynthia A, Tsen WC, Lawrence C, et al. Endocrine disorders: Chestnut's Obstetric Anesthesia Principles and Practice, 5th ed. pp 1040–57.

2. Casey BM, Leveno KJ. Thyroid disease in pregnancy. Obstet Gynecol 2006;108:1283–92.

3. Glinoer D, de Nayer P, Bourdoux P, et al. Regulation of maternal thyroid during pregnancy. J Clin Endocrinol Metab 1990;71:276–87.

4. Bartalena L, Robbins J. Variations in thyroid hormone transport proteins and their clinical implications. Thyroid 1992;2:237–45.

5. Pearce EN. Diagnosis and management of thyrotoxicosis. Br Med J 2006;332:1369–73.

6. Weetman AP. Graves' disease. N Engl J Med 2000; 343:1236–48.

7. Marx H, Amin P, Lazarus JH. Hyperthyroidism and pregnancy. Br Med J 2008;336:663–7.

8. Kaplan MM, Meier DA, Dworkin HJ. Treatment of hyperthyroidism with radioactive iodine. Endocrinol Metab Clin North Am 1998;27:205–23.

9. Cooper DS. Antithyroid drugs. N Engl J Med 2005; 352:905–10.

10. Bahn RS, Burch HB, Cooper DS, et al. Hyperthyroidism and other causes of thyrotoxicosis: management guidelines of the American Thyroid Association and American Association of Clinical Endocrinologists. Endocr Pract 2011;17:456–520.

11. Schussler-Fiorenza CM, Bruns CM, Chen H. The surgical management of Graves' disease. J Surg Res 2006;133:207–14.

12. American College of Obstetricians and Gynecologists. Thyroid disease in pregnancy. ACOG Practice Bulletin No. 37. Washington DC, August 2002. Obstet Gynecol 2002;100:387–96.

13. Kung AW, Lau KS, Kohn LD. Epitope mapping of TSH receptorblocking antibodies in Graves' disease that appear during pregnancy. J Clin Endocrinol Metab 2001;86:3647–53.
14. Lockwood CM, Grenache DG, GronDevdhar M, Ousman YH, Burman KD. Hypothyroidism. Endocrinol Metab Clin North Am 2007;36: 595–615.
15. Gaitonde DY, Rowley KD, Sweeney LB. Hypothyroidism: an update. Am Fam Physician 2012;86:244–51.
16. Zulewski H, Muller B, Exer P, et al. Estimation of tissue hypothyroidism by a new clinical score: evaluation of patients with various grades of hypothyroidism and controls. J Clin Endocrinol Metab 1997;82:771–6.

14.4 PHEOCHROMOCYTOMA (Pathophysiology, Clinical Presentation, Interaction with Pregnancy and Anesthetic Management)

INTRODUCTION

Pheochromocytomas are paragangliomas that arise in the adrenal medulla (90%) or in the adjacent sympathetic nervous system tissues. Paragangliomas are a heterogeneous group of tumors that develop from neural crest-derived chromaffin cells.[1,2] Extra-adrenal paragangliomas may develop from sympathetic or parasympathetic tissues and include such diverse neoplasms as glomus tumors, chemodectomas, carotid body tumors, and jugulotympanic tumors.[3]

EPIDEMIOLOGY

Pheochromocytomas occur in 0.1 to 0.2% of hypertensive adults.[2] Pheochromocytoma is rare during pregnancy, with an overall incidence estimated to be less than 0.2 per 10,000 pregnancies.[6] It occurs bilaterally in 5 to 10% of cases.[4] Approximately 10% of them are malignant.[4,5] Large tumor size, extra-adrenal location, and certain tumor susceptibility gene mutations (e.g. succinate dehydrogenase subunit B) are associated with malignant pheochromocytomas.[3]

Diseases associated with pheochromocytoma
1. Multiple endocrine neoplasia (MEN) syndromes—MEN 2A and MEN 2B.
2. Von Recklinghausen's disease
3. Von Hippel Lindau disease
4. Sturge-Weber syndrome
5. Tuberous sclerosis

PATHOPHYSIOLOGY

The pathophysiology of pheochromocytoma is related almost entirely to the systemic effects of its endocrine secretory products, typically norepinephrine and epinephrine. Some pheochromocytomas may, however, secrete other catecholamines like dopamine, dihydroxyphenylalanine [DOPA] or peptide hormones. As strong vasoactive compounds, catecholamines, such as noradrenaline and adrenaline, have a plethora of physiological functions, even far beyond cardiovascular homeostasis.

The plasma concentrations of neurotransmitter and hormone reflect global sympathoadrenomedullary function and in many clinical conditions plasma catecholamines are elevated, wherein the sympathoadrenomedullary activity is enhanced. Differentiating these conditions from those that are the consequence of a pheochromocytoma is particularly a challenging task.

Effect of Excessive Catecholamines on Pregnancy

In healthy pregnant women, plasma and urinary catecholamine levels are normal or only slightly increased.[7–11] Catecholamine metabolism is not changed in pregnant women. Excessive maternal levels of catecholamines in pheochromocytoma can cause extreme vasoconstriction and compromise the uteroplacental circulation. This can lead to placental abruption and intrauterine hypoxia, thus imposing a serious risk to the fetus.

Effect of Excessive Maternal Catecholamines on Fetus

Maternal catecholamines do not cross the placental barrier. Even in patients with pheochromocytoma, the umbilical cord blood contains <10% of the maternal catecholamine concentrations.[12,13] A protective barrier for the fetus against excessive catecholamine exposure is formed by the placental cells containing catecholamine-metabolizing enzymes such as monoamine oxidase and catechol-*O*-methyltransferase.

Eventhough fetus has a high basal catecholamine secretion rate, the circulating concentrations of catecholamines are low due to a high clearance.[14] This high secretion is needed for its stressful journey through the parturient birth canal during.[15]

SIGNS AND SYMPTOMS

Patients typically have **paroxysmal symptoms** because of the episodic nature of hormone secretion by the tumor. The symptoms may be headache, sweating, palpitations, pallor, nausea, tremor, anxiety, abdominal pain, chest pain, weakness, dyspnea, weight loss, flushing, and visual disturbances. The prevalence of these symptoms is probably slightly lower than in non-pregnant patients.[16]

The most common symptoms are sweating, tachycardia, and headaches; one study suggested that the diagnosis of pheochromocytoma can be excluded with 99.9% certainty, if a patient does not have these symptoms.[17]

Pallor is common and flushing is uncommon in patients with pheochromocytoma. In addition to their systemic endocrine, effects, pheochromocytomas can occasionally cause local abdominal symptoms.[18]

Effect of Gravid Uterus on Pheochromocytoma

The symptoms in many patients increase along with further progress of pregnancy, including the growing uterus and fetal movements.[19] The abdominal palpation and uterine contractions may also account for a sudden precipitation of a pheochromocytoma crisis, often mimicking into a real cardiovascular emergency.

There is similarity of some signs and symptoms of pheochromocytoma with pregnancy-related hypertension, such as nausea and hypertension. To diagnose the tumor, close attention has to paid to other symptoms.

Orthostatic hypotension occurs in 70% of patients.[5,20] If it occurs in a pregnant hypertensive patient should immediately cause suspicion of a pheochromocytoma. The presumed mechanisms for orthostatic hypotension are chronic vasoconstriction with intravascular volume depletion and impaired reflex responses secondary to receptor down-regulation or synaptic effects of circulating catecholamines.[5,20]

DIAGNOSIS

The current approach to the diagnosis of pheochromocytoma involves the following three steps:

1. Biochemical testing for increased catecholamine secretion,
2. Anatomic imaging, and
3. Functional imaging.[1,2]

Certain medications alter the normal catecholamine secretion and interfere with the results. If possible a tapering or cessation of medication is suggested before the diagnostic tests (Table 14.4.2).

Biochemical Tests

1. Catecholamines excretion for 24 hours of epinephrine norepinephrine and dopamine. Urinary total and fractionated metanephrines normetanephrine and metanephrine.
2. Plasma fractionated metanephrines to be measured, if normal excludes pheochromocytoma (except dopamine secreting tumors). A plasma test is done as

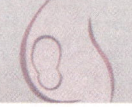

Table 14.4.1: Pheochromocyatema vs pre-eclampsia

S.no	Clinical feature	Pre-eclampsia	Pheochromocytoma
1.	Onset of symptoms	Usually after 20 weeks of gestation	Anytime during pregnancy
2.	Nature of the symptoms	Continuous	Episodic
3.	Pedal edema, proteinuria and elevated plasma uric acid	Not present	Usually present
4.	Orthostatic hypotension	Not present	Almost always present
5.	Maternal catecholamine levels	Raised in moderate pre-eclampsia twofold raise in eclampsia	Raised

Proteinuria and hypertension may occur in pregnancy confusing pheochromocytoma.

Table 14.4.2: Factors altering the plasma and urinary concentrations of catecholamine metabolites

Medical conditions[28]	Drugs[29]
Congestive heart failure	Tricyclic antidepressants
Acute myocardial infarction	Acetaminophen
Stroke	Hydralazine and methyldopa
Cocaine abuse	Beta-antagonist—labetalol
Sleep apnea (OSAS)	Epinephrine, phenylephrine
Ethanol or clonidine withdrawal	Phencyclidine
	Terbutaline

confirmatory after 24 hours urinary catecholamines or as the firstline test in cases where 24-hr urine collection may not be possible. Though sensitivity is high (96 to 100%), the specificity of plasma fractionated metanephrines is poor at 85 to 89%.

3. Other biochemical tests:
   a. **Plasma catecholamines**—poor accuracy no longer has a role.
   b. **Chromogranin A** (CGA)—Chromogranin A is a protein stored and released from secretory granules of neuroendocrine cells. Elevation in serum CGA is found in 80% of patients with pheochromocytoma but may also be seen with other neuroendocrine tumors, and in a variety of other conditions.[25,26]
   c. **Neuropeptide Y**—are increased but are less accurate than 24-hour urinary fractionated metanephrines and catecholamines.
   d. **Vanillylmandelic acid** (VMA)—The 24-hour urinary VNA excretion is not

preferred in view of poor sensitivity and specificity compared to 24-hour urinary fractionated metanephrines.
   e. **Provocative testing and suppression testing** are not used in pregnancy due to increased risk to mother and the fetus.

Radiological Diagnosis

Both CT and MRI are sensitive in localizing the tumor. Risk of radiation is high especially with pelvic CT. Tumor localization in the antenatal period is best done with MRI without gadolinium. MRI is without radiation risk to the fetus. High-intensity signals on T2-weighted image provide the best sensitivity without fetal exposure to ionizing radiation.

CT is done in the postpartum period. There is no risk of exacerbation of hypertension with CT alone or with the low osmolar contrast.

[123]I-metaiodobenzylguanidine (^{123}I-MIBG) scintigraphies are not considered safe for pregnant women. An MIBG scan can be done

in the postpartum period to detect, if multiple tumors are detected in CT or MRI. Fludeoxy-glucose-positron emission tomography (**FDG-PET**) is more sensitive to detect metastatic disease.

MANAGEMENT OF PHEOCHROMOCYTOMA IN PREGNANCY

The initially reported maternal mortality in undiagnosed and untreated patients was as high as 50%.[16,21–23] The mortality depends on the time of diagnosis, whether antepartum or postpartum.[23] Early antepartum recognition of the tumor and appropriate management has decreased the maternal mortality to <5% over the last 50 years.[16,24]

The highest risk of cardiovascular complications is during the peripartum period[21,22] due to labor, abdominal palpation, anesthesia, delivery or by using certain medications like analgesics. All these factors may precipitate a pheochromocytoma crisis by invoking a sudden release of catecholamines from the tumor. Proper evaluation and medical management can prevent the morbidity.

Medical Management

Initially managed with alpha-blockade using phenoxybenzamine, phentolamine, prazosin. A combined alpha and beta blocker labetalol is safe in pregnancy.

Phenoxybenzamine: It is a long-acting non-competitive α_1- and α_2-adrenoceptor antagonist. Phenoxybenzamine crosses the placental barrier but is generally considered safe. The starting dose is 10 mg twice a day with titration up to 1 mg/kg per day. Most prominent side effects include orthostatic hypotension, tachycardia, and nasal congestion. Neonates should be monitored for respiratory distress and hypotension in the first 72 hours following delivery.

Doxazosin: It is a competitive adrenoceptor blocker with α_1-adrenoceptor specificity. It causes less reflex tachycardia due to lack of presynaptical α_2-adrenoceptor blockade. It is short-acting than phenoxybenzamine and hence causes less postoperative hypotension. The usual dose of doxazosin is 2 to 16 mg per day.

Beta-blockers: The role of beta-blockers in pheochromocytoma is to treat maternal tachycardia or arrhythmias. Beta blockade has to be resorted to only after adequate alpha blockade and volume replacement. There is a risk of IUGR with long-term beta blockade use in the antenatal period. Labetalol which is a combined alpha and beta blocker is safe to be used in pheochromocytoma complicating pregnancy.

Surgical Management

The timing of surgery for pheochromocytoma depends upon the location of the tumor, gestational age and the success of the medical management. Surgery may be contemplated in the first and second trimesters of pregnancy once adequate alpha blockade is achieved. Risk of fetal loss is less in second trimester surgeries. The surgical excision can be combined with cesarean delivery in the third trimester or tumor resection may be scheduled at a later date in the postpartum period. Laparoscopy has lesser catecholamine surge, lower complication rate, and better maternal and fetal output compared to the open approach.

Mode of delivery: Labor, uterine contractions and vaginal delivery can cause uncontrolled catecholamine surge, severe maternal hypertension, placental ischemia and fetal compromise. Nevertheless in well-controlled patients on a good alpha blockade vaginal delivery may be contemplated with epidural labor analgesia and cut shortening of second stage of labor. In patients in whom the tumor has been removed in the first trimester of pregnancy, vaginal delivery can be an option.

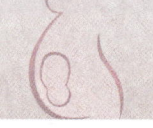

ANESTHETIC MANAGEMENT

A pregnant patient with pheochromocytoma can be posted for cesarean section alone or combined with tumor resection, or for tumor resection during antenatal period. Regional anesthesia has been used alone or in combination with general anesthesia. Through preoperative preparation and careful prevention of intraoperative hemodynamic surge leads to a good outcome.

Regional anesthesia: Low thoracic epidural gives good anesthesia and analgesia for both cesarean delivery and tumor resection, also provides postoperative pain relief.

General anesthesia: Drugs causing catecholamine release (morphine, atracurium) and those causing muscle twitching (succinylcholine, etomidate) should be avoided. Rocuronium is preferred for RSI (rapid sequence induction) .

Management of Hypertensive Emergencies

Hypertensive crisis can be precipitated in pregnant patients under conservative medical management during periods of acute stress like labor and delivery. Crisis may be precipitated during cesarean delivery without tumor removal. Crisis can be seen during surgical removal of the tumor. Hypertensive emergencies should be treated with phentolamine (1–5 mg) or nitroprusside. In antenatal patients, the duration of sodium nitroprusside should be limited due to potential fetal cyanide toxicity.

Lower segment cesarean section (LSCS) combined with tumor resection is more challenging. The fluid shifts due to cesarean delivery should be balanced with the fluid shifts during tumor resection. Intraoperative management can be further complicated, if PPH occurs during cesarean delivery (Table 14.4.3).

Postoperative Pain Relief

Effective pain management should be done with multimodal approach with a combination of low dose local anesthetic via epidural catheter, opioids, and paracetamol.

SUMMARY

1. Pheochromocytoma during pregnancy though rare can have varied presentation.
2. Uncontrolled pressures in pregnancy should always arouse the suspicion of pheochromocytoma.

Table 14.4.3: Perioperative management of pheochromocytoma

Event	Treatment
Hypertension during manipulation of tumor	Sodium nitroprusside (SNP), phentolamine, prazosin, nitroglycerine, magnesium sulfate, beta-blockers
Tachycardia/tachyarrhythmias	Beta-blockers—esmolol or metaprolol
Hypotension after ligation of veins	Discontinue vasodilators and blocker
	Modest fluid bolus
	Infusion of a vasopressor—norepinephrine or phenylephrine
Postoperative hypertension	Continue antihypertensives
	R/o residual tumor
Postoperative hypotension	Fluids, vasopressors
	R/o intra-abdominal bleed
Postoperative hypoglycemia	Closely monitor sugars, dextrose infusions

3. 24-hour urinary fractionated metanephrines and plasma metanephrine levels are used for diagnosing pheochromocytoma in pregnancy.

4. MRI without gadolinium can be used for localization of the tumor.

5. Phenoxybenzamine is the drug of choice in pregnancy.

6. Surgical management is the best in the second trimester of pregnancy done through laparoscopic approach.

7. Mode of delivery is usually cesarean section to avoid catecholamine surge during labor and delivery.

8. Anesthetic technique should be individualized. Epidural or general anesthesia or a combination of both can be used.

9. Preoperative alpha blockade must be optimized before surgery.

10. The goal of anesthesia should be to prevent fluctuations in hemodynamics during tumor manipulation and resection.

11. Three important postoperative complications to be dealt with are hypertension, hypotension and hypoglycemia.

12. Early diagnosis, meticulous preoperative optimization, anticipation and management of intraoperative hemodynamic fluctuations and a good postoperative care can decrease the maternal morbidity and mortality in pheochromocytoma complicating pregnancy.

REFERENCES

1. Tischler AS. Pheochromocytoma and extra-adrenal paraganglioma: updates. Arch Pathol Lab Med 2008;132:1272–84.

2. Chen H, Sippel RS, O'Dorisio MS, et al. The North American Neuroendocrine Tumor Society consensus guideline for the diagnosis and management of neuroendocrine tumors: pheochromocytoma, paraganglioma, and medullary thyroid cancer. Pancreas 2010;39:775–83.

3. Eisenhofer G. Screening for pheochromocytomas and paragangliomas. Curr Hypertens Rep 2012; 14:130–7.

4. Sutton MG, Sheps SG, Lie JT. Prevalence of clinically unsuspected pheochromocytoma. Review of a 50-year autopsy series. Mayo Clin Proc 1981;56:354–60.

5. Ross EJ, Griffith DN. The clinical presentation of phaeochromocytoma. Q J Med 1989;71:485–96.

6. Harper MA, Murnaghan GA, Kennedy L, et al. Phaeochromocytoma in pregnancy: five cases and a review of the literature. Br J Obstet Gynaecol 1989;96:594–606.

7. Natrajan PG, McGarrigle HH, Lawrence DM, Lachelin GC. Plasma noradrenaline and adrenaline levels in normal pregnancy and in pregnancy-induced hypertension. Br J Obstet Gynaecol 1982;89:1041–5.

8. Jaffe RB, Harrison TS, Cerny JC. Localization of metastatic phaeochromocytoma in pregnancy by caval catheterization. Including urinary catecholamine values in uncomplicated pregnancies. American Journal of Obstetrics and Gynecology 1969;104:939–44.

9. Zuspan FP. Urinary excretion of epinephrine and norepinephrine during pregnancy. Journal of Clinical Endocrinology and Metabolism 1970;30: 357–60.

10. Goodall M, Diddle AW. Epinephrine and norepinephrine in pregnancy. A comparative study of the adrenal gland and catechol output in different species of animals and man. American Journal of Obstetrics and Gynecology 1971;111: 896–904.

11. Peleg D, Munsick RA, Diker D, Goldman JA, Ben-Jonathan N. Distribution of catecholamines between fetal and maternal compartments during human pregnancy with emphasis on L-dopa and dopamine. Journal of Clinical Endocrinology and Metabolism 1986;62:911–4.

12. Saarikoski S. Fate of noradrenaline in the human foetoplacental unit. Acta Physiologica Scandinavica Supplementum 1974;421:1–82.

13. Dahia PL, Hayashida CY, Strunz C, Abelin N, Toledo SP. Low cord blood levels of catecholamine from a newborn of a phaeochromocytoma patient. European Journal of Endocrinology 1994;130:217–9.

14. Bzoskie L, Blount L, Kashiwai K, Tseng YT, Hay WW Jr, Padbury JF. Placental norepinephrine clearance: in vivo measurement and physiological role. American Journal of Physiology 1995;269: E145–E149.

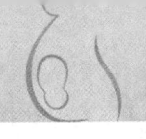

15. Slotkin TA, Seidler FJ. Adrenomedullary catecholamine release in the fetus and newborn: secretory mechanisms and their role in stress and survival. Journal of Developmental Physiology 1988;10:1–16.

16. Ahlawat SK, Jain S, Kumari S, Varma S, Sharma BK. Phaeochromocytoma associated with pregnancy: case report and review of the literature. Obstetrical and Gynecological Survey 1999; 54: 728–37.

17. Bravo EL, Gifford RW Jr. Current concepts. Pheochromocytoma: diagnosis, localization and management. N Engl J Med 1984;311:1298–1303.

18. Counselman FL, Brenner CJ, Brenner DW. Adrenal pheochromocytoma presenting with persistent abdominal and flank pain. J Emerg Med 1991;9:241–6.

19. Oliva R, Angelos P, Kaplan E, Bakris G. Phaeochromocytoma in pregnancy: A case series and review. Hypertension 2010;55:600–6.

20. Carney JA. Familial multiple endocrine neoplasia: the first 100 years. Am J Surg Pathol 2005;29: 254–74.

21. Schenker JG, Chowers I. Phaeochromocytoma and pregnancy. Review of 89 cases. Obstetrical and Gynecological Survey 1971;26:739–47.

22. Schenker JG, Granat M. Phaeochromocytoma and pregnancy—an updated appraisal. Australian and New Zealand Journal of Obstetrics and Gynaecology 1982;22:1–10.

23. Harper MA, Murnaghan GA, Kennedy L, Hadden DR, Atkinson AB. Phaeochromocytoma in pregnancy. Five cases and a review of the literature. Br J Obstet Gynaecol 1989;96:594–606.

24. Oishi S, Sato T. Phaeochromocytoma in pregnancy: a review of the Japanese literature. Endocrine Journal 1994;41:219–25.

25. d'Herbomez M, Forzy G, Bauters C, et al. An analysis of the biochemical diagnosis of 66 pheochromocytomas. Eur J Endocrinol 2007; 156:569–75.

26. Algeciras-Schimnich A, Preissner CM, Young WF Jr, et al. Plasma chromogranin A or urine fractionated metanephrines follow-up testing improves the diagnostic accuracy of plasma fractionated metanephrines for pheochromocytoma. J Clin Endocrinol Metab 2008;93:91–5.

27. Timmers HJ, Taieb D, Pacak K. Current and future anatomical and functional imaging approaches to pheochromocytoma and paraganglioma. Horm Metab Res 2012;44:367–72.

28. Makino S, Iwata M, Fujiwara M, et al. A case of sleep apnea syndrome manifesting severe hypertension with high plasma norepinephrine levels. Endocr J 2006;53:363–9.

29. Eisenhofer G, Goldstein DS, Walther MM, et al. Biochemical diagnosis of pheochromocytoma: how to distinguish true- from false-positive test results. J Clin Endocrinol Metab 2003;88: 2656–66.

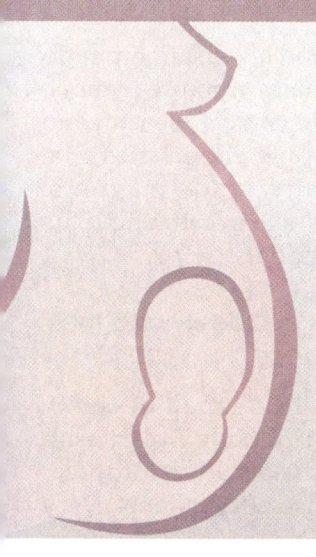

15 CHAPTER

Obesity and Pregnancy

Rakesh Garg, Anju Gupta

The perioperative management of a pregnant woman has peculiar concerns because of various physiological changes and its clinical variations. Also it requires considerations of two lives. These challenges are further aggravated, if the parturient is obese. In this chapter, we will discuss various implications of obesity in pregnant women regarding perioperative anesthetic management.

World Health Organization has considered obesity as a 'global epidemic' posing a serious health threat to people all over the world.[1] Obesity and its consequent morbidity and mortality contribute significantly not only to cost of health care but have significant socio-economic impact as well. With the increasing prevalence of obesity, it is likely to replace under-nutrition and infectious diseases as the leading health concern worldwide.[2] In United States, 30–40% of females are obese and it is estimated that by 2050, 50% of females will be obese.[3–5]

OBESITY IN INDIA

The global wave of obesity has hit developing country such as India alike. Five percent of Indian population are obese.[6] A recent study

in the Lancet has ranked India third in global obesity.[7] Developing nations are facing over nutrition as well as under-nutrition as a health threat. In India, more women are overweight (6.6%) than men (3.5%).[8] The percentage of women aged 15–49 years who are overweight or obese rose from 11% in *National Family Health Survey* (NHFS)-2 to 15% in NHFS-3.[9,10] Data from 2001 NFHS show that Punjab tops the list of states with most obese people (30.0% males and 37.5% females) followed by Kerala and Goa.[11]

OBESITY IN PREGNANCY

Prevalence of obesity has seen a parallel rise among women of reproductive age group worldwide.[12] The number of obese parturients has doubled in last decade.[13] Obesity has been described as one of the most important contributors to maternal death.[14] Confidential enquiry into maternal and child health (CEMACH) report for the triennium 2003–2005 highlighted obesity as a direct factor in four out of eight anesthesia-related maternal deaths.[15] As the epidemic of obesity continues to grow, anesthesiologists all over the world are likely to face challenges related to peripartum management of an obese parturient.

Definition

The word obesity is derived from the Latin word *'obesus'* meaning fattened by eating. Obesity can be defined as a condition in which body fat exceeds beyond that compatible with physical and mental health and normal life expectancy.[16] It may thus be categorized as a disease in itself. The underlying etiology may be environmental, genetic or endocrine. Body mass index (BMI) or 'Quetlet's index' can be used as a tool to quantify its severity (Table 15.1). BMI is defined as equal to weight (kg)/height(m^2).

Morbid obesity is BMI >40 kg/m^2 and supermorbid obesity is BMI >50 kg/m^2. Individuals with a BMI > 35 kg/m^2 have double the risk of premature death.[17,18] For obese parturients, BMI used for stratify them is their pre-pregnancy BMI or BMI recorded at their first antenatal visit. The WHO classification of obesity and risk of morbidity and mortality in relation to increasing BMI and waist circumference in a female is shown in Table 15.1.[1,19] Also, abdominal obesity is known to be associated with more significant health risk than an absolute BMI value. It can be detected by a waist circumference of >102 cm or waist to hip ratio of >1 in males and a waist circumference >88 cm and a waist to hip ratio of more than 0.9 in females (pre-pregnancy). In addition to the above clinical measures to estimate obesity, imaging modalities like computed tomography and magnetic resonance imaging may help in estimating the body fat and its distribution.[20]

Physiological Changes in Obesity and their Interaction with Pregnancy

Obesity is associated with a gamut of pathophysiological changes in the body which result in multiple comorbidities. Physiological changes in pregnancy also affect almost every organ system in the mother. Coexistence of obesity with pregnancy thus intensifies the magnitude of systemic changes when compared with either condition alone.

Airway

The pregnant patient is considered to have difficult airway and obesity further increases the difficulty in airway management. Airway management is difficult in obese due to presence of chubby cheeks, large tongue, short neck, increased palatal and pharyngeal soft tissue, high and anterior larynx, reduced mouth opening, restricted neck movements (fat pad at the nape of neck) and large breasts.[21] Pregnancy accentuates all these changes due to estrogen and increased blood volume

Table 15.1: Classification of obesity and associated health risk[1,19]

Classification	BMI (kg/m^2)	Waist circumference (cm)	Health risk
Underweight	<18.5	–	Increased
Normal weight	18.5–24.9	<88	Least
Obesity			
• Class I	30–34.9	<88	High
		>88	Very high
• Class II	35–39.9	<88	Very high
		>88	Very high
• Class III (morbid obesity)	≥40	<88	Extremely high
		>88	Extremely high
Super morbid obesity	≥50	–	Extremely high

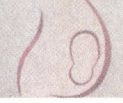

leading to upper airway mucosal edema and nasal congestion. Increased vascularity makes them prone to bleeding during airway instrumentation. The pregnant patients have increased risk of obstructive sleep apnea (OSA), which in turn increases the risk of airway obstruction and difficult airway management in obese patients.[22]

> **Pearl**
> Pregnancy increases the risk of obstructive sleep apnea (OSA).

Respiratory System

The pregnancy affects the various parameters of respiratory mechanics and they are further altered in presence of increased weight (Table 15.2).[13] Decreased chest wall compliance and splinting of diaphragm in morbidly obese patients leads to significant reductions in functional residual capacity (FRC), expiratory reserve volume (ERV) and total lung capacity (TLC). The ERV is the most sensitive indicator

of effect of obesity on respiratory system.[23] The decrease in FRC is proportional to increase in BMI.[24] Similar reductions are seen in pregnant patient when at term, FRC is reduced by 15–20% of non-pregnant state. However, the reduction in FRC may not be additive in an obese parturient.[25] This might be due to progesterone-induced airway smooth muscle relaxation counters, some of the negative effects of obesity.[26]

Obese parturients typically have a rapid shallow breathing pattern. Also, their oxygen consumption and carbon dioxide production are increased. Hence, their ventilatory requirements are higher and the work of breathing increases linearly with increased BMI.[27,28] These changes are further exaggerated by induction of general anesthesia in supine or lithotomy position and they may experience a 50% reduction in FRC under general anesthesia.[29] FRC may fall within the closing capacity in obese subjects leading to atelactasis, intrapulmonary shunting and hypoxemia. In

Table 15.2: Effect of pregnancy with morbid obesity on respiratory system[13]

Parameter	Pregnant patient	Obese patient	Obese parturient
Tidal volume	↑	↓	↑
Respiratory rate	↑	↓ or ↑	↑
Minute volume	↑	↓ or ↔	↑
Residual volume	↓	↓ or ↔	↑
FRC	↓↓	↓↓↓	↓↓
VC		↓	↓
FEV$_1$	↔	↓ or ↔	↔
FEV$_1$/ FVC	↔	↔	↔
Lung compliance	↔	↓↓	↓
WOB	↑	↑↑	↑
Resistance	↓	↑	↓
V/Q mismatch	↑	↑	↑↑
PaO$_2$	↓	↓↓	↓
PaCO$_2$	↓	↑	↓

(Adapted from Sravankumar et al.[13]: ↑=increase; ↓=decraese; ↔=no change (multiple arrows indicte the severity) CO_2=carbon dioxide; O_2=oxygen; FEV$_1$=forced expiratory volume in 1s; WOB: work of breathing; V/Q=ventilation perfusion ratio; PaO$_2$=partial pressure of oxygen PaCO$_2$=partial pressure of carbon dioxide)

fact, the intrapulmonary shunt may be as high as 10–25% in obese parturients under general anesthesia as compared to 2–5% in lean patients.[30] Deposition of fat tissue around the cheat wall, diaphragmatic breathing and increased intrapulmonary blood flow decrease lung compliance in obese by up to 30% of normal for that age.[31,32] Presence of large uterus in pregnant patients at term is likely to compound above changes because of additional diaphragm splinting.

Obese parturients are at an increased risk for OSA despite the ventilatory stimulant action of circulating progesterone.[33] In obese pregnant patients with long-standing OSA, obesity hypoventilation syndrome (Pickwickian syndrome) can be present in 8% of cases.[34] These patients have chronic hypoventilation, hypoxemia, polycythemia, cardiomegaly and right heart failure.[34] The work of breathing may be four times normal in these patients and mortality is increased significantly.

Pearl

Expiratory reserve volume (ERV) is the most sensitive indicator of effect of obesity on respiratory system.

Cardiovascular Changes

The occurrence of cardiovascular disease is seen in 37% of obese patients as compared to only 10% of normal adults.[35] Cardiovascular changes in obese parturient are summarized in Table 15.3.[13]

The pregnant patients have increased prevalence of hypertension, hyperlipidemia, ischemic heart disease and heart failure. 50–60% of obese patients have chronic hypertention.[36] Morbidly obese patients have five times the risk of developing pre-eclampsia.[5,14,36] Hypertension in obesity is associated with increased circulating blood volume and increase in cardiac output. Hypertension leads to gradual hypertrophy of left ventricle which becomes less compliant.

Cardiac output increases by 30–40 mL/min per 100 gm of excess fat tissue.[5,23] Non-obese pregnant patients experience an increase in cardiac output up to 50% during pregnancy. It peaks at 75% of prepartum value in immediate postpartum period.[37] In parturient with normal body weight, there is a decreased peripheral vascular resistance which reduces afterload. In obese parturient, however, afterload reduction fails to occur because of greater conduit artery stiffness.[38] This factor combined with non-compliant left ventricle in obese patients makes them especially prone to LVF especially in immediate post-partum period. In OSA and obesity hypoventilation syndrome (OHS), right ventricle failure can also develop because of pulmonary hypertension. Obese parturients are prone to cardiac arrhythmias because of increased circulating catecholamines, hypoxemia, hypercapnia, ventricular hypertrophy, fatty infiltration of the conducting system.[39,40] Incidence and severity of supine hypotension syndrome is increased in obese parturients because the weight of large panniculus adds to uterine aortocaval compression to the extent that two cases of sudden death have been reported in morbidly obese parturients on positioning them supine.[41] Also, sudden circulatory changes associated with positioning are poorly tolerated because of cardiomyopathy.[23] Hence, morbidly obese parturients should never be positioned supine without placing a wedge for leftward tilt.

Pearl

Morbidly obese patients have five times the risk of developing pre-eclampsia.

Clinical pearl

In obese parturient, due to absence of afterload reduction due to greater conduit artery stiffness and non-compliant left ventricle makes them prone to left ventricular failure especially in immediate postpartum period.

Table 15.3: Effect of pregnancy with morbid obesity or cardiovascular system[13]

Parameter	Pregnant patient	Obese patient	Obese parturient
Tidal volume	↑	↓	↑
Heart rate	↑	↑↑	↑↑
Stroke volume	↑↑	↑	↑
Cardiac output	↑↑	↑↑	↑↑↑
Hematocrit	↓↓	↑	↓
Blood volume	↑↑	↑	↑
SVR	↓↓	↑	↔ or ↓
MAP	↑	↑↑	↑↑
Supine hypotension	Present	Present	Markedly increased
CVP	↔	↑	↑↑
PAH	Not present	May be present	May be present
Pre-eclampsia	↔	Not applicable	↑↑

(Adapted from Sravankumar et al.[13]: ↑=increase, ↓=decraesc; ↔=no change (multiple arrows indicte the severity); SVR=systemic vascular resistance; CVP=central venous pressure; PAH=pulmonary arterial hypertension)

Metabolic and Endocrine Changes

Obese patients are at a higher risk of having type II diabetes mellitus, hyperlipidemia and hypothyroidism even in non-pregnant period.[5,23,42] During pregnancy, many circulating hormones, like human placental lactogen, human chorionic gonadotropin, and estrogen, lead to insulin resistance and hyperinsulinemia. Obesity increases insulin resistance further due to increased proinflammatory cytokines secreted by visceral adipocytes. Risk of developing gestational diabetes mellitus is four times higher in obese patients.[42] Leptin secreted by adipose tissue stimulates sympathetic nervous system leading to hypertension, sodium and water retention. Fetal macrosomia and associated morbidity is increased in fetus and mother.[5,13,20,22]

Pearl

Risk of developing gestational diabetes mellitus is four times higher in obese parturients.

Gastrointestinal Systemic Effects

Lower esophageal sphincter (LES) tone is reduced in pregnancy because of the effect of progesterone. Placental gastrin increases acidic gastric secretions. Obesity also reduces LES tone and precipitates hiatus hernia and leads to increased gastrointestinal reflux disease. Gastric emptying is also delayed in labor and gastric volume is considered to be higher in obese parturient. The risk of pulmonary aspiration is thus considered to be increased in pregnant obese patient.[43,44]

Pearl

Obese parturients have increased risk of gastrointestinal reflux and thus aspiration.

Hematological and Coagulation

Obesity and pregnancy lead to increased fibrinogen and inhibit fibrinolysis increasing the risk of deep vein thrombosis (DVT) and thromboembolism.[22] Polycythemia may be associated with OSA and OHS syndrome.

Musculoskeletal

Osteoarthritis, immobility and low back pain may lead to difficulty in positioning for regional block and surgery. Rhabdomyolysis may occur in prolonged surgery because of ischemia of large muscle group.[19]

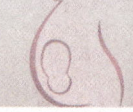

Psychological

The pregnancy induces some psychological changes. These may be related to hormonal changes. The presence of obesity may also have impact on psychological parameters which primarily may be related to social and physical barriers. There is an increased risk of suicide and depression.[5,22]

Pharmacokinetic and Pharmacodynamic Alterations

Obesity increases fat mass so the volume of distribution (V_D) for lipid-soluble drugs increases, so the loading dose is increased. But maintenance dose is based on clearance which may be normal or even increased in obese patients.[45] Levels of free fatty acid, triglycerides and $\alpha 1$ acid glycoprotein are increased and may affect the protein binding in obesity while pregnancy leads to fall in serum albumin levels.[5] Thus, complex interaction of various factors can lead to uncertainty in drug effects. In pregnancy, pseudocholinestrase levels are decreased slightly but succinylcholine metabolism is not much affected.

Anesthetic Management of Labor and Operative Delivery

Obstetric facility taking care of obese patients should be equipped with specialized equipment[23,46] compatible with their body weight (Table 15.4).

A BMI >30 kg/m² in a pregnant patient has been recognized as an important factor for maternal mortality.[14] Also, cesarean section is three times more common than normal delivery.[5,20,22] Hence, pregnancy in an obese patient is considered as high risk. Anesthetic concerns in obese parturient include:

- Increased prevalence of chronic hypertension and diabetes mellitus (type 2)
- Increased risk of gestational diabetes mellitus and pregnancy-induced hypertension.
- Peripartum cardiomyopathy and ischemic heart disease

Table 15.4: List of equipment for obstetric facility providing care to obese parturients

1. Large gowns
2. Large sphygmomanometer cuffs (up to 60 cm arm circumference)
3. Sit on weighing scale
4. Large chairs without arms
5. Bariatric wheelchairs (>450 lb limit)
6. Ultrasound scan couches
7. Ward and delivery beds (650–1000 lb limit)
8. Theatre trolleys
9. Operating theatre tables (600 lb limit)
10. Lifting and lateral transfer equipment
11. Long regional block needles
12. Difficult airway cart
13. Extra large thromboelastic stockings
14. Troop's elevation pillow

- Increased risk of difficult and prolonged labor and failed induction of labor
- Increased risk of instrumental delivery and cesarean section
- Prolonged duration of surgery with increased blood loss and postpartum hemorrhage
- Increased risk of deep vein thrombosis and pulmonary embolism
- Increased wound infection
- Failed/difficult intubation
- Gastric aspiration
- Difficult/failed central neuraxial block placement
- Increased risk of dural puncture during epidural in sitting position
- Increased supine hypotension syndrome and hypoxemia
- Increased cephalad spread of local anesthetic during epidural and spinal block
- Obstructive sleep apnea
- Difficult external fetal monitoring

All obstetric facilities taking care of obese parturient should have environmental risk assessment including safe working loads for floors and equipment (up to 250 kg), accessibility, transportation and staffing.[46] Guidelines from various obstetric societies recommend that antenatal consultation should be sought for all morbidly obese patients from an obstetric anesthetist so that the difficulties with their anesthetic management can be assessed and a plan for the labor and delivery can be chalked out and documented.[46,47] Such facilities should have a skilled anesthesiologist present round the clock and admission of an obese parturient should be informed to the duty anesthesiologist at the earliest.[46] Early involvement of other specialities for multi-disciplinary management of such patients is desirable including anesthesiologist, obste-trician, endocrinologist, general physician, neonatologist, physiotherapist and radiologist for optimum care. Such cases mandate the involvement of consultant anesthesiologists.

> **Clinical pearl**
>
> Antenatal evaluation of obese should be sought from an obstetric anesthetist to assess and a plan for the safe and uneventful labor and delivery.

Pre-Anesthesia Check-Up

Pre-anesthetic examination of such patients should elicit history of exercise intolerance, gastro-oesophageal reflex disease (GERD), OSA, gestational diabetes mellitus (GDM) and pre-eclampsia. Any pre-existing or pregnancy-related cardiopulmonary co-morbidities should be identified and relevant investi-gations done. An electrocardiogram should be done to screen for any cardiac involvement (e.g. ischemic heart disease, arrhythmias, heart failure, etc.) as these patients have a sedentary lifestyle and may not give any history suggestive of a cardiac disease. The patients who are symptomatic or have other risk factors (diabetes mellitus, hypertension, coronary artery disease, OHS) should under-go additional non-invasive cardiac testing, e.g. echocardiogram and also a cardiology consultation to optimize the cardiac status.[13,40] Preoperative arterial blood gas analysis and pulmonary function tests (PFT) can be done in these patients to evaluate lung functions. A fall in oxygen saturation from sitting to supine position can indicate a high risk for basal atelectasis and hypoxemia and such candidate may benefit from postpartum continuous positive airway pressure (CPAP) administration.[5,22]

Any obese patient with BMI >35 kg/m² and neck circumference >16 inches with frequent awakening during sleep and snoring may have OSA and should undergo polysomnography. Patients with severe OSA (apnea/hypopnea index >30) on polysomnography can undergo rapid arterial desaturation on induction.[17] Patients of preoperative CPAP levels of more than 10 cm H₂O may be at increased risk of difficult bag mask ventilation.[17] Patients should be instructed to bring their CPAP machine as preoperative initiation and postoperative continuation of CPAP has been shown to be beneficial.[22,34]

One should also identify venous cannu-lation sites and examine the back in view of anticipated difficulty in regional blocks. All these patients should be informed about high-risk nature of pregnancy and anesthesia and other appropriate consent should be taken. The patients should be informed regarding invasive procedures (e.g. fiberoptic intubation, central and arterial cannulation) and possibility of a postoperative stay in high dependency unit (HDU) or intensive care unit (ICU). DVT prophylaxis should be started as per policy in all such patients.

> **Pearl**
>
> Obese parturient may have difficult venous cannulation and difficult placement of regional blocks.

Increased BMI is known to correlate with increased incidence of difficult airway and appropriate assessment should be done (Table 15.5). Neck circumference of ≥15 inches and a Mallampati score of 3 or more are highly predictive of difficult intubation.[48] Harmen has

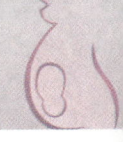

Table 15.5: The tests for airway assessment in obese parturient
1. History: Snoring, change in voice, previous history of a difficult airway
2. Oral cavity: Interincisor gap, Mallampati class, buck teeth
3. Receding mandible
4. Neck distances: Thyromental, sternomental distance
5. Neck circumference at the level of cricoid cartilage
6. Neck movements

described a simple obstetric assessment checklist of six questions with yes/no answers (obesity >90 kg, neck mobility <90°, mouth opening <5 cm, lack of temporomandibular joint mobility, posterior pharyngeal wall not seen in pharyngeal view and risk of airway edema—upper respiratory tract infection/recent voice change/PIH).[49] He suggested that if two or more are present, then awake intubation or regional anesthesia should be considered. Detailed airway assessment to predict difficult intubation should be repeated after labor because airway parameters are dynamic in labor and Mallampati grades may worsen during labor due to airway edema.[22]

Detailed airway assessment to predict difficult intubation should be done keeping in mind that airway changes are dynamic in labor and Mallampati grades may worsen during labor due to airway edema. Hence, the airway assessment should be repeated prior to anesthetizing these patients.

Women who have conceived post-bariatric surgery have been found to have a better maternal and fetal outcome in terms of decreased pregnancy-induced hypertension (PIH), gestational diabetes mellitus (GDM) and macrosomia.[50] Consideration should be given to nutritional supplementation in these women. Active band management by removing fluid from adjustable gastric band can help by allowing adequate gestational weight gain and decrease nausea and vomiting in early pregnancy in these females.[50,51]

Labor Analgesia and Instrumental Delivery

Obese parturients are at increased risk of fetal macrosomia, dysfunctional uterine contractions, shoulder dystocia and instrumental vaginal delivery.[5,20] Most obese women ask for labor analgesia.[52] Modalities for pain relief remain the same as in case of non-obese parturients, e.g. inhalational, parenteral and regional blocks. Entonox and patient-controlled analgesia with opioids have been used with variable efficacy.[5] However, inhalational and parenteral analgesics may lead to loss of airway reflexes in a potentially difficult airway, so neuraxial blockade remains the most efficient form of pain relief in such patients. In addition to excellent pain relief, epidural analgesia has multiple beneficial effects like decreased oxygen consumption, improved maternal oxygenation, decreased work of breathing, decreased plasma catecholamines and subsequent decreased cardiac work.[53,54] Also, since obese parturients have an increased risk of cesarean delivery and have a potentially difficult airway, presence of a functional epidural catheter allows anesthesiologist to provide surgical anesthesia thus avoiding airway manipulation. In fact, it is advisable to place a prophylactic epidural in obese parturient before active labor to increase the margin of safety for cesarean section and maximize patient cooperation. Sitting position is preferred to lateral position in obese patients due to:[55,56]

- Difficulty in positioning these patients in knee chest position
- Gravity dragging down the pad of fat and obliterating the midline
- Increased epidural depth in lateral position
- Decreased cardiac output in lateral position with maximal spine flexion as compared to sitting position in obese patients.

Technical challenges in successful epidural catheter placement in these patients include difficulty in positioning, increased epidural space depth requiring specialized block needles, difficult midline and iliac crest identification, increased risk of dural puncture, catheter displacement and high failure rate.[57] In a study by Perlow et al on 43 morbidly obese patients, 75% patients required more than one attempt for successful placement of epidural catheter.[58] This may be due to increased depth of epidural space from skin which leads to exaggerated directional errors even with slight lateral deviation from midline.

Various methods have been described to correctly identify midline and insertion point for successful epidural placement (Table 15.6).[5,22,59-61]

There is a positive correlation between increasing BMI and epidural space depth.[62] Hamza et al found that the distance from the skin to the epidural space is significantly higher in lateral position as compared to sitting position.[63] Even obese parturits rarely have epidural space depth more than 8 cm, making standard epidural needles feasible for use in this population.[60,64] Large epidural needles of up to 15 cm are available and may be necessary in some morbidly obese patients. A scout US scan prior to the procedure can help identify the correct landmark and epidural depth and hence the length of the epidural needle to be chosen.[60] There is increased risk of catheter dislodgement due to skin movement (up to 3 cm)[65] and position change from sitting to lateral position (up to 2.5 cm).[66] Hence,

increased length of catheter is placed inside (5–7 cm) the epidural space. Many investigators have suggested securing the epidural catheter by suturing to the skin or after making the patient lateral decubitus from sitting position. It is also prudent to ensure functional epidural catheter before securing it so that any failed or partial epidural block is avoided in case of emergency cesarean section. Local anesthetic requirements are 25% less in obese parturients because of fatty infiltration of epidural space and engorged veins due to increased abdominal pressure.

Incidence of dural puncture (up to 4%) is also increased significantly in morbidly obese patients,[67] though the risk of PDPH is low.[68,69] In case of inadvertent dural tap, epidural catheter can be threaded 2–3 cm into intrathecal space and used as continuous spinal analgesia (CSA) or anesthesia.[52] CSA provides fast, reliable and predictable block but one should be cautious in maintaining the sterility in handling it. The catheter should be clearly labeled as subarachnoid catheter to be handled by anesthesiologists only because in case the catheter is mistaken as an epidural catheter and full local anesthetic dose is injected high/total spinal can result with devastating consequences. So, CSA use should be limited to scenarios of accidental dural puncture or in cases of failed epidural where the risks of general anesthesia are prohibitive.

Combined Spinal Epidural Anesthesia

Combined spinal efridural anesthesia (CSEA) is increasingly being preferred for labor analgesia due to its advantage of faster onset of effective pain relief combined with flexibility of presence of an epidural catheter. The concerns of initial uncertainty of correct positioning of epidural catheter have been unfounded.[70,71] In fact, it has been seen that such epidural catheter may be more reliable as ability to achieve subarachnoid block through the same needle indirectly confirms its correct placement.[72]

Table 15.6: Methods to identify midline and insertion point in obese parturient

- Line dropped from occiput or C1 spinous prominence to gluteal cleft approximates midline
- Fetal heart rate monitor belt, if in place, usually rests on iliac crest and hence its intersection with vertical line dropped from C7 spinous process is a reasonable landmark
- Strapping of fat pads away from midline
- Guidance of the patient herself in directing the needle towards the center by asking whether the feel of the needle is towards right or left
- Use of an ultrasound to aid in block, paramedian longitudinal approach provides superior images

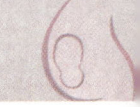

ANESTHESIA FOR OPERATIVE DELIVERIES

There is a significant correlation between increasing BMI and risk of cesarean section.[13,14,73] Weiss et al documented a cesarean section rate of 50%, 33% and 20.7%, respectively in morbid obese, obese and non-obese parturient.[74] Obesity and cesarean section are both known risk factors for maternal morbidity and mortality.[14,74,75]

Regional Anesthesia

Seventy-five percent of all deaths in pregnant women under anesthesia have been reported to occur in obese patients and inability to secure the airway was found to be the biggest contributor.[76] Confidential enquiry report on maternal mortality in United Kingdom (1979–2005) also documented that majority of deaths happened under general anesthesia as compared to regional anesthesia.[37] Hence, regional anesthesia should always be preferred over general anesthesia.

Epidural place for labor analgesia can be extended to provide anesthesia for cesarean section using carefully titrated doses of local anesthetic such as lignocaine 2% with adrenaline or bupivacaine 0.5% following injection of the test dose to achieve the desired level. The local anesthetic requirements for epidural block are reduced by around 25% in obese parturients. If labor epidural is not in place, CSEA is preferable to single shot spinal as cesarean section is generally difficult and prolonged in these patients. A CSEA allows extension of block, if required. Excellent postoperative analgesia can also be achieved with an epidural catheter. Single shot spinal anesthesia is appropriate when the duration surgery is expected to be less than 90 minutes. Since the risk of hypotension and high spinal block is there with spinal anesthesia (requiring emergency airway access), one should ensure that cardiopulmonary reserves are adequate and backup plans are ready. In case the surgery outlasts the duration of spinal block,

one may need to induce general anesthesia in emergency manner and can lead to devastating consequences. Long spinal needles (12, 15 and 17.5 cm) are commercially available and may be required. Tuohy needle can be used as an introducer to these spinal needle. Standard 8 cm Tuohy needle can be used with 12 cm spinal needle.[19] Obese patients can have excessive cephalad spread of intrathecal local anesthetic drug because of decreased cerebrospinal fluid (CSF) volume and large buttocks which place spinal column in a relative Trendelenburg position.[77] High spinal block may be poorly tolerated in obese patient because of poor chest compliance and decreased FRC.

Even regional blocks are fraught with more complications in a morbidly obese patients. In a retrospective study of 142 morbidly obese patients, authors concluded that patients with peripartum BMI >40 kg/m² and delivery BMI >45 kg/m² are particularly at risk for regional anesthesia-related complications such as intraoperative hypotension, difficult placement and conversion to general anesthesia.[78]

General Anesthesia

Premedication

All obstetric patients should receive acid aspiration prophylaxis as a rule. Obesity increases the risk of acid aspiration further and thus it is mandatory to give a combination of H_2 blockers, e.g. ranitidine or a proton pump inhibitor, such as omeprazole along with a prokinetic agent, e.g. metoclopramide night prior and 1–2 hours before surgery.[79] Thirty milliliters of 0.3 M sodium citrate should also be given 15 minutes prior to induction. Opioid and sedative premedication can lead to maternal and fetal respiratory depression especially in OSA patients and should be avoided. Prophylactic antibiotics and thromboprophylaxis should be given as indicated.

Pearl

Aspiration prophylaxis is mandatory for all obese parturients.

Transfer to Operating Room and Positioning

Transfer of morbidly obese patients within the hospital can be best done on their own hospital bed. Operating room staff should be alerted and adequate manpower should be available for safe positioning of such patients. The operating room staff should be trained in lifting and moving of heavier patients. Lateral transfer equipment should be available. In awake patients, self-transfer to the operating room table may be safer. Specially designed operating room tables should be available or two tables should be placed side by side.[79] Arm boards can also be used to extend the table. The patients should be placed in left lateral tilt and secured to the table with straps.[46]

Clinical pearl

Shifting obese parturient on left lateral position in hospital bed is a good option. Also, use lateral transfer equipment for shifting such women.

Monitoring

Standard sphygmomanometer cuffs can over estimate the blood pressure and the cuff should be at least two-thirds of the circumference of arm to be reliable. Invasive arterial pressure monitoring can be useful in morbidly obese patients, if appropriate size cuff is not available and it will also allow for frequent arterial blood gas analysis. Central venous catheter should be considered in cases where peripheral venous access cannot be secured or where significant cardiopulmonary disease is present. Neuromuscular monitoring will also be helpful in guiding appropriate doses of muscle relaxant during surgery.

Airway Management

Both pregnancy and obesity are potential difficult airway situations. Systematic airway assessment is of paramount importance in obese parturient as inadequate airway management is the most important risk factor leading to morbidity and mortality in these patients.[76,80] This may be due to difficulty because of anatomic and physiologic changes of pregnancy and obesity, increased risk of aspiration, potential urgent nature of situation and lack of experience among residents in managing an obstetric airway because of increasing utility of regional anesthesia for cesarean section. Incidence of difficult intubation in morbidly obese pregnant patient was reported to be as high as 33% in a study by Hood and Dewan.[81] This is almost double the incidence (15.5%) in obese non-pregnant patients.

Pearl

Difficult airway in pregnancy is compounded by problem of obesity.

In addition to the airway changes, obese parturients have reduced FRC and increased oxygen consumption which predisposes them to rapid desaturation following induction of anesthesia. These factors increase the likely hood of airway catastrophe in this patient population. Hence, the importance of meticulous airway assessment, planning and preparation cannot be overstated. It is important to note that in morbidly obese patients, increasing neck circumference (≥ 15 inches) rather than actual BMI has been found to correlate with difficult intubation.[83] Interestingly, gestational weight gain of more than 15 kg has been found to be associated with 3 times more incidence of difficult intubation in obese as compared to non-obese parturients.[84] If airway is predicted to be difficult by previously described methods, regional anesthesia or awake intubation should be planned instead of rapid sequence induction. A back up airway management plan should always be kept ready for emergency even if regional anesthesia is chosen for operative delivery. Maternal safety should be the prime concern of anesthesia provider. Even presence of fetal distress should not coerce anesthetist to opt for general anesthesia in a predicted difficult airway and thereby subjecting the mother to the dreaded risk of failed intubation. Rather a clear communication with the obstetrician regarding the risks involved will facilitate their cooperation for regional anesthesia in most of the cases. When regional anesthesia is contraindicated in emergency situation, rapid sequence induction intubation (RSII) should be instituted after adequate preoxygenation, with a skilled assistant and surgical airway backup. For controlled condition, awake fiberoptic intubation (FOI) after adequate preparation will be the safest option. FOI should be done with utmost care as nasal mucosa in pregnant patient is very prone to bleeding.

Adequate preparation and anticipation of difficulty are the key to success in the management of difficult airway. Obstetric anesthesiologist should be trained in managing difficult and failed intubation using simulation and repeated drills. Alternate airway management plans should be formulated before anesthetizing such patients and should be rehearsed. The difficult airway cart should be stocked with following equipment:

- Oral and nasopharyngeal airway
- Flexible fiberoptic bronchoscope
- At least one of the advanced laryngoscopes: Bullard laryngoscope, Bonfils intubation fiberoscope, videolaryngoscope, C-Mac, Glidescope, King vision, etc.
- At least any two of the following supraglottic devices: LMA, ProSeal laryngeal mask airway, I-Gel, LMA supreme, laryngeal tube, etc.
- Jet ventilation apparatus
- Cricothyroidotomy seldinger kit

Difficulty in managing the airway of such patients and possible solutions have been highlighted in Table 15.7.

> **Clinical pearl**
>
> In obese parturient, adequate preparation and anticipation of difficulty are the key to success in the management of airway. Short handle laryngoscope is useful in obese parturients.

Table 15.7: Airway-related problems with solutions in obese parturient

Change in patient	Effect	Implication	Suggestion
Physiological changes in the respiratory system	Upper airway mucosal edema (fluid retention and fat deposition)	Poor oropharyngeal visualization	Gentle in handling maternal airway
	Nasal congestion	↑ Bleeding during airway handling	Avoid nasal intubation
	Increased oxygen consump; decreased FRC	Rapid desaturation post-induction shorten the allowable time from induction to intubation	Preoxygenation is must Try awake intubation
Physiological changes all in the GI tract	Relaxation of the LES	Increased risk for reflux of	Aspiration prophylaxis in
	and displacement of the stomach	gastric contents and aspiration	patients irrespective of LMT
	Delayed gastric emptying (labor, opioids)		
Increased fat deposition all over the body	Poor positioning Breasts engorgement Restricted chest wall movement	Difficult to achieve sniffing position Placement of the laryngoscope difficult	Ramp (ensure ear at level of sternum) use of a short handle/insert the blade first and then connect the handle

Patient should be positioned in ramped position using either commercial pillow (e.g. Troop Elevation Pillow) or blankets or pillows are placed under head and shoulders so as to align the tragus of the ear with sternal notch (Fig. 15.1). This position has been found to improve laryngeal views by better alignment of oropharyngeal axis.[85] In addition, head elevation leads to improved respiratory function and reduced gastric reflux as compared to supine position. Videolaryngoscope has been found to improve glottis view in morbidly obese non-pregnant patients and find increased utility in managing difficult obstetric airway as well in future.

In obese patients, apnea time after onset of paralysis is reduced and may be just 40 seconds.[86] Thus, importance of adequate preoxygenation to improve oxygen reserves cannot be over emphasized in such patients. Three minute tidal volume preoxygenation or 8 vital capacity breaths over 1 minute have been found to be better than 4 vital capacity breaths over 30 seconds.[87] Effective preoxygenation is considered as end tidal oxygen concentration of 90% which corresponds to about 2 litres of oxygen, i.e. ten times basal requirement. Head up position improves preoxygenation efficacy.[86] In OSA patients, use of CPAP during preoxygenation has been found to be effective in prolonging apnea times.[22] Nasal oxygen insufflations during airway instrumentation, i.e. co-oxygenation has also been effective in prolonging the time to desaturation.[88] Senior anesthetists should conduct the case of morbidly obese parturient with anticipated difficult airway. Skilled help should be available to assist with bag mask ventilation, application of cricoids pressure and drug injection. Doses for thiopentone (4 mg/kg of total body weight up to a maximum dose of 500 mg) and succinylcholine (1–2 mg/kg up to a maximum of 200 mg) should be pre-calculated and loaded in syringes.[89] Lower doses of both the drugs are preferable so as to fasten the awakening in case of failed intubation. Tracheal intubation should be confirmed with both auscultation and capnography. Ultrasonography is a useful adjunct for airway management in obese patients. It is useful to quickly identify esophageal intubation prior to initiation of ventilation, thereby avoiding gastric insufflation and consequent regurgitation and aspiration.[90] It is also useful to correctly identify cricoids cartilage and cricothyroid membrane in these patients.[00] In case of a failed intubation during RSI, alternative intubation plans should be put into action while maintaining maternal oxygenation all the time.

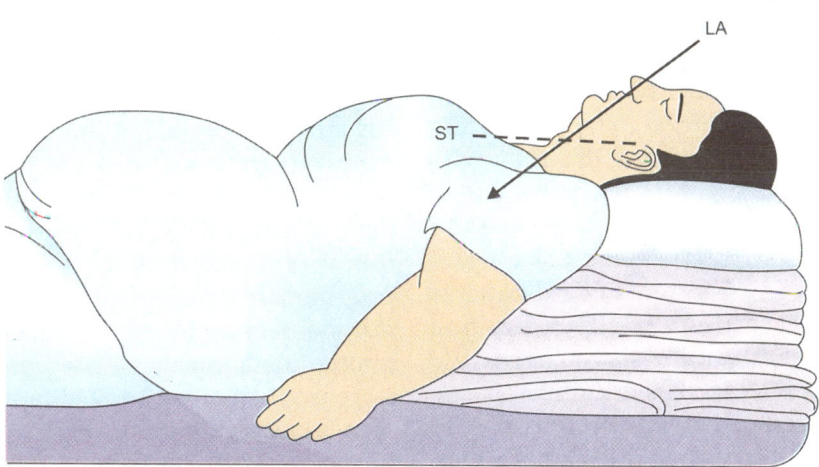

Fig. 15.1. Positioning of obese parturient using ramp

Bag mask ventilation can prove difficult in obese patients because of heavy chest wall and diaphragmatic splinting with gravid uterus. In such situation, supraglottic device can be inserted to maintain oxygenation while cricoid pressure is in place. Though studies have shown that laryngeal mask airway (LMA) classic can be safely used in fasted non-obese pregnant patient,[91] current evidence is limited in their use in obese parturients. In case the patient cannot be ventilated with both bag-mask and LMA and intubation fails (cannot intubate, cannot ventilate [CICV]), emergency pathway of difficult airway algorithm should be activated immediately.[92] CICV setting in obstetric anesthesia is the most feared emergency as reserves are less and it endangers two lives. Situation is worse in an obese parturient where margin of safety (apnea time) is even less. If ventilation becomes possible but fatal distress is present, anesthetist may choose to get the case done with mask anesthesia while maintaining cricoid pressure or may choose surgical airway. However, even in the presence of fetal distress, maternal safety should be the priority of anesthetist.

Short handle laryngoscope will be especially useful in obese parturients with heavy chest and pendulous breast which preclude the insertion of a routine laryngoscope. Alternatively, laryngoscope blade can be disarticulated from its handle and inserted first into the mouth and then reattached to its handle. Placement of patient's arms on the arm board will usually cause the breast to fall away from center on chest, thus reducing obstruction to laryngoscopy. Placing the patient in left lateral tilt to avoid aortocaval compression and simultaneously in ramp position can compromise glottis view.[5,52] Morbidly obese patients experience decrease in FRC in supine position for surgery. General anesthesia can aggravate the decrease in FRC further and thus airway closure can occur in dependant zones of lung, leading to hypoxemia. Measures which has been suggested to improve oxygenation involve use of high inspired oxygen concentration, increased tidal volumes (12–15 mL/kg), propped up position, application of positive end-expiratory pressure (PEEP) and panniculus suspension.[93] Use of PEEP to improve oxygenation has recently been challenged. It was seen that PEEP administration may actually worsen hypoxemia by reducing cardiac output.[94] Tidal volumes of 10–12 mL/kg of ideal body weight are recommended. End tidal capnography may not reflect arterial $PaCO_2$ in these patients and arterial blood gas (ABG) analysis may be a better guide to adequacy of ventilation.[22]

Anesthetic Agent and Dosages

Appropriate drug dosing is one of the challenges faced in anesthetizing these patents due to the complexity of pharmacokinetic alterations in the presence of obesity with pregnancy. Maintaining depth of anesthesia is desirable to avoid awareness and hemodynamic fluctuations while overdosing of drugs can lead to delayed recovery. Both lean body weight and fat reserve increase in obese patients and volume of distribution is increased for most anesthetic drugs, while clearance may be normal or increased. However, since fat has poor blood supply, doses based on total body weight (TBW) can lead to accumulation in body and delayed recovery.[23] Hence calculating the initial doses using lean body weight (LBW) and subsequent doses based on pharmacological response to it is advisable. Among opioids, fentanyl is the drug of choice as there is no change in elimination and dose is unchanged.[95] Atracurium and cis-atracurium are non-depolarizing muscle relaxants of choice as their metabolism and dose are unchanged in pregnancy. Among inhalation agents, isoflurane may be the agent of choice due to its limited metabolism. Obese patients may have increased reductive and oxidative metabolism of inhalational agents leading to accumulation of metabolites and increased risk of hepatotoxicity and nephrotoxicity.[96] Sevoflurane despite its large hepatic metabolism has been

Table 15.8: Pharmacokinetics of anesthetic agents in obese patient

Drugs	Dosage	Rationale
Thiopentone	LBW	Highly lipophilic. $\uparrow V_D$, delayed clearance
Propofol	LBW (induction)	Initial V_D same as non-obese
	TBW(maintenance)	$\uparrow V_D$ and clearance at steady state
Succinylcholine	TBW	Large ECF and $\uparrow$ pseudocholinesterase levels
Rocuronium and vecuronium	LBW	$\uparrow V_D$, impaired hepatic clearance
Atracurium and *cis*-atracurium	TBW	V_D, clearance and elimination half-life unchanged
Fentanyl	LBW	$\uparrow V_D$, clearance unchanged
Sufentanyl	LBW	$\uparrow V_D$, prolonged elimination half-life, clearance unchanged
Remifentanyl	LBW	$\downarrow V_D$ and $\downarrow$ clearance
Dexmedetomidine	TBW	V_D, clearance and elimination half-life unchanged

LBW=lean body weight; TBW=total body weight; V_D =volume of distribution; ECF=extracellular fluid

find to be safe. Among newer inhalation agents, desflurane leads to faster recovery than sevoflurane in obese patients. Pharmacokinetics of various anesthetic agents and dose calculation is shown in Table 15.8.[17,23,97]

It should be remembered that obese parturients are as much risk of aspiration during extubation as during intubation. Residual anesthetic agents can predispose to airway obstruction in patients with OSA. Hence, extubation should be done only after patient is completely awake and neuromuscular monitor shows complete recovery.

Role of Dexmedetomidine

Dexmedetomidine has been shown to be useful in non-obstetric obese patients because of its opioid-sparing action, thus decreasing incidence of respiratory depression in postoperative period.[98] However, literature is lacking on its use in obstetric patients.

Postoperative Analgesia

Effective postoperative analgesia is important in obese parturients to encourage early ambulation and deep breathing. Multimodal analgesia using non-steroidal anti-inflammatory drugs (NSAIDs), paracetamol, opioids, local infiltration and regional blocks is most effective and reduces the dose of opioids. Patient-controlled analgesia, wound infiltration, continuous wound infusion of local anesthetic,[99] transverse abdominis plane (TAP) blocks[100] and ilioinguinal blocks have also been described as useful adjunctive modalities when central neuraxial blocks are contraindicated.[101] American Society of Anesthesiologists (ASA) task force has recommended regional blocks instead of systemic opioids for OSA patients.[102] Continuous epidural analgesia and patient-controlled epidural analgesia improves quality of dynamic postoperative pain relief and thus may help in early mobilization.[103] Epidural analgesia improved respiratory function in morbidly obese patient having undergone abdominal surgery.[104] However, even epidural opioids should be used with extreme vigilance as potential for respiratory depression exists with neuraxial use also especially in patients with OSA.[105]

POSTOPERATIVE CARE AND COMPLICATIONS

Morbidly obese patients are at an increased risk of cardiopulmonary complication in postoperative period and should be continuously monitored in intensive care unit/high dependency unit (ICU/HDU) settings, in

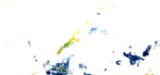

propped up position with oxygen supplementation.[106] Patients who were on CPAP preoperatively should continue to receive it in postoperative period. Risk of postoperative pulmonary complication, such as hypoxemia, atelactasis, pneumonia, pulmonary thromboembolism and pulmonary edema, is doubled in obese parturients even after regional anesthesia.[81,107] The OSA patients are at risk of airway obstruction and apneic episodes during recovery and should receive supplemental oxygen and be monitored with pulse oxymetry even after discharge from recovery.[102] Mhyre et al reported that all anesthesia-related maternal deaths in obese patients from airway obstruction or hypoventilation occurred during recovery period.[34] There is risk of intraoperative blood loss and postpartum hemorrhage in obese patients. Infectious complications, such as urinary tract infection, wound infection and wound dehiscence, are more common. Hence, antibiotic prophylaxis must be given in these patients.

Thromboembolic complications are more frequent and major cause of maternal mortality in obese parturients.[108] So, early mobilization should be encouraged. It has been recommended that pneumatic compression devices should be used in all such patients in perioperative period.

The Royal College of Obstetricians and Gynaecologists (RCOG) recommends thromboprophylaxis with low molecular weight heparin (LMWH) for all morbidly obese patients who are hospitalized antenatally.[109] In pregnant patients with pre-pregnancy BMI >30 kg/m², use of LMWH is recommended for 3–5 days after vaginal delivery and for CS it should be started preoperatively and continued 3–5 days later.[109] It has been suggested that dose of LMWH should be based on actual body weight in obese parturient.[110] Postoperatively physiotherapy and incentive spirometry should be started as soon as feasible. Morbidly obese patients have been increased length of hospital stay, irrespective of mode of delivery and thus consume significantly more heath care resources than non-obese parturients.[111]

SUMMARY

Obesity constitutes a significant risk factor for anesthesia-related maternal mortality and adverse perinatal outcomes. Pre-emptive approach of antenatal assessment, placement of a functional epidural catheter in early labor and keeping alternative plans for airway management in mind while anesthetizing such high-risk patients, appears to be most beneficial approach. Newer technologies, such as ultrasonography, videolaryngoscopy, etc., can help us provide safer anesthesia to obese parturients. A multidisciplinary care would provide better outcome in obese parturients. Continuous vigilant monitoring well into postoperative period is desirable.

REFERENCES

1. World Health Organization. Obesity: preventing and managing the global epidemic. Geneva: World Health Organization, 2000.

2. Obesity: Preventing and Managing a Global Epidemic. WHO Technical Support Series 894. Geneva, Switzerland: World Health Organization, 2000.

3. Baskin ML, Ard J, Franklin F, et al. Prevalence of obesity in United States. Mayo Clin Proc 2006;81:S5–S10.

4. Canoy D, Buchan I. Challenges in obesity epidemiology. Obes Rev 2007;8(Suppl1):1–11.

5. Shah N, Latoo Y. Anaesthetic management of obese patient. BJMP 2008;1(1):15–23.

6. India facing obesity epidemic: experts. The Hindu, 2007, p. 10–2.

7. Ng M, Fleming T, Robinson M, et al. Global, regional, and national prevalence of overweight and obesity in children and adults during 1980-2013: a systematic analysis for the Global Burden of Disease Study 2013. Lancet 2014;384:766–81.

8. Saha UC, Saha KB. A trend in women's health in India–what has been achieved and what can be done. Rural Remote Health 2010;10:1260.

9. Regional Medical Research Centre for Tribals (ICMR), Jabalpur, MP, India. Available from: http://www.rmrct.org. [last submitted on 2009 Jun 25].

10. International Institute for Population Sciences. National Fact Sheet. India National Family Health Survey (NFHS)-3, 2005–6. Mumbai: IIPS; 2006.

11. Third National Family Health Survey. International Institute for Population Sciences, Mumbai. Available from: http://www.nfhsindia. orgnfhs3_national_report.html [last cited on 2005–2006].

12. Chu SY, Kim SY, Bish CL. Prepregnancy obesity prevalence in United States, 2004–2005. Matern Child Health J 2009;13:614–20.

13. Saravankumar, et al. Obesity and obstretic anaesthesia. Anaesthesia 2006;61:36–48.

14. Confidential Enquiry into Maternal and Child Health (CEMACH). Why mothers die? The sixth report into maternal deaths in the United Kingdom. London: RCOG Press; 2004.

15. Cooper GM, McClure JH. Anaesthesia chapter from Saving Mothers' Lives; reviewing maternal deaths to make pregnancy safe. Br J Anaesth 2008;100:17–22.

16. National Institutes of Health Consensus Development Conference Statement. Health Implications of Obesity. Ann Int Med 1985;103:147–51.

17. Sinha AC, Eckmann DM. Anaesthesia for Bariatric surgery. In: Miller RD (Ed). Miller's Anesthesia, 7th ed. Philadelphia: Churchill Livingstone pp. 2089–2104.

18. Garrison RJ, Castelli WP. Weight and thirty-year mortality of men in the Framingham study. Ann Int Med 1985;103:1006–9.

19. Nortcliffe SA. Obstretic Anaesthesia and Obesity. Anaesthesia tutorial of the week 2009, p. 141.

20. Chin JR, Murtaugh MA, Silver R. Obesity: Implications for Women's health. Current Epidemiology Reports 03/2014;1(1).

21. Brodksy JB. Anesthetic management of the morbidly obese patient. Int Anesthesiol Clin 1986; 24:93–103.

22. Ankichetty SP, Angle P, Joselyn AS, Chinnappa V, Halpern S. Anesthetic considerations of parturients with obesity and obstructive sleep apnea. J Anaesthesiol Clin Pharmacol 2012;28:436–43.

23. Ogunnaike BO, Whitten CW. Anaesthesia and Obesity. In: Barasch, Clinical Anesthesia, 6th ed.

Philadelphia: Lippincott Williams and Wilkins. pp. 1230–46.

24. Biring MS, Lewis MI, Liu JI, Mohsenifar Z. Pulmonary physiologic changes of morbid obesity. Am J Med Sci 1999;318:293–7.

25. Eng M, Butler J, Bonica JJ. Respiratory function in pregnant obese women. Am J Obstet Gynecol 1975;123:241–5.

26. Unterborn J. Pulmonary function testing in obesity, pregnancy, and extremes of body habitus. Clin Chest Med 2001;22:759–67.

27. Parmeswaran K, Todd DC, Soth M. Altered respiratory physiology in obesity. Can Respir J 2006;13:203–10.

28. Chang AB. Physiologic changes of pregnancy. In: Chestnut DH (Ed). Obstetric Anesthesia: Principles and Practice, 3rd ed. Philadelphia: Elsevier Mosby, 2004; pp.15–36.

29. Damia G, Mascheroni D, Croci M, Tarenzi L. Perioperative changes in functional residual capacity in morbidly obese patients. Br J Anaesth 1988; 60; 574–8.

30. Soderberg M, Thomson D, White T. Respiration, circulation and and anaesthetic management in obesity. Investigation before and after jejunoileal bypass. Acta Anaesthesiol Scand 1977;21:55–61.

31. Luce JM. Respiratory complications of obesity. Chest 1980;78:626–31.

32. Pelosi P, Croci M, Ravgnan I, et al. The effect of body mass on lung volumes, respiratory mechanics, and gas exchange during general anesthesia. Anesth Analg 1998;87:645–60.

33. Lefcourt LA, Rodis JF. Obstructive sleep apnea in pregnancy. Obst Gynecol Surv 1996;51:503–6.

34. Mhyre JM, Rienser MN, Polley LS, Naughton NN. A series of anesthesia related maternal deaths in Michigan, 1985–2003. Anaesthesiology 2007;106: 1096–1104.

35. Lean ME. Obesity and cardiovascular disease: the waisted years. Br J Cardiol 1999;6:269–73.

36. Alexander JK. Obesity and cardiac performance. Am J Cardiol 1964;14:860–1865.

37. Duvekot JJ, Peeters LL. Maternal cardiovascular hemodynamic adaptation to pregnancy. Obstet Gynecol Surv 1994;49(12 Suppl):S1.

38. Vasan RS. Cardiac function and obesity. Heart 2003;89:1127–9.

39. Bharati S, Lev M. Cardiac conduction system involvement in sudden death of obese young people. Am Heart J 1995;129:273–81.

40. Hubert HB, Feinleib M, McNamara PM, Castelli WB. Obesity as an independent risk factor for cardiovascular disease: A 26-year follow-up of participants in the Framingham heart study. Circulation 1983;67:968–77.

41. Tsueda K, et al. Obesity supine death syndrome: reports of two morbidly obese patients. Anesthesia and Analgesia 1979;58:345–7.

42. Chu SY, Callaghan WM, Kim SY, et al. Maternal obesity and risk of gestational diabetes mellitus. Diabetes care 2007;30(8):2070–6.

43. Mendelson CL. The aspiration of stomach contents into the lungs during obstetric anesthesia. Am J Obstet Gynaecol 1995;52:191–204.

44. Olsson GL, Hallen B, Hambraeus-Jonzon K. Aspiration during anaesthesia: a computer-aided study of 185358 anaesthestics. Acta Anaesthesiol Scand 1986;30:84–92.

45. Casati A, Putzu M. Anesthesia in the obese patient: Pharmacokinetic considerations. Journal of Clinical Anesthesia Vol-17, Issue 2, pp. 134–45

46. Fitzsimons K J, Modder J. Setting maternity care standards for women with obesity in pregnancy. Seminars in Fetal and Neonatal Medicine. 2010; 15:100–7.

47. Davies GA, Maxwell C, McLeod L, et al. Society of Obstetricians and Gynaecologists of Canada. SOGC Clinical Practice Guidelines: Obesity in pregnancy. No. 239, February 2010. Int J Gynaecol Obstet 2010;110:167–73.

48. Merah NA, et al. Prediction of difficult laryngoscopy in a population of Nigerian obstetric patients. West African Journal of Medicine 2004; 23:38–44.

49. Harmer M. Difficult and failed intubation in obstetrics. Int J Obstet Anesth 1997;6:25–31.

50. Weiss JL, Malone FD, Emig D, et al. Obesity, obstetric complications and caesarean delivery rate: a population-based screening study. Am J Obstet Gynecol 2004;190:1091–7.

51. Maggard MA, Yermilov I, Li Z, et al. Pregnancy and fertility following bariatric surgery: A systematic review. JAMA 2008;300:2286–96.

52. D'Angelo R, Dewan DD. Obesity. In: Chestnut DH (Ed.) Obstetric Anesthesia: Principles and Practice 2004;pp. 893–903.

53. Howell CJ. Epidural versus non-epidural analgesia for pain relief in labour (Cochrane Review). In: The Cochrane Library, Issue 4. Chichester: John Wiley & Sons, Ltd., 2004.

54. Cascio M, et al. Labour analgesia with intrathecal fentanyl decreases maternal stress. Canadian Journal of Anaesthesia 1997;44:605–9.

55. Hamza J, et al. Parturient's posture during epidural puncture affects the distance from skin to epidural space. Journal of Clinical Anesthesia 1995;7:1–4.

56. Vincent RD, Chestnut DH. Which position is more comfortable for the parturient during identification of the epidural space? International Journal of Obstetric Anesthesia 1991;1:9–11.

57. Eappen S, Blinn A, Segal S. Incidence of epidural catheter replacement in parturients: a retrospective chartreview. Int J Obstet Anesth 1998;7: 220–5.

58. Perlow JH, Morgan MA. Massive maternal obesity and perioperative cesarean morbidity. Am J Obstet Gynecol 1994;170:560–5.

59. Badve M, Shah T, Jones-Ivy S, Vallejo MC. Ultrasound guided epidural analgesia for labor in a patient with an intrathecal baclofen pump. Int J Obstet Anesth 2011;20:370–2.

60. Soens MA, Birnbach DJ, Ranasinghe JS, van Zundert A. Obstetric anesthesia for the obese and morbidly obese patient: An ounce of prevention is worth more than a pound of treatment. Acta Anaesthesiol Scand 2008;52:6–19.

61. Maitra AM, Palmer SK, Bachhuber SR, Abram SE. Continuous epidural analgesia for cesarean section in a patient with morbid obesity. Anesth Analg 1979;58:348–9.

62. Hamza J, Smida M, Benhamou D, Cohen SE. Parturient's posture during epidural puncture affects the distance from skin to epidural space. J Clin Anesth 1995;7:1–4.

63. Bahk JH, Kim JH, Lee JS, Lee SC. Computed tomography study of the lumbar (L3–4) epidural depth and its relationship to physical measurements in young adult men. Reg Anesth Pain Med 1998;23:262–5.

64. Watts RW. The influence of obesity on the relationship between body mass index and the distance to the epidural space from the skin. Anaesth Intensive Care 1993;21:309–10.

65. Iwama H, Katayama T. Back skin movement also causes 'walking' epidural catheter. J Clin Anesth 1999;11:140–1.

66. Hamilton CL, Riley ET, Cohen SE. Changes in the position of epidural catheters associated with patient movement. Anesthesiology 1997;86: 778–84.

67. Faure E, Moreno R, Thisted R. Incidence of postdural puncture headache in morbidly obese parturients. Reg Anesth 1994;19:361–3.

68. Coker LL. Continuous spinal anaesthesia for Caesarean section for a morbidly obese patient: a case report. AANA J 2002;70:189–92.

69. Faure E, et al. Incidence of postdural puncture headache in morbidly obese parturients. Reg Anesth 1994;19:361–3.

70. Eappen S, Blinn A, Segal S. Incidence of epidural catheter replacement in parturients: a retrospective chart review. Int J Obstet Anesth 1998;7:220–5.

71. van de Velde M, Teunkens A, Hanssens M, van Assche FA, Vandermeersch E. Post-dural puncture headache following combined spinal epidural or epidural anesthesia in obstetric patients. Anaesth Intensive Care 2001;29:595–9.

72. Pan PH, Bogard TD, Owen MD. Incidence and characteristics of failures in obstetric neuraxial analgesia and anesthesia: a retrospective analysis of 19 259 deliveries. Int J Obstet Anesth 2004;13:227–33.

73. Young TK, Woodmansee B. Factors that are associated with caesarean delivery in a large private practice: the importance of pre pregnancy body mass index and weight gain. Am J Obstet Gynecol 2002;187(2):312–8 discussion 318–20.

74. Weiss JL, Malone FD, Emig D, Ball RH, Nyberg DA, Comstock CH, et al. Obesity, obstetric complications and cesarean delivery rate—a population-based screening study. Am J Obstet Gynecol 2004;190:1091–7.

75. Sheiner E, Levy A, Menes TS, Silverberg D, Katz M, Mazor M. Maternal obesity as an independent risk factor for caesarean delivery. Paediatr Perinat Epidemiol 2004;18:196–201.

76. Vallejo MC. Anesthetic management of the morbidly obese parturient. Curr Opin Anaesthesiol 2007;20:175–80.

77. Greene NM. Distribution of local anesthetics within the subarachnoid space. Anesthesia and Analgesia 1985;64:715–30.

78. Vricella LK, Louis JM, mercer BM, Bolden N. Anesthesia complications during scheduled caesarean delivery for morbidly obese women. Am J Obstet Gynecol 2010;203:276.e1–5.

79. Cooper JR, Brodsky JB. Anesthetic management of the morbidly obese patient. Semin Anesth 1987;6:260–70.

80. Schneider MC. Anaesthetic management of high-risk obstetric patients. Acta Anaesthesiol Scand 1997;41(1 Suppl 111):163–5.

81. Hood DD, Dewan DM, Kashtan K. Anesthesia outcome in the morbidly obese parturient. Anesthesiology 1993;79:1210–8.

82. Juvin P, et al. Difficult tracheal intubation is more common in obese than lean patients. Anesthesia and Analgesia 2003;97:595–600.

83. Bell RL, et al. Postoperative considerations for patients with obesity and sleep apnea. Anaesthesiol Clin N Am 2005;23:493–500.

84. Shankar KB, et al. Airway changes during pregnancy. Anaesthesiology 1997;87:A895.

85. Collins JS, Lemmens HJ, Brodsky JB, et al. Laryngoscopy and morbid obesity: a comparison of the 'sniff' and 'ramped' positions. Obes Surg 2004;14:1171–5.

86. Altermatt FR, Munoz HR, Delfino AE, Cortinez LI. Pre- oxygenation in the obese patient: effects of position on toler- ance to apnoea. Br J Anaesth 2005;95:706–9.

87. Baraka AS, Taha SK, Aouad MT et al. Preoxygenation–comparison of maximal breathing and tidal volume breathing techniques. Anesthesiology 1999;91:612–6.

88. Baraka AS, Taha SK, Siddik-Sayyid SM, Kanazi GE, El-Khatib MF, Dagher CM, et al. Supplementation of pre-oxygenation in morbidly obese patients using nasopharyngeal oxygen insufflation. Anaesthesia 2007;62:769–73.

89. Bray GA. Complications of obesity. Ann Intern Med 1985;103:1052–62.

90. Kristensen MS, Teoh WH, Graumann O, Laursen CB. Ultrasonography for clinical decision-making and intervention in airway management: from the mouth to the lungs and pleurae. Insights Imaging 2014;5:253–79.

91. Halaseh BK, Sukkar ZF, Hassan LH, Sia ATH, Bushnaq WA, Adarbeh H. The use of ProSeal laryngeal mask airway in caesarean section-experience in 3000 cases. Anaesth Intensive Care 2010;38:1023–8.

92. Apfelbaum JL, Hagberg CA, Caplan RA, et al. Practice guidelines for management of the difficult airway: an updated report by the American Society of Anesthesiologists Task Force on Management of the Difficult Airway. Anesthesiology 2013;118:251–70.

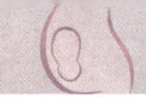

93. Wyner J, Brodsky JB, Merrell RC. Massive obesity and arterial oxygenation. Anesth Analg 1981; 60:691–3.

94. Santesson J. Oxygen transport and venous admixture in the extremely obese: influence of anaesthesia and artificial ventilation with and without positive end–expiratory pressure. Acta Anaesthesiol Scand 1976;20:387–94.

95. Marik P, Varon J. The obese patient in the ICU. Chest 1998;113:492–8.

96. Strube PJ, Hulands GH, Halsey MJ. Serum fluoride levels in morbidly obese patients: Enfurane compared with isofurane anaesthesia. Anaesthesia 1987;42:685–9.

97. Sjostrom LV. Mortality of severely obese subjects. Am J Clin Nutr ÈÈ 1992;55:516S-23S.

98. Hofer RE, Sprung J, Sarr MG, Wedel DJ. Anesthesia for a Patient with Morbid Obesity using Dexmedetomidine without Narcotics. Can J Anaesth 2005;52:176–80.

99. Liu SS, Richman JM, Thirlby RC, Wu CL. Efficacy of continous wound catheters delivering local anesthetic for postoperative analgesia. A quantitative and qualitative systemic review of randomised controlled trials. J Am Coll Surg 2006;203; 914–32.

100. Eslamian L, Jalili Z, Jamal A, Marsoosi V, Movafegh A. Transversus abdominis plane block reduces postoperative pain intensity and analgesic consumption in elective cesarean delivery under general anesthesia. J Anesth 2012;26: 334–8.

101. McDonnell NJ, Keating ML, Muchatuta NA, Pavy TJG, Paech MJ. Analgesia after caesarean delivery. Anaesth Intensive Care 2009;37:539–51.

102. American society of Anesthesiologists Task force on Perioperative guidelines for the perioperative management of patients with Obstructive Sleep Apnea. Practise guidelines for perioperative management of patients with obstructive sleep apnea. Anesthesiology 2006;104:1081–93.

103. Wheatley RG, Schug SA, Watson D. Safety and efficacy of postoperative epidural analgesia. Br J Anaesth 2001;87:47–61.

104. Rawal N, Sjostrand U, Christoffersson E, et al. Comparison of intramuscular and epidural morphine for postoperative analgesia in the grossly obese: Influence on postoperative ambulation and pulmonary function. Anesth Analg 1984;63:583–92.

105. Lamarche Y, Martin R, Reiher J, Blaise G. The sleep apnoea syndrome and epidural morphine. Can Anaesth Soc J 1986;33:231–3.

106. Manuel C Vallejo. Anaesthetic management of the morbidly obese parturient. Current Opinion in Anaesthesiology 2007;20:175–80.

107. Perlow JH, Morgan MA. Massive maternal obesity and perioperative caesarean morbidity. Am J Obstet Gynecol 1994;170:560–5.

108. Lewis G (Ed). The Confidential Enquiry into Maternal and Child Health (CEMACH). Saving Mother's Lives: Reviewing Maternal Deaths to Make Motherhood Safer 2003–2005. The Seventh Confidential Enquiry into Maternal Deaths in the United Kingdom. RCOG Press, London 2007.

109. Nelson-Piercy C. Thromboprophylaxis during pregnancy, labour and after vaginal delivery. RCOG Guideline No. 37, 2004.

110. Michota F, Merli G. Anticoagulation in special patient populations: are special dosing considerations required? Clev Clin J Med 2005;72(Suppl. 1): S37–42.

111. Heslehurst N, Simpson H, Ells LJ, et al. The impact of maternal BMI status on pregnancy outcomes with immediate short-term obstetric resource implications: a meta-analysis. Obes Rev 2008;9: 635–83.

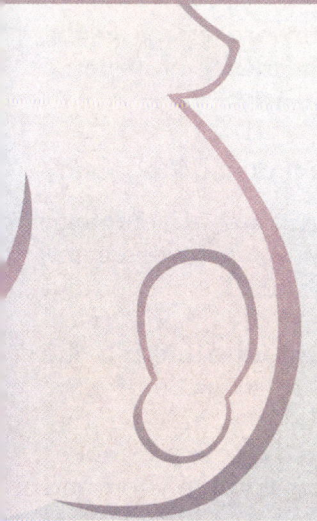

Neurologic, Neuromuscular, and Renal Diseases in Pregnancy

Sushama Tandale

16.1 NEUROLOGIC AND NEUROMUSCULAR DISEASES (Pathophysiology, Clinical Presentation, Interaction with Pregnancy and Anesthetic Management)

Neuromuscular and neurological disease influences obstetric outcome due to involvement of nervous and musculoskeletal systems. Multidisciplinary team work, specific precautions and preanesthetic optimization help to improve outcome in peripartum period.

MULTIPLE SCLEROSIS

Optimal anesthetic management of multiple sclerosis requires careful preoperative assessment, awareness of perioperative hazard and risk of postoperative exacerbation.

Pathophysiology

Multiple sclerosis is an autoimmune demyelinating disorder of central nervous system characterized by multifocal areas of inflammation and demyelination in the brain and spinal cord resulting in wide variety of neurological impairment with progressive disability as time passes.[1–6] It affects genetically susceptible young individuals with female preponderance.[1–6] Prevalence is 30–100 cases per 1,00,000 individuals.[2] Disease course includes periods of exacerbations and remissions at unpredictable interval.[1]

The disease is characterized by immunologic (mediated by autoreactive T cell) destruction of myelin brain protein throughout nervous system.[2] Damage to the myelin sheath results in formation of scar tissue resulting in decreased conduction of nerve impulse. This produces diminished function of central nervous system including muscle weakness, loss of coordination, fatigue and cognitive impairment.[5] During the period of remission, myelin undergoes partial regeneration leading to resolution of symptoms. But as the disease becomes progressive, more and more myelin gets destroyed leading to worsening of symptoms.[5] Relapses are subacute in onset and occur due to activation of myelin reactive T cells producing acute inflammation and edema which shows better clinical response to steroid due to its anti-inflammatory activity.[2]

Types of Disease[2,5]

1. **Relapsing-remitting:** It is most common type, characterized by periodic relapse and remissions.
2. **Primary progressive:** It is characterized by steady and progressive deterioration of neurological function without relapses and remission.
3. **Secondary progressive:** Progressive deterioration of neurological function occurs with remission.

Clinical Presentation

It includes motor complaints like cerebellar sign, spasticity, fatigue ability and sexual dysfunction, sensory complaints like numbness and paresthesia over face and extremity, visual complaints like temporary loss of vision, diplopia and blurred vision and bladder, bowel dysfunction, mood disorder and cognitive impairment.[5]

Exacerbation of disease is known to occur following emotional stress, trauma, surgery, infection and postoperative pain.[1,2]

Medical management aims at reducing the progress of disease which includes immuno-suppressive therapy, immunotherapy and corticosteroid. Symptomatic treatment includes use of gabapentin and carbamazepine for paroxysmal pain, baclofen and diazepam for spasticity, anticholinergic drugs for bowel and bladder dysfunction and antidepressant for depression.[2,5]

Interaction with Pregnancy

The effect of pregnancy on disease is poorly understood. Usually, a reduction in relapse rate is seen during pregnancy[2,4,7] and exacerbation is common in first three months following delivery, three times higher than the non-pregnant woman.[1,2,4,7] In mild cases and remissions, pregnant patient does well.

Pregnancy has no untoward effect on the course of disease and incidence of obstetric complications is not increased.

Anesthetic Management during Pregnancy

1. Preoperative documentation of neurological deficit, respiratory system involvement, autonomic nervous system dysfunction and current drug therapy is essential. Cervical motor root involvement affecting the diaphragm contractility, may compromise the breathing of patient in preoperative period.[1] Autonomic dysreflexia makes patient susceptible to hypotension and reduced response to intravenous fluid and vasopressor therapy in perioperative period. Hence adequate preloading should be done prior to neuraxial block.[1,8] Preoperative counseling regarding exacerbation of disease in postpartum period should be done.

2. Perioperative steroid supplement is essential in patients with steroid therapy to avoid adrenal insufficiency. Chronic steroid intake results in muscle wasting and osteoporosis which increase the risk of injury during positioning.[1]

3. Recurrence following use of general anesthesia and neuraxial anesthesia in pregnant patients with multiple sclerosis is still matter of controversy. Use of spinal anesthesia has been implicated in postoperative recurrence.[5,6] General anesthesia and epidural anesthesia with low concentration (<0.25%) of bupivacaine are considered safer option.[1] Lowest concentration of local anesthetics should always be used whenever possible as demyelinated neurons are more susceptible to injury when exposed to mechanical trauma, neuronal ischemia and neurotoxicity of local anesthetics resulting in aggravation of conduction blockade.[2-6] Addition of opioid to epidural anesthesia is useful for postoperative pain control to minimize the relapse.[1]

4. During general anesthesia, succinylcholine is better to avoid as it can result in hyperkalemia due to up regulation of acetylcholine receptor (extrajunctional) following demyelination. This also causes increase resistance to action of non-depolarizing muscle relaxant.[1,2,5,6] On the other hand, patients on baclofen have muscle weakness and decease muscle mass, which may increase sensitivity to non-depolarizing muscle relaxant. Hence dose titration for lowest necessary dose needs to be done with neuromuscular monitoring.[1,2,5,6]

5. Perioperative hyperthermia is capable of reducing the neurological function by slowing the conduction along demyelinated segment. Hence use of intravenous fluid at room temperature, use of antipyretic is suggested along with temperature monitoring in perioperative period.[1,2,5,6]

6. Deep venous thrombosis may occur in patients who are bedridden in postoperative period. Prophylactic measures, like compression stocking, intermittent external pneumatic compression, use of anticoagulant and early ambulation, should be considered in these patients.[1]

Pearls

- Whenever possible use lowest concentration of local anesthetics in neuraxial anesthesia.
- Avoid depolarizing muscle relaxant.
- Use neuromuscular monitoring, if using nondepolarizing muscle relaxant.
- Avoid perioperative hyperthermia

MYASTHENIA GRAVIS

Course of myasthenia gravis during pregnancy and postpartum period is variable and unpredictable. Anesthetists are involved in the conduct of anesthesia as well as management of myasthenic and cholinergic crises. Multidisciplinary approach, appropriate selection and administration of anesthesia and close monitoring for complications in postoperative period contribute to improve outcome in peripartum period.

Pathophysiology

Myasthenia gravis is an acquired autoimmune disorder caused by autoantibodies against nicotinic acetylcholine receptor on postsynaptic membrane at neuromuscular junction resulting in weakness and fatigability of voluntary muscles.[9–12] Incidence of the disease is 3–7 in 1,00,000 population.[10] It affects individuals of all age and exhibits bimodal peak of incidence, first in third decade of life predominantly affecting female and second in sixth decade of life predominantly affecting male.[13]

Inactivation of postsynaptic receptors results in reduced number of receptors, loss of fold on postsynaptic membrane and widening of synaptic cleft.[11] Disease is most commonly associated with thymic abnormality in 85% (thymus hyperplasia, thymoma) and thyroid disorder in 13% (hyperthyroidism, hypothyroidism, and goiter) of individuals. Other less common associated conditions are rheumatoid arthritis, systemic lupus erythematosus, sarcoidosis, polymyositis, scleroderma, pernicious anemia and lymphofollicular hyperplasia.[9,13]

Types of Disease

1. **Seropositive myasthenia gravis:** It is the commonest type. 85% of generalized myasthenia gravis and 60% of ocular myasthenia gravis are positive for antiacetylcholinergic receptor antibodies by radioimmunoassay.[13]

2. **Seronegative myasthenia gravis:** 10–20% of patients will have antimuscle specific kinase (MUSK) antibody. These patients have localized muscle weakness and reduced response to immunosuppressive therapy.[13]

3. **Transient neonatal myasthenia gravis:** Only 10–15% of newborns of mother having myasthenia gravis are affected.[14] It occurs

due to transplacental passage of maternal anti-acetylcholinergic receptor antibody in newborn and reacting with their acetylcholine receptor. Newborn usually manifests weak cry, sucking and breathing difficulty and hypotonia within few hours of life. Symptoms usually resolves spontaneously within 1–3 weeks of life though pyridostigmine therapy along with supportive treatment may required in some neonates.[13]

Myasthenia Crisis

It is defined as respiratory failure requiring ventilatory assistance or delayed postoperative extubation for more than 24 hours due to myasthenic weakness. Precipitating factors are infection, aspiration, surgery, rapid tapering of immunomodulation, beginning treatment with steroid, exposure to certain drugs and pregnancy.[10, 15] Treatment with neostigmine improves the muscle strength.[11]

Cholinergic Crisis

It is characterized by muscle weakness resulting from over dosage of anticholinesterase drug. Patient will present with generalized weakness and muscarinic symptoms like salivation, diarrhea, bradycardia and miosis. Edrophonium test will differentiate between these two crises as its administration will increase the weakness in cholinergic crisis and will improve the muscle strength in myasthenic crisis.[16] Atropine is drug of choice for treatment of cholinergic crisis.[11]

Clinical Presentation

Patient will present with ptosis, diplopia, and extremity weakness, breathing and swallowing difficulty. Symptoms fluctuate in severity, worsen with exertion and relieved with rest.[13] In most patients, weakness progresses from ocular muscle to other muscles in craniocaudal direction. The weakness of intercostal muscle and diaphragm may lead to exertional dyspnea. In severe cases, respiratory failure may necessitate mechanical ventilation.[13] Factors which exacerbate weakness are emotional stress, exertion, infection, hot temperature, pregnancy and drug exposure with aminoglycoside, local anesthetics, phenytoin, magnesium, etc.[12–14]

Treatment

As the disease has no permanent cure, treatment aims at reducing the severity of symptoms. Medical management includes use of drugs like cholinesterase inhibitors, namely pyridostigmine and neostigmine which improve the muscle strength. Corticosteroid helps in decreasing the antibody production. Azathioprine and cyclosporine act as immunosuppressant. Plasmapheresis helps in removing antibody from the circulation and its effect lasts for 2–3 weeks. Intravenous immunoglobulin G is used in dose of 0.4–1 mg/kg and its effect lasts up to 3 months.[13]

Interaction with Pregnancy

During pregnancy, one-third of patients show improvement in symptoms, one-third experience exacerbation of disease and remaining one-third do not exhibit any change. Exacerbation of disease is common during first trimester and first month postpartum.[9,11–15,17] Improvement of symptoms during second and third trimesters has been attributed to immunosuppression during late pregnancy.[14] Maternal mortality is highest within one year of diagnosis of disease due to severity of symptoms hence it is advised to delay the pregnancy for at least one year after onset of disease. Risk is lowest after seven years of diagnosis.[12,14] Vaginal delivery is recommended as disease does not involve uterine smooth muscle but assistance may require during bearing down effort as abdominal striated muscles are involved during second stage of labor.[9,13,14] Cesarean delivery should be reserved only for obstetric indications as

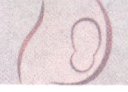

surgery is stressful in patient with myasthenia gravis.[14] Preoperative thymectomy decreases the disease exacerbations during pregnancy, need of medication during pregnancy and also the risk of neonatal myasthenia gravis in newborn.[14,15]

Anesthesia Management

1. It is important for anesthetist to assess preoperatively the extent of respiratory or bulbar muscle involvement, frequency and severity of myasthenic attack, type and dose of anticholinesterase drug and other medication and coexisting illness. In patients with respiratory muscle involvement, PFT should be asked and on clinical suspicion of thyroid disorder TFT should be undertaken. Perioperative steroid supplement is essential in patients with steroid therapy to avoid adrenal insufficiency. Anticholinesterase drug should be continued in perioperative period by any route to avoid exacerbation of disease.[11]

2. General anesthesia and regional anesthesia both have been used successfully in these patients. General anesthesia is more appropriate in presence of bulbar or respiratory muscle involvement as it ensures protection of airway and helps to provide adequate ventilation.[9,11] Patients with mild generalized disease or ocular myasthenia gravis are suitable for regional anesthesia.[9,11]

3. These patients are highly sensitive to action of non-depolarizing muscle relaxant even in period of remission. 1/5th to 1/10th of paralyzing dose is often sufficient to induce muscle paralysis in both seronegative and seropositive patients. Hence neuromuscular monitoring is essential to avoid problems of prolonged neuromuscular block.[10,11,13] Depolarizing muscle relaxant should be avoided due to its variable effect. Patient may manifest resistance to their action or prolonged block.[11,16] In severely compromised patient, use of thiopentone or inhalational agent alone can produce good intubating conditions.[11,16] Use of inhalational agent should be kept to minimum as it can aggravate the muscle weakness. Low dose of short-acting opioid and benzodiazepine should be used for intraoperative maintenance as these patients are sensitive to respiratory depressant effect.[11] Reversal should be achieved with incremental intravenous dose of neostigmine with monitoring of response with nerve stimulator. Overenthusiastic efforts at reversal may precipitate cholinergic crisis.[11] Use of sugammadex can rapidly reverse neuromuscular block regardless of its depth and reduces the incidence of postoperative residual curarization.[10]

4. Spinal anesthesia (with limitation of upper level of block) is preferable over epidural anesthesia as the requirement of local anesthetic is small. In case of epidural anesthesia where large quantity of local anesthetics is required, amide group of local anesthetics are preferred which do not require pseudocholinesterase for its metabolism.[11,14,15] Elevated blood levels of local anesthetics in patients on anticholinesterase therapy may interfere with neuromuscular transmission.[9,15] Epidural opioid should be used judiciously in patients with respiratory and bulbar muscle involvement.

5. Anticholinesterase drug, steroid, azathioprine and plasmapheresis should be used during exacerbation of disease in pregnancy.[11] Drugs, like magnesium sulfate, are contraindicated as they produce neuromuscular block by inhibiting release of acetylcholine from prejunctional membrane.[11] Other drugs to be avoided are phenytoin, local anesthetics, quinidine, antibiotic like aminoglycoside, macrolide and penicillamine as they aggravate muscle weakness.

Table 16.1.1:	Equivalent doses of anticholinesterase drug in perioperative period by other route[18]		
Anticholinesterase	Intramuscular (mg)	Intravenous (mg)	Oral (mg)
Neostigmine	0.5	0.7–1	15
Pyridostigmine	2	3–4	60

6. Postoperatively patient should be continuously monitored for exacerbation of symptoms by repeated evaluation of breathing, swallowing and speech. Anticholinesterase drug requirement may vary and it should be continued in postoperative period by best possible route to avoid aggravation of muscle weakness.[9] In severely compromised patients, postoperative ventilation should be considered.

Pearls

- Anticholinesterase drug should be continued in perioperative period by possible route (Table 16.1.1).
- Neuraxial blocks are preferred in presence of mild generalized disease and general anesthesia is preferred in severe disease with systemic manifestations.
- Intraoperative neuromuscular monitoring is essential.

EPILEPSY

Epilepsy is most common neurological disorder. Anesthesia care of patient with neurological disease require expertise in neuroanesthesia and obstetric anesthesia care, detailed examination of neurological system preoperatively, safe choice and conductance of anesthesia, avoidance of unfavorable drug effect for fetus and nervous system of mother and intraoperative neuromonitoring with control of fetal heart rate.

Pathophysiology

Epilepsy is recurrent seizure activity resulting from congenital or acquired factors and usually associated with certain behavioral and neurological effects.[19] It occurs due to repetitive synchronous electrical discharges in cerebral cortex.[20] International classification of seizure disorder is as follows:[20]

1. Generalized seizures: They are subclassified into absence seizure, tonic clonic seizure, tonic seizure and myoclonic seizure.
2. Partial seizures: They are subclassified into simple seizure, complex seizure and partial seizure with secondary generalized activity.
3. Unclassified

Clinical Presentation

When seizure occurs for first time in peripartum period, it becomes difficult to differentiate the eclampsia from new onset or late relapse of epilepsy. Simultaneous institution of treatment for eclampsia and evaluation of etiology should be done. Patient with history of epilepsy are at increased risk of seizure during pregnancy and postpartum period. Maternal seizures, particularly generalized tonic clonic seizure, result in fetal hypoxia and acidosis.[20] Physiologic changes during pregnancy and alteration in drug therapy may result in status epilepticus.

Interaction with Pregnancy

Approximately 0.5% of pregnant patients will have chronic seizure disorder.[21] Pregnancy exerts variable effect on frequency of seizure. Approximately one-third of patient experiences increase in frequency whereas half of the patients do not show any change.[20–22] Few possible etiologies for decreased threshold of seizure during pregnancy are increased estrogen concentration, increased sodium and water retention, respiratory alkalosis secondary to hyperventilation due to labor pain, sleep deprivation, stress and anxiety.[19] Blood level of anticonvulsant drug are affected by multiple factors like nausea and vomiting during morning sickness, altered protein binding, delayed gastric emptying, folic acid supplementation, increase in plasma volume and distribution, increased renal clearance and noncompliance with drug due to fear of congenital malformation. Hence careful titration of medication to attain therapeutic blood levels is needed.[18,21]

These patients experience increased incidence of pre-eclampsia, placental abnormality, bleeding in peripartum period and preterm labor during their pregnancy.[21,22] Neonatal adverse outcomes are low birth weight, fetal distress, fetal loss, hemorrhages and congenital malformations (4–6%) like cleft lip, cleft palate, cardiac defect, neural tube defect and urogenital defect.[20,21] They should be given vitamin K at birth as maternal anticonvulsant therapy produces transient depression of prothrombin and factors V, VII. Mother should also receive vitamin K supplement during late pregnancy.[18,21] Mother should be given monotherapy during pregnancy to avoid the risk of teratogenicity. Newer drugs, like gabapentin, are preferred.[20]

Status epilepticus requires immediate attention with standard anticonvulsant therapy, airway protection and aspiration prophylaxis.[18] Controlled ventilation with oxygen in these patients decreases metabolic and respiratory acidosis and ensures adequate oxygenation of mother and fetus.[18] The dose of phenytoin to terminate seizure is 13–18 mg/kg by continous intravenous drip. Patient should be monitored for hypotension and first degree atrioventricular heart block. Alternative drugs, like lorazepam (4 mg IV), diazepam (10 mg IV) and midazolam, can be given in incremental doses. Phenobarbitone can also be used in dose of 10–20 mg/kg IV but it has potential for respiratory depression.[18,22]

Anesthesia Management

1. In pregnant patient with epilepsy, one must consider the cause of epilepsy, obstetric course and treatment for same. Serum level of anticoagulant should be checked to ensure therapeutic level, if patient is already on anticonvulsant.[21]

2. If seizure occurs during pregnancy, the primary goal of treatment should be termination of seizure followed by airway protection, support of ventilation and aspiration prophylaxis. Persistence of fetal bradycardia during seizure warrants immediate delivery.[21] In such event, small doses of benzodiazepine, propofol and sodium thiopentone will stop most of seizure. If seizure occurs just before the delivery of fetus, propofol 1% can be given in aliquots of 3–4 mL in repeated bolus with acceptable level of consciousness till normal delivery occurs and after delivery diazepam 10 mg should be given.[22]

3. Regional anesthesia is not a contraindication in patient with epilepsy. It is safe and appropriate choice in well-controlled epileptic patient.[18,20,21] Labor analgesia is indicated in as it suppresses the pain and stress of delivery and helps to prevent maternal hyperventilation and respiratory alkalosis that provoke seizure.[18,22]

4. Succinylcholine and sodium thiopentone have been used safely during induction of general anesthesia.[21] It is better to avoid drugs which lower the seizure threshold like ketamine, etomidate, enflurane and meperidine.[18,20] Sevoflurane has epileptogenic property (>1.5 MAC) but coadministration of nitrous oxide and hyperventilation may counteract this property.[19,21] Low dose propofol results in activation of electrocorticogram but higher dose causes burst suppression.[21] Anesthesia can be maintained with oxygen, nitrous oxide and volatile agent like isoflurane. Patients on phenytoin (enzyme inducer) are resistant to action of non-depolarizing muscle relaxant

particularly vecuronium.[20,21] Use of meperidine for analgesia may cause myoclonic seizure.[21]

5. Patients with recent activity of seizure are at increased risk in postpartum period also. Hence, it is essential to be prepared to treat seizure activity regardless of anesthetic and analgesic technique.

Pearls

- Antiepileptic should be continued in perioperative period.
- Regional anesthesia is not contraindicated.
- Seizure activity needs to be treated on priority basis irrespective of anesthesia technique.

MYOTONIA AND MYOTONIC DYSTROPHY

Pathophysiology and Clinical Presentation

Myotonic dystrophy is most common cause of myotonia (difficulty in initiating muscle movement with delayed muscle relaxation following contraction) and shows autosomal dominant pattern of transmission.[16,18,21] Its prevalence is 5 in 1,00,000 population. The affected gene is located on chromosome 19 locus q12.3. It manifests in second to third decade of life but patients can presents in infancy also.[18,21] As disease progresses, muscle weakness and atrophy becomes prominent particularly of hand, facial, masseter and pretibial muscles.[16,21] Pharyngeal, laryngeal and diaphragm also get involved with advancement of disease. Cardiac and uterine muscles are also involved in myotonic dystrophy.[21]

Its multisystemic involvement is evidenced by presenile cataract, premature frontal baldness, hypersomnolence with sleep apnea and endocrine dysfunction leading to pancreatic, adrenal, thyroid and gonadal insufficiency.[16] Alveolar hypoventilation due to pulmonary dysfunction results in chronic hypercapnia, hypoxia and cor pulmonale.[16,18,21] Gastrointestinal hypomoti-lity can predispose them to pulmonary aspiration.[16,18] Cardiac arrhythmia includes atrial arrhythmia, prolonged PR interval, heart block and depressed ventricular function.[16,18,21] Phenytoin, quinine sulfate and procainamide are used in treatment of myotonia. Patients on quinine therapy have decreased requirement of non-depolarizing muscle relaxant.

Myotonia congenita is a milder familial disorder caused by mutations of gene on chromosome 7q35 encoding a chloride channel of skeletal muscle fiber surface membrane.[16] Disease affects only skeletal muscles and smooth muscles are never affected.[21] In some cases, muscle hypertrophy rather than wasting occurs.[18,21] Multisystem involvement does not occur, unlike with myotonic dystrophy. Cardiac abnormality is not present.[18,21] This disorder can be compatible with long life. Drugs, such as quinine and procainamide, are most commonly used to relieve myotonic symptoms. Corticosteroid, phenytoin and tocainide have also been used.[18,21]

Paramyotonia congenita is rare autosomal dominant disorder localized to chromosome 17q. Symptoms include transient stiffness (myotonia) and occasionally weakness after exposure to cold temperatures. Stiffness worsens with activity in contrast to true myotonia. Seum potassium level may rise following an attack.[21]

Interaction with Pregnancy

Obstetric problems have not been described in patients with myotonia congenita as disease affects only smooth muscles.[21] Though temporary worsening of symptoms during pregnancy has been reported in these patients.[21] In patients with myotonic dystrophy, muscle weakness and myotonia may remain unchanged or worsen during pregnancy.[21] These patients are at increased risk of spontaneous abortion and preterm labor.[21]

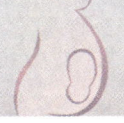
Anesthesia Management

1. Preoperative estimation of cardio-respiratory function with help of pulmonary function test and electrocardiogram should be done. Anesthesia management is complicated by abnormal response to succinylcholine, troublesome intraoperative myotonic contractions and need to avoid hypothermia.

2. Concerns during general anesthesia are same as those described in patients with muscular dystrophy. In patients with myotonic dystrophy, use of succinylcholine may precipitate the intense myotonic contractions of respiratory, chest wall and laryngeal muscles which make ventilation difficult. Trismus can also occur which prevent mouth-opening and makes intubation difficult.[16,18] Shivering triggers myotonic contractions in these patients hence appropriate warming measures to be instituted.[16,21]

3. Regional anesthesia is safe and avoids the risk of respiratory depression. Neither regional anesthesia nor non-depolarizing muscle relaxant prevents myotonic spasm.[16, 18] They will become flaccid on injection of local anesthetics. They can also be treated with intravenous quinine (300–600 mg). Use of steroid and dantrolene has also been suggested.[16,18,21] Uterine myotonia at cesarean section can be treated with topical local anesthesia to relax the uterus.[18]

Pearls

- Avoid depolarizing muscle relaxant.
- Regional anesthesia is safe.

MUSCULAR DYSTROPHY

These groups of patients require highly individualized care with team of surgeon, anesthetist, physician, intensivist and if required pulmonologist and cardiologist for safe conduct of anesthesia.

Pathophysiology

Muscular dystrophies are heterogeneous group of disorders characterized by muscle fiber necrosis and regeneration leading to progressive weakness and degeneration of muscle.[16]

Duchenne muscular dystrophy is common but severe form of muscular dystrophy. Affected individuals produce abnormal dystrophin, a protein found on the sarcolemma of muscle fibers.[16] Disease is characterized by symmetric proximal muscle weakness with pseudohypertrophy of muscles.[16] Degeneration of respiratory and cardiac muscles is common.[16]

Becker muscular dystrophy is less common X-linked recessive muscular dystrophy. It occurs due to deletion or point mutation in the dystrophin gene.[16] Manifestations are similar to Duchenne muscular dystrophy except that they progress slowly.[16]

Above two mentioned dystrophies affect male gender exclusively.[21] The most common muscular dystrophies that affect females include fascioscapulohumeral dystrophy and limb-girdle dystrophy. Fascioscapulohumeral dystrophy is an autosomal dominant, slowly progressive disorder involving the muscles of the shoulders and face. As the disease advance, pelvic and pretibial muscles are also affected. Infrequently, cardiac tachycardia and arrhythmias have been reported.[21]

Limb girdle dystrophy primarily affects the muscles of shoulder and pelvis. Cardiac conduction abnormality is also associated.[21]

Clinical Presentation

Manifestations during infancy include difficulty in respiration, swallowing and sucking. With the progression of disease, muscles become thin and weak.[16] Proximal muscle involvement manifests as gait disturbance. Respiratory muscle involvement leads to ineffective coughing with retention of secretions resulting into recurrent pulmonary infections. Restrictive airway disease can occur due to severe kyphoscoliosis and muscle wasting.[16] Cardiac manifestation includes arrhythmia, heart block and sudden death.[16] Death may occur from bulbar involvement, cardiac defect and aspiration pneumonia.[16]

Interaction with Pregnancy

Patients with muscular dystrophy can have uterine atony resulting in increased incidence of retained placenta and obstetric hemorrhage.[16,18,21] Other associated findings are ovarian insufficiency, amenorrhea, infertility, polyhydramnios and spontaneous abortion.[16] Abdominal muscle weakness may result in prolonged stage of labor and increased incidence of instrumental delivery.[21]

Anesthesia Management

1. Anesthesia management of these patients is not only complicated by presence of muscle weakness but also perioperative respiratory and cardiac manifestations. Preoperative evaluation should note the extent of disease, potential for untoward response to otherwise routine anesthetic agent and obstetric course of patient. Cardiorespiratory function should be assessed with PFT and echocardiography with Holter monitoring respectively in preoperative period.[21]

2. It is better to avoid general anesthesia as exaggerated response is seen to commonly use anesthetic agent. They are very sensitive to circulatory and respiratory depressant effects of opioid, benzodiazepine, inhalational agent and intravenous induction agent hence minimum effective dose to be used and sedative premedication should be avoided.[16,18,21] Aspiration prophylaxis might be beneficial as these patients are prone for pulmonary aspiration.[16] Intraoperative positioning should be gentle and careful in patients with muscle contracture and kyphoscoliosis.[16]

Use of succinylcholine is to be avoided due to its unpredictable response. It carries the risk of inducing severe hyperkalemia or triggering malignant hyperthermia.[16] Association with malignant hyperthermia has been suggested but unproven.[16] For rapid sequence induction, small doses of non-depolarizing muscle relaxant should be used in place of succinylcholine.[18] Some patients exhibit normal response to non-depolarizing muscle relaxant (NDMR) whereas some patients are sensitive to it hence neuromuscular monitoring is essential during its use.[16] Anesthesia can be maintained with use of oxygen, nitrous oxide and low dose of inhalational agent.[18] Extubation should be attempted when patient is fully alert and able to maintain spontaneous and effortless breathing.[18]

3. Regional anesthesia is preferable in this group of patients for labor analgesia and cesarean delivery as it helps to avoid the complications associated with general anesthesia.[16]

Pearls

- Regional anesthesia is preferable.
- Avoid depolarizing muscle relaxant.
- Neuromuscular monitoring is essential.

NEUROFIBROMATOSIS

Anesthetist must be aware of multisystemic involvement of patient with neurofibromatosis (NF) while evaluating and managing patient for surgery. Guideline for pregnant patient is not well documented hence anesthetist should have comprehensive anesthetic plan.

Pathophysiology

It is an autosomal dominant neurocutaneous disorder affecting 1 in 3000 births.[18] Type I NF is characterized by café au lait macule (CALM) and benign cutaneous neurofibroma and is more common than type II.[18,23,24] Type II NF affects central nervous system and incidence of spinal cord tumor and bilateral vestibular schwannoma is high.[23,24] NF is caused by mutation of NF gene that results in loss of activity or in nonfunctional neurofibromin protein.[25] NF1 gene is located on chromosome 17q11.2 and for type II located on 22q12.1.[25] Neurofibromin plays role in the control of cell division and possesses certain tumor suppression qualities.[25] Neurofibroma arises from neurilemma sheath, fibroblast of peripheral nerve and melanocytes.[18] Tumor may involve nerve roots, blood vessels and arise in and around most organ and body cavity.[18]

Clinical Presentation

The presence of two or more of following supports the diagnosis of neurofibroma (National Institute of Health)[25]

1. Six or more café au lait macules of more than 5 mm size in prepubertal children and more than 15 mm size in postpubertal children.
2. Presence of two or more of any type of neurofibromas or one plexiform neurofibroma
3. Presence of axillary or inguinal freckling
4. Two or more Lisch nodule of iris
5. Distinct bony lesion, optic nerve glioma
6. First degree relative with NF I

Various systemic manifestations are as follows:[18,25]

1. Respiratory system—presence of neurofibroma over tongue, larynx, trachea, bronchi and cystic lesion of lung.
2. Cardiovascular system—hypertension (due to pheochromocytoma, renal artery stenosis or diffuse vascular changes), vasculopathy, arteriovenous malformation, aneurysm and cardiomyopathy.
3. Central nervous system—astrocytoma, cerebellar glioma, optic pathway glioma, malignant peripheral nerve sheath tumor.
4. Musculoskeletal system—scoliosis, kyphoscoliosis, osteoporosis, spinal cord tumor, rhabdomyosarcoma.

5. Gastrointestinal system—gastrointestinal stromal tumor, pheochromocytoma, carcinoid.

Interaction with Pregnancy

Patient often experiences increase in number and size of neurofibroma during pregnancy with potential for hemorrhage in lesion.[18] Tumor growth regresses after pregnancy suggesting that they may be hormone responsive.[18,25] Paravertebral and spinal neurofibromas are often present hence pregnant patient should also be observed for change in neurological function.[18] Obstruction from pelvic neurofibroma may cause dystocia in labor or preterm labor.[18,25] The incidence of spontaneous abortion, stillbirth, HELLP syndrome and hypertension is high in these patients.[23–25]

Anesthesia Management

1. Initial evaluation with careful history to elicit sign and symptoms indicative of multisystemic involvement is vital. Based on symptomatology, appropriate diagnostic evaluation should be done. Simple café au lait spot and cutaneous neurofibroma do not warrant further diagnostic procedure.[18] History of labile hypertension may indicate pheochromocytoma or renal vascular disease.[18] Airway examination for laryngeal and neck involvement should be done.[18]
2. Regional anesthesia is acceptable particularly in patients with type I NF due to rare involvement of CNS.[18,23] It is better to avoid regional anesthesia in presence of intracranial neurofibroma or spinal cord tumor.[18] Presence of spinal deformity makes regional anesthesia technically difficult.[25]
3. General anesthesia is a better choice in patients with NF II as CNS involvement is common.[23,24] These patients may exhibit abnormal response to non-depolarizing muscle relaxant due to dennervation phenomenon produced in generalized NF.[18] Effect of depolarizing muscle relaxant is also unpredictable, either resistant or

prolonged.[18] Hence minimal effective dose of muscle relaxant is to be used with neuromuscular monitoring.[18,25] Presence of neurofibroma in trachea, larynx or bronchi interfere in laryngoscopy or intubation.[18,23,25] The possibility of cystic lung lesion leading to pneumothorax should be considered, if intubation is required.[18]

> **Pearl**
> Regional anesthesia is preferable in type I NF and general anesthesia is preferable in type II NF.

POLIO

Poliomyelitis, a neuromuscular disease almost eliminated from most parts of world but still found in some tropical countries. Patient suffers from acute illness as well as sequelae-like chronic neurological and respiratory insufficiency. Choice of anesthesia technique depends upon clinical assessment and individual judgment and it is a challenging task in these patients in various aspects as mentioned below.

Pathophysiology

The disease is caused by polio virus with feco-oral route of transmission.[26,27] It affects the motor and autonomic nervous system with involvement of neurons in anterior horn of spinal cord, vital center in medulla, cranial nerve nuclei and nuclei in roof of cerebellum.[26,27] During the initial phase of disease, virus destroys motor neurons resulting in muscle weakness and paralysis. When the recovery begins, surviving neurons sprouts collaterals and reinnervate the motor unit giving rise to new motor neurons which are larger and fewer in numbers. This results in improvement in muscle strength during recovery phase.[27,28]

Clinical Presentation

Infection with polio virus results in muscle weakness followed by paralysis. During recovery, patient may show improvement in upper extremity but usually damage persists in lower extremities.[27] Poliomyelitis is associated with scoliosis in 30% of patients[26,27] and is more common in adolescent. Females are more affected than males in ratio of 3:1.[26]

Disease is classified into following subtypes:[28]

1. Abortive poliomyelitis—is minor form of disease and presents with flu-like symptoms.
2. Non-paralytic poliomyelitis—here disease presents like viral meningitis.
3. Paralytic poliomyelitis—is most severe form of disease with incidence 1–2%. It presents with muscle pain and paralysis. 60% of affected individuals experience postpolio syndrome.

Postpolio syndrome refers to condition in which recurrence of neuromuscular symptoms occurs in patient with past history of paralytic polio with neurologic recovery.[28,29] Patient presents with new, gradual onset muscle weakness, muscle pain, intolerance to cold, dysphagia and respiratory system dysfunction.[28] Degeneration, decreased number or overuse of motor neurons during ageing process are possible explanations behind the occurrence of postpolio syndrome.[28]

Interaction with Pregnancy

Literature search reveals very limited data on how polio affects pregnancy and how pregnancy affects polio. Patients with muscle weakness may experience prolonged labor.

Anesthesia Management

1. Preoperative evaluation should document extent of neuromuscular involvement, associated disease and presence of postpolio syndrome. Patients at risk of aspiration and likely postoperative respiratory dysfunction should be identified.

2. Anesthetist may have hesitancy to use regional anesthesia because of pre-existing neuromuscular deficit and medicolegal issues in polio patient. But numerous studies have shown no significant adverse events associated with its use in these patients.[27,28] Central neuraxial blocks are challenging because of difficulty in identifying intervertebral space, performing lumbar puncture and prediction of extent of block.[26] Patient may demonstrate asymmetry in spread of sensory block particularly when has coexisting with scoliotic spine.[27]

3. There are numerous concerns while administering general anesthesia to these patients. These patients are sensitive to opioid and non-depolarizing muscle relaxant. Patients with preoperative respiratory tract involvement or dysphagia are prone for delayed awakening, postoperative apnea and aspiration. Hence careful titration of opioid along with neuromuscular monitoring is required.[26–29] Use of depolarizing muscle relaxant is controversial due to associated risk of hyperkalemia, severe myalgia and prolonged duration of action but no specific data is available on its use in these patients.[28,29] Another concern is dysfunctional autonomic nervous system hence drug should be titrated to its desired clinical effect.[26,27] Careful positioning is required under anesthesia due to contracture, spinal deformity and possible neuropathic pain postoperatively.[28,29] They often experience cold intolerance hence warming method should be instituted in perioperative period.[27,28] Extubation may be difficult in patient with respiratory muscle involvement.[26,27]

4. Postoperative vigilant monitoring for sedation and respiration is required particularly in patients with affected muscles of respiration.

Pearl
Regional anesthesia has been found safe.

BRAIN NEOPLASM

Intracranial tumor presenting for neurosurgery during pregnancy, labor and puerperium requires understanding of maternal and fetal physiology, fetal drug pharmacology and principles of neuroanesthesia for safe perioperative management. Close communication between neurosurgeon, neuroanesthetist, obstetrician and patient is crucial. The decision to proceed with neurosurgery during pregnancy depends upon site, size, type of tumor, neurological sign and symptoms, age of fetus and patient consent.

Pathophysiology

Intracranial neoplasms vary in histology, clinical presentation and prognosis.

Gliomas are most common tumors. They are derived from astrocytes with varied invasive potential.[21] Low grade glioma, like astrocytoma, presents with nonspecific symptoms and grow slowly which usually requires conservative treatment. On the other hand, aggressive glioma, like glioblastoma multiforme, grows rapidly with progressive neurological deficit which requires definitive treatment.[30]

Meningioma is next common benign tumor which originates from dura mater or arachnoid.[21] It continues to grow during pregnancy. Definitive treatment is required only in presence of neurological deterioration.[30]

Pituitary adenoma is also common. Patients present with either mass lesion or hypopituitarism. Posterior pituitary involvement manifests as diabetes insipidus.[18] Pituitary infarction can also occur in patients with peripartum hemorrhage due to hypotension. Clinical manifestations include hypopituitarism, failure to lactate, amenorrhea and orthostatic hypotension.[18]

Schwannoma originates from Schwann cell surrounding the nerve. Clinical presentation depends on tumor location. Acoustic neuroma results when eighth nerve is involved and it presents with loss of hearing.[21]

Metastatic carcinoma can also present during pregnancy and their prognosis depends upon the tumor of origin.[21] High incidence is seen with brain metastasis which needs surgical excision prior to chemotherapy due to hemorrhagic and neoplastic potential.[18]

Neurologic deficit can result from mass effect even if tumor is benign. Brain edema is prominent feature of brain neoplasm due to vasogenic or cytotoxic mechanism.[21] Potential for herniation must be considered in any patient with mass lesion. Whenever possible neurosurgical intervention is usually deferred until after delivery when maternal physiology returns to non-pregnancy state and fetal risk is non-existent.[18]

Clinical Presentation

Intracranial neoplasm presents with signs of raised intracranial pressure like headache, vomiting, seizures and visual impairment. Morning sickness, pre-eclampsia and eclampsia during pregnancy may cause delay in diagnosis.[18,20, 1] MRI is procedure of choice as it avoids radiation exposure and confirms the diagnosis. Pregnant patient with rapidly progressing headache, vomiting persisting beyond first trimester, new onset seizure and visual defect should be evaluated accordingly.[20,30]

Interaction with Pregnancy

Incidence of primary brain tumor appearing in pregnancy is same as non-pregnant patient.[18, 21] But some tumors appear to grow faster during pregnancy like meningioma, some gliomas and pituitary adenoma.[18,21] Edema due to salt and water retention, increase in blood volume of vascular tumor, hormonal changes and immunotolerance to foreign tissue antigen that occurs during pregnancy are possible explanation for the same.[18,20,21,32]

In pregnant patient, CSF pressure increases significantly with painful uterine contractions which further ads to risk of herniation in patients with already elevated ICP.[20,21] In patient with intracranial mass lesion, this could result in increased risk of herniation. Hence, it is advised to cut short the second stage of labor.[21]

Treatment of cerebral edema during pregnancy involves the use of a mannitol, antiepileptic, and irradiation of skull or chemotherapy. This increases the fetal adverse effects like abortion, growth retardation and congenital malformation.[21,31] Steroids are useful during pregnancy as they decrease vasogenic edema, improve patient's symptoms and increase fetal surfactant production but also have risk of fetal adrenal hypoplasia.[30]

Anesthesia Management

1. Perioperative management of pregnant patient with intracranial lesion should include avoidance of further neurological injury from rebleed, delayed cerebral ischemia, increase in ICP, metabolic complications and maintenance of maternal and fetal wellbeing.

2. Choice of analgesia during labor is controversial. Parenteral analgesic, particularly opioid, may result in sedation, respiratory depression and hypercarbia which further elevate ICP. Epidural analgesia is good alternative as it attenuates raised ICP due to painful contraction and allows pain free second stage of labor for instrumental vaginal delivery. But inadvertent dural puncture is always risk with epidural procedure which may result in transtentorial brain herniation particularly in patient with compromised neurological function.[20,21] Hence neuraxial block is to be avoided in patients with raised ICP.[20]

3. General anesthesia is better choice in patients with raised ICP as it gives better hemodynamic stability, allows hyperventilation to reduce ICP and induction agents, like thiopentone and propofol, help in reducing ICP.[20] Aggressive hyperventilation results in uteroplacental vasoconstriction with leftward shift of maternal oxyhemoglobin dissociation curve and fetal hypoxia hence its duration and extent should be limited to minimum.[18,20,21] Along with fetal monitoring during surgery, injection fentanyl or lignocaine can be used to attenuate raised ICP during laryngoscopy and intubation.[20] Succinylcholine should be avoided as it raises ICP momentarily. Use of nitrous oxide is controversial as its use may cause cerebral vasodilatation and postoperative nausea and vomiting.[20,21] Anesthesia can be maintained with volatile agent preferably isoflurane and short-acting opioid like fentanyl.[20]

4. Use of osmotic diuretics like mannitol during surgery to decrease intracranial edema is associated with maternal hypovolemia and fetal injury due to uterine hypoperfusion. It also crosses placenta and accumulates in fetus.[18] Hence, it should be used with caution and in low dose 0.25 gm/kg. Furosemide, a loop diuretic, has been used without any adverse maternal and fetal effects. However, it can also cause dose dependant fetal diuresis.[18]

5. Deliberate hypotension used in neurosurgery to reduce intraoperative hemorrhage with the use of high concentration of volatile agent and venodilator may cause fetal asphyxia.[18] However, low concentrations of volatile agent (0.5 MAC) are well tolerated and not associated with significant reduction in blood flow.[18]

6. Pregnant patient posted for neurosurgery should have wide bore intravenous line along with central venous pressure and intra-arterial blood pressure monitoring. External Doppler can be used to monitor fetal heart rate and its variation can detect abnormality in maternal ventilation, uterine perfusion and fetal wellbeing.[18] Maternal systolic blood pressure should be maintained above 100 mm Hg with prompt recognition and treatment of hypotension and hypoxia, if occurs intraoperatively.[18] If fetal distress persists during surgery and not responding to conservative measures like increase in inspired oxygen, change in position, blood pressure changes, etc., then neurosurgery should be stopped and emergency cesarean delivery should be performed.[18] Neonatologist should be always stand by for resuscitation as he will be anesthetized.[18]

Pearls

- General anesthesia is preferred in patients with raised intracranial pressure
- Avoid deliberate hypotension.
- Judicious use of osmotic diuretics intraoperatively
- Mild hypocapnia is accepted.
- Anticipate blood loss.

MATERNAL HYDROCEPHALOUS WITH SHUNT

Shunting of CSF out of brain to extracranial site is the most common treatment modality of hydrocephalous. Due to recent technology and advances in treatment, patients of hydrocephalous are now reaching reproductive age and considering pregnany. Careful management by team of obstetrician, neurosurgeon and anesthetist enables these patients to go through pregnancy and delivery without major adverse effects.

Pathophysiology

Patient may have shunt catheter for variety of reasons like intracranial infection of childhood, intracerebral hemorrhage in preterm infant, aqueductal stenosis, Arnold-Chiary malformation and Dandy-Walker syndrome, etc.[20] During the placement of catheter, its proximal end is kept in ventricular cavity and distal end is placed in extracranial site like peritoneal cavity or atrium after subcutaneous tunneling of remaining catheter. It helps to relieve intracranial pressure by diverting the flow of CSF.

Clinical Presentation

Patients with functioning shunt are neurologically stable. As the pregnancy advances, increase in intra-abdominal pressure may cause impairment of drainage and malfunction of shunt due to occlusion of distal end of catheter. Hence, patients should be observed for signs and symptom of raised ICP. Patients may need further diagnostic evaluation of pre-existing intracranial lesion in event of neurological deterioration. Ideally preconception counseling along with pre pregnancy MRI image for ventricular size should be done.

Interaction with Pregnancy

VP shunt in pregnant patient with hydrocephalus does not affect the mode of delivery. Cesarean delivery should be reserved for patient with obstetric indication or malfunction of shunt.[20,33] With the advancement of pregnancy, impairment of drainage occurs leading to symptoms of raised ICP like headache, nausea, vomiting and neurological deficit.[33] Neurosurgical evaluation of shunt is indicated in such patients.[33] Pregnancy, labor and delivery are safe in patient successfully treated for hydrocephalus.[34] Women with normal ICP and shunt dependant are not at risk of sudden neurological decompensation. Shortened second stage is preferred to obviate straining and raised ICP during cesarean section. Risk

of intra-abdominal infection and adhesion formation around distal end of shunt remains hence distal end is always to be inspected for occlusion.[34]

Anesthesia Management

1. In patients without raised ICP and well-functioning shunt, very few anesthetic considerations exist. Patient's detailed neurological evaluation, functional status of shunt and prior neuroimaging records should be documented in preoperative visit. Patients with severe symptoms or unresponsive to conservative treatment may warrant urgent delivery followed by shunt revision surgery.[34]

2. Patients may be given prophylactic antibiotic prior to surgery to prevent shunt infection.[20]

3. Neuraxial block has been used safely with certain precautions in these patients.[20,22,33] Individual case management is advised according to surgical as well as neuro-anesthesia requirement and gestational age.[33] Possibility of drainage of intrathecal medication into peritoneum or atrium resulting in inadequate anesthesia exists at least theoretically.[20]

4. General anesthesia is required in patients with deteriorating neurological function with care to prevent further rise in ICP along with maintenance of fetoplacental unit perfusion.

Pearls

- Neuraxial blocks are preferred in presence of well functioning shunt.
- General anesthesia is preferred with malfunction of shunt and deterioration of neurological status.

16.2 RENAL DISEASES (Pathophysiology, Clinical Presentation, Interaction with Pregnancy and Anesthetic Management)

ACUTE RENAL FAILURE (ARF)

ARF is uncommon but serious complication of pregnancy. Rapid deterioration of renal function leads to accumulation of fluid and nitrogenous waste products with impaired electrolyte regulation. Steady decline in incidence of ARF in obstetric cases is noted due to improved obstetric care and fewer septic abortions.[21] The early detection and management of renal diseases during pregnancy can have successful pregnancy outcome.

Pathophysiology

In ARF, sharp elevation in plasma creatinine and BUN is seen. Patient may have oliguria (<400 mL/day) or anuria.[21] Causes of ARF have been divided into prerenal, intrarenal and postrenal. Few of the common obstetric causes are septic abortion, severe pre-eclampsia–eclampsia, acute pyelonephritis of pregnancy and bilateral renal cortical necrosis.[21]

Prerenal Cause

Most common causes are hyperemesis gravidarum and obstetric hemorrhage.[21] Obstetric hemorrhage leads to hypovolemia and inadequate renal perfusion. Plasma volume expansion is essential for successful pregnancy outcome. Investigations include urinary osmolality >500 mosm/kg H_2O, urine sodium <20 mEq/L, fractional sodium excretion <1% and urinary to plasma creatinine ratio >40.[21] Woman with pre-eclampsia is more prone for ARF due to pre-existing intravascular volume contraction, prostacyclin deficiency, and hyperactivity to catecholamine and coexisting coagulopathy.[21]

Postrenal Cause

Postrenal causes include nephrolithiasis and ureteral obstruction by gravid uterus. Pre-existing ureteral dilatation and impaired peristalsis increase risk of obstructive uropathy during pregnancy.[21] Patient presents with flank pain, hematuria and decrease urine output.[21]

Intrarenal Cause

Oliguric intrarenal ARF is not easily reversed. Common causes include interstitial nephritis, acute tubular nephritis, acute glomerulonephritis and causes unique to pregnancy are renal cortical necrosis, acute pyelonephritis, severe pre-eclampsia–eclampsia, acute fatty liver of pregnancy and idiopathic postpartum renal failure.[21] Detailed history taking, review of medications and urine analysis help to determine specific initiating factor.[21]

Acute tubular necrosis: It is major cause of ARF and results from nephrotoxic drug, amniotic fluid embolism, rhabdomyolysis, intrauterine fetal death and prolonged renal ischemia secondary to hemorrhage or septic shock.[21] Urine analysis reveals dirty brown epithelial cell cast and coarse granular cast. Other investigations include urine osmolality <350 mosm/kgH_2O, urine sodium >40 mEq/L, fractional sodium excretion >1%, and urinary to plasma creatinine ratio <20.[21]

Acute interstitial nephritis (AIN): NSAIDs and various antibiotics cause AIN. These patients typically have fever, rash, eosinophilia and urine eosinophils.[21]

Acute glomerulonephritis: It is a rare condition and urine analysis shows hematuria, red cell cast and proteinuria. Urinary indices are similar to prerenal ARF.[21]

Bilateral renal cortical necrosis: It is the common (10–38%) obstetric cause of ARF seen during early or late pregnancy. Placental abruption is most common precipitating event.[21] Underlying cause is the renal hypo-perfusion or endothelial damage by endotoxin imposed on the normal hypercoagulable state of pregnancy.[21] Extensive microthrombi is seen within glomeruli and renal arterioles. Selective renal arteriography reveals absent or patchy cortex. Renal biopsy can be performed in absence of coagulopathy for confirmation of diagnosis.[21]

Acute pyelonephritis: It is most common infectious complication of pregnancy and responsible for 5% of ARF amongst parturient. Kidneys are more sensitive to bacterial endotoxin during pregnancy.[21] It shows marked decrease in GRF in pregnant patient.

Severe pre-eclampsia–eclampsia: It is responsible for obstetric ARF in almost 20% of parturients. Majority of the patients show derangement of multiple organ system and obstetric complications like placental abruption, IUFD, DIC, sepsis, postpartum hemorrhage.[21] Renal histology reveals thrombotic microangiopathy and acute tubular necrosis.[21]

Acute fatty liver of pregnancy: It is rare but life-threatening event and characterized by abdominal pain, vomiting, fever, progressive jaundice and hepatic failure.[35] Hypertension is seen in about 20% of patient. Investigations will reveal marked hyperbilirubinemia with mild elevation of liver enzymes.[35]

Idiopathic postpartum renal failure: This syndrome is characterized by ARF, micro-angiopathic hemolytic anemia and thrombo-cytopenia with high mortality. It occurs 2 days to 10 weeks after an uncomplicated delivery.[21] Presentation is closely related to hemolytic uremic syndrome.[21] Typically preceded by upper respiratory or gastrointestinal viral infection that rapidly progress to ARF. Generalized endothelial dysfunction is the key pathological feature.[35] Spontaneous bleeding, congestive heart failure, hypertension and seizures can also occur. Treatment includes infusion of plasma and antiplatelet therapy.[21,35]

Clinical Presentation

Patient presents with signs of volume overload such as dyspnea, edema, hypertension and generalized malaise. As toxins accumulate, without treatment, patients become lethargic, nauseated, and confused. Salt and water excess leads to pulmonary edema and hypoxia, while hyperkalemia and acidosis affect cardiac rhythm and contractility. Encephalopathy, coma, seizures, and death may ensue.

Other signs and symptoms of ARF may be associated with the etiology, such as hypotension, jaundice, hematuria, and urinary retention.

Rapid recognition of underlying abnormality is important. Reversible causes, such as hypovolemia, concealed uterine hemorrhage, UTI, ureteral obstruction, drug-induced ARF, must be excluded.[21] Urine to plasma osmolality ratio is useful lab test to identify reversible prerenal causes.[21] Intravascular volume should be optimized. Electrolytes and acid base should be monitored carefully. Hypertension should be aggressively treated. ARF can cause DIC hence coagulation abnormality to be excluded. Because urea and other metabolite product cross placenta, hemodialysis and peritoneal dialysis should be directed towards maintaining post-dialysis BUN concentration <30 mg/dL. Fluid shift during dialysis should be minimized by short but frequent period of dialysis. Pediatrician should be alerted to high fetal BUN level which may lead to osmotic diuresis and neonatal dehydration, if patient is considered for urgent delivery.[21]

Interaction with Pregnancy

Maternal mortality due to ARF is up to 34%. Fetal prognosis is bad in presence of severe renal dysfunction. More than 40% pregnancy will have IUFD.[21] Good outcome is seen in patients with mild renal dysfunction (creatinine <1.4 mg/dL) without nephrotic proteinuria and minimal or absent hypertension. The impact on long-term renal functions is minimal in this subset of patients.[35]

Anesthesia Management

1. Level of azotemia, electrolyte balance and hematologic status should be assessed in preoperative period. If BUN is >80 mg/dL and potassium >5.5 mEq/L, then dialysis is indicated before elective vaginal delivery or cesarean delivery.[21] Intravascular volume is to be monitored with CVP or pulmonary artery pressure monitoring.[21]

2. Regional anesthesia can be given in absence of thrombocytopenia, coagulopathy and hypovolemia.[21] Epidural anesthesia is preferred over spinal anesthesia as sympathetic block is established slowly while appropriate volume of intravascular fluid is being administered. IV fluid containing no potassium like normal saline can be used for resuscitation.[21] As sympathetic block wears off, mother should be monitored for evidence of volume overload or pulmonary edema.[21]

3. General anesthesia is indicated in presence of urgent indication of delivery or in presence of coagulopathy or hemorrhage.[21] Drugs dependent on renal elimination should be avoided. Short-acting opioid should be used for analgesia. Throughout surgery urine output and CVP should be monitored meticulously.

Pearl

Regional anesthesia is safe in absence of coagulopathy.

RENAL TRANSPLANTATION

Large number of patients with chronic kidney disease undergo renal transplant surgery and the resultant improved survival and quality of life give opportunities to many of these patients to become pregnant and experience motherhood. For successful perioperative outcome in parturient with renal transplantation, close communication between nephrologist, obstetrician, and anesthesiologist is essential, as these patients have altered physiology and are immune-compromised. Main goal of anesthetic management is to maintain optimum perfusion pressure of renal allograft to preserve its function.

Pathophysiology

Renal hyperfiltration (a response which attempts to bring GFR towards the rate of binephric system following transplantation) leads to glomerular sclerosis and increase glomerular pressure resulting in loss of renal function.[21] In normal parturient, RBF and GFR increase significantly during first and second trimesters along with dilation of ureter and renal pelvis.[18,21] In patient with well-functioning renal allograft, GFR also increases. This additional hyperfiltration of pregnancy may predispose patient to loss of renal function.[21] In most of the patients with renal transplantation, allograft function is enhanced during early pregnancy with slight deterioration in late pregnancy.[21] Only 15% of patients experience persistent renal impairment.[21]

Mean serum creatinine and creatinine clearance remains stable throughout pregnancy and up to one year postpartum. However, mean urinary protein increases from 0.45 gm/24 hr at onset of pregnancy to 1.11 gm/24 hr at delivery with return to baseline by 3 months postpartum.[21] In absence of hypertension, it is not significant.[18] HTN, pre-eclampsia, diabetes and multiple pregnancy do not increase the risk of graft loss, however, rejection is increased in parturient with pre-existing or deteriorating renal function or proteinuria.[18]

Clinical Presentation

Renal allograft does not confer normal kidney function and any improvement should be noted.[18] An evaluation for autonomic and peripheral neuropathy should include an assessment for silent MI, delayed gastric emptying and lower limb sensory and motor changes.[18]

Extraperitoneal location of kidney makes it prone for compression by enlarging uterus leading to obstruction and pelvic pain. Obstruction may become so severe that it may necessitate placement of nephrostomy tube.[18] Preoperative blood investigations should include CBC, blood chemistry, RFT, LFT, serum protein, calcium, phosphate, electrolytes, coagulation profile, and echocardiography.[18,21]

Interaction with Pregnancy

Successful renal transplantation improves the fertility rate.[21] Many reports confirm no deleterious effect of pregnancy on a renal graft that was functioning well before pregnancy and 94% of pregnancies that go beyond first trimester end successfully.[18]

Pregnancy in parturient with renal allograft is complicated by abortion, IUGR, preterm delivery and pre-eclampsia.[21,35] Use of immunosuppressant drugs, like cyclosporine, tacrolimus, azathioprine, sirolimus and corticosteroid in post-transplantation protocol, results in fetal congenital malformation.[21] Intrauterine exposure to cyclosporine is associated with impaired function of T, B, NK cell and immunoglobulin resulting in suboptimal response to vaccination. Hence, delayed vaccination (>6 months) is advised in these infants.[21] Infection with CMV in transplant recipient during pregnancy leads to congenital anomaly like cerebral cyst, microcephaly and mental retardation.[21]

Residual renal impairment leads to false biochemical screening for trisomy 21. Hence, in such patients, measurement of nuchal translucency with serial obstetric USG is more helpful for antenatal detection of malformation.[21]

Anesthesia Management

1. Parturient with renal transplantation should be intensively monitored for acute or chronic allograft rejection, presence of infection, ureteral or renal artery obstruction, fluid and electrolyte disturbance and presence of hypertension or anemia. Appropriate definitive measures should be instituted immediately with the consultation of nephrologists and physician. Recombinant human erythropoietin has been used without any adverse effects and should be continued during pregnancy.[21]

2. Immunosuppressive drugs used in renal transplantation have important side effects. Drug, like cyclosporine, is known to cause hypertension, hyperlipidemia, nephrotoxicity, neurotoxicity and hepatotoxicity. Azathioprine use is associated with bone marrow suppression. Side effects with glucocorticoid therapy include sodium retension, hypertension, diabetes, peptic ulcer disease, osteoporosis and delayed wound healing.[36] Anesthetist should be aware of above side effects and appropriate investigations should be asked to rule out drug toxicity. Neurological examination along with documentation of paresthesia is important, if regional anesthesia is planned.[36]

3. Vaginal delivery is preferred.[21] Number of per vaginal examinations should be kept to minimum and done with strict aseptic precaution.[21] Patient undergoing any operative intervention should receive appropriate dose of corticosteroid and prophylactic antibiotic in preoperative period.[21,36] Presence of active genital infection, such as herpes virus infection, is contraindication for vaginal delivery.[21]

4. Choice of anesthesia technique depends on renal function, associated cardiovascular and hematological disorder and urgency of delivery. In absence of hypertension or renal dysfunction, anesthesia management is similar to that in normal parturient.[21] stric

aseptic precautions should be taken while placing intravascular catheter and performance of central neuraxial block.[21,36] Patient positioning and intravenous cannula insertion should be done in consideration with AV fistula.[18] Parturients with significant myocardial dysfunction and ischemia that requires meticulous fluid management need invasive hemodynamic and continuous ECG monitoring.[18]

5. Regional anesthesia is better option in absence of contraindications.[18] Fluid loading should be cautious. Cesarean delivery can be prolonged and difficult due to previous abdominal surgery.[18]

6. During general anesthesia, drug selection should depend upon existing renal function. Drugs, like vecuronium, morphine, local anesthetics, can have prolonged action in presence of deranged RFT. Isoflurane is preferred inhalational agent as it undergoes minimal metabolism.[18] For analgesia, shorter-acting drugs, like fentanyl, alfentanyl and sufentanyl, should be preferred.[18] Non-steroidal anti-inflammatory drugs should be avoided due to its nephrotoxic potential.[18] Solubility agent of cyclosporine augments the action of muscle relaxant hence neuromuscular monitoring is advocated intraoperatively.[36] Perioperative hypotension may make transplanted kidney susceptible to acute tubular necrosis hence patient hydration and urine output should be maintained carefully.[36]

Pearls

- Anesthesia should be administered under all aseptic precautions.
- Prophylactic antibiotics should be given.
- Neuraxial anesthesia is safe in well-functioning graft.

UROLITHIASIS

t is one of the common causes of non-obstetrical abdominal pain and often poses diagnostic and therapeutic challenge. Radiation exposure through imaging modality and anesthesia for surgical procedure may adversely affect the fetus as well as its clinical presentation can mimic other conditions like appendicitis, ectopic pregnancy, diverticulitis and abruption of placenta, preterm labor, pyelonephritis and benign hematuria of pregnancy.[21]

Pathophysiology

Urolithiasis is abnormal formation of calculi within renal calyces or pelvis which may lodge in ureter or bladder. Symptomatic urolithiasis occurs during 1 in 240 to 1 in 3,300 pregnancies.[21] Various physiological changes of pregnancy, such as elevated levels of 1,25-dihydroxyvitamin D which promotes hypercalciuria, increase in urinary pH and increased excretion of uric acid, sodium and oxalate, promote stone formation during pregnancy.[21,37] Whereas increased excretion of calcium stone inhibitors like citrate, magnesium and glycoprotein offsets the stone forming tendency.[21] Patient with history of urolithiasis with or without pancreatitis, hyperemesis beyond first trimester, history of recurrent spontaneous abortion or IUFD, neonatal hypocalcemia or tetany should be screened for primary hyperparathyroidism.[21]

Clinical Presentation

Patients most commonly present during second or third trimester with symptoms of flank pain, urgency, dysuria, nausea and fever. Examination reveals costovertebral tenderness, abdominal tenderness, pyuria and hematuria.[21] Urolithiasis should be considered in parturients who give history of renal calculi, pyelonephritis, fever and continued bacteriuria despite of 48 hours of parenteral antibiotics. Urine microscopy will reveal presence of RBC. Initial imaging modality should be transabdominal ultrasonography but, however, 40% of calculi are missed with its use.[21] In such patients, limited IVP can be done which gives less (<1.5 rad) fetal radiation exposure.[21] MRI with strongly T2-weighed sequence shows the site and type of obstruction without exposing fetus to ionizing radiation.[21] During pregnancy, 70% of calculi pass spontaneously with conservative management (hydration, antibiotic if patient is febrile, bed rest, analgesia).[21] Urologic intervention is indicated in presence of persistent pyelonephritis, deterioration of renal function, massive hydronephrosis, persistant pain or sepsis.[21] Available treatment options are ureteral stent placement with ureteroscopy, percutaneous nephrostomy and open ureterolithotomy.[21] Extracorporeal lithotripsy is not approved for use during pregnancy.[21]

Interaction with Pregnancy

Pregnancy does not alter the activity or severity of stone disease.[21] Obstetric complications, such as premature rupture of membrane, preterm labor and spontaneous abortion, are more in patients with renal colic possibly due to abnormal calcium homeostasis causing myometrial hyperirritability.[21,37]

Calcium supplementation should be avoided in patients with recurrent history of urolithiasis.[21] Maternal use of certain drugs, like thiazide, results in fetal hyponatremia, hypoglycemia and thrombocytopenia and D-penicillamine which is used to treat cystinuric urolithiasis is associated with congenital connective tissue defect.[21] Use of NSAID also to be avoided because of their teratogenic potential.[21]

Anesthesia Management

1. In any pregnant patient presenting for definitive surgery for urolithiasis, one must consider the maternal and fetal safety. During first trimester of pregnancy, main fetal concern is teratogenicity and risk of abortion and during third trimester of pregnancy main maternal concern is

preterm delivery.[38] Fetal heart rate monitoring is advocated in perioperative period along with use of prophylactic tocolytic particularly after 20th week of gestation.[21,38]

2. Use of epidural analgesia for renal colic provides significant pain relief and facilitates passage of calculus by relieving spasm. Use of parenteral drugs, like opioid, impairs normal peristalsis of ureteral smooth muscle and passage of stone hence better to be avoided.[21] Better pain control with regional anesthesia decreases the catecholamine release and improves the uteroplacental blood flow.[21]

3. Usual obstetric considerations, like avoidance of hypotension, aspiration prophylaxis, left uterine displacement, and adequate oxygenation, should be followed regardless of technique of anesthesia.

Pearl

Use of epidural analgesia is therapeutic in renal colic.

SUMMARY

Neuromuscular and neurological diseases influence obstetric outcome due to involvement of nervous and musculoskeletal systems. Anesthesia in such patients requires multidisciplinary team work. Specific precautions and preanesthetic optimization help to improve outcome in peripartum period in obstetrics.

REFERENCES

1. Sethi S, Kapil S. Anesthetic management of a patient with multiple sclerosis undergoing cesarean section with low dose epidural bupivacaine. Saudi J Anaesth 2014;8:402–5.

2. Malhotra D, Alex M, Bengtsson J. Anesthetic management of pregnant patient with multiple sclerosis. The Internet Journal of Anesthesiology 2010;28:2.

3. Christopher QRA. Management of anaesthesia during caesarean section of a multiple sclerosi

pregnant woman: case report and literature review. Rev Colomb Anesthesiol 2015;43:104–6.

4. Lorenzi AR, Ford HL. Multiple sclerosis and pregnancy. Postgrad Med J 2002; 78:460–4.

5. Schneider KM. An overview of multiple sclerosis and implications for anaesthesia. AANA Journal 2005;73:217–24.

6. Lata M Kulkarni, Sanikop CS, Shilpa HL, Anupama Vinayan. Anaesthetic management in patient with multiple sclerosis. Indian J Anaesth 2011;55(1):64–7.

7. Celia Oreja Guevara. Specific aspect of modern life for people with multiple sclerosis: considerations for the practitioner. Ther Adv Neurol Disord 2014; 7(2):137–49.

8. Fragoso YD. Multiple Sclerosis and Pregnancy. International Encyclopedia of Rehabilitation. Available online: http://cirrie.buffalo.edu/encyclopedia/en/article/248/

9. Surbhi DM, Bharat S, Sukriti A. Emergency caesarian section in a patient of myasthenia gravis: Is neuraxial anesthesia safe? Saudi J Anaesth 2012;6(4):430–1.

10. Alina RN, Mariusz P. Anaesthetic management of a patient with myasthenia gravis for abdominal surgery using sugammadex. Arch Med Sci 2011;7(2): 361–4.

11. Sanwal MK, Baduni N, Jain A. Caesarean section in a patient with Myasthenia Gravis: A bigger challenge for the anesthesiologist than the obstetrician. J Obstet Anaesth Crit Care 2012;2: 34–7.

12. Sebastian B, Benjamin T, Saskia S, Marc S, Regine S. Myasthenia gravis in pregnancy: A case report. Case Reports in Obstetrics and Gynecology 2012, Article ID 736024, 4 pages.

13. Thanvi BR, Lo TCN. Update on myasthenia gravis. Postgrad Med J 2004; 80:690–700.

14. Shahnaz AC, Biruthvie V, Gideon K. Myasthenia Gravis during pregnancy. Canadian Family Physician 2012;58(12): 1346–9.

15. Nidhi K, Gaurav C, Rohit G. Anaesthesia in a parturient with myasthenia gravis—transient myasthenia in newborn. IOSR-JDMS 2013;4(6): 73–5.

16. Edward G Morgan, Maged SM, Michael JM, (Eds). Clinical Anaesthesiology, 4th ed. Lange medical books: McGraw Hill, Health Professions Division, 2006.

17. Almeida C, Coutinho E, Moreira D, Santos E, Aguir J. Myasthenia gravis and pregnancy: anaesthetic management—a series of cases. Eur J Anaesthesiol 2010; 27(11):985–90.

18. Samuel C Hughes. Shnider and levinsons (Eds). Anaesthesia for obstetrics. Philadelphia: Lippincott, Williams and Wilkins 2001.

19. Maria Hirsch. Intrapartum seizure in a patient undergoing cesarean delivery: Differential diagnosis and causative factors. AANA Journal 2011;79(5):403–7.

20. Brenda AB, David RG, David JW, (Eds). A Practical Approach to Obstetric Anaesthesia, 4th ed. Philadelphia: Wolters Kluwer, Lippincott, Williams and Wilkins; 2009.

21. David H, Chestnut, Donna M (Eds). Obstetric Anaesthesia: Principles and Practice, 3rd ed. Philadelphia, Pennsylvania: Elsevier Mosby, the Curtis center; 2004.

22. Nesrine Abd El-Rahman El-Retai. Anesthetic management for parturient with neurological disorders. Anesth Essays Res 2013;7(2):147–54.

23. Wang YL, Yong SS, Chae SI, Woo SC, Byung MK Spinal anaesthesia for emergency caesarean section in a preeclampsia patient diagnosed with type I neurofibromatosis. Korean J Anesthesiol 2013;65(6):S91–S92.

24. Singh T, Hooda S, Anand A, Kaur K, Bala R. Anesthetic consideration in a preeclamptic parturient with Von Recklinghausen's neurofibromatosis. J Obstet Anaesth Crit Care 2014;4: 38–40.

25. Charles JF, Samir T, Aaron JK, Stephanie R, Jacqueline VA, Alan DK. Perioperative management of neurofibromatosis type I. Ochsner J 2012; 12(2):111–21.

26. Shrestha AB, Shrestha S, Sharma KR, Gurung T. Anesthetic management of a parturient with poliomyelitis associated with kyphoscoliosis. NJOG 2014;17(1):67–70.

27. Ballarapu G, Aloka S, Veldurti AKK, Padmaja D, Gudaru J. Spinal anaesthesia in poliomyelitis patients with scoliotic spine: A case control study. Indian J Anaesth 2013;57(2):145–9.

28. Donna Wheeler. Anaesthetic considerations for patients with postpolio syndrome: A case report. AANA Journal 2011;79(5):408–10.

29. Kulshrestha A, Bajwa SK, Bajwa SS, Mathur M, Kaur J. Critical issues in a parturient with preexisting neurological deficits with severe anaemia: A clinical challenge to anesthesiologist and intensivist!. Int J Crit Illn Inj Sci 2013; 3:164–5.

30. Subramanian R, Sardar A, Mohanaselvi S, Khanna P, Baidya DK. Neurosurgery and pregnancy. J Neuroanaesthesiol Crit Care 2014;1:166–72.

31. Hala M Goma, Terry Lichtor (Ed). Clinical Management and Evolving Novel Therapeutic Strategies for Patients with Bbrain Tumors. ISBN 978-953-51-1058-3; 2013.

32. Abd-Elsayed AA, Díaz-Gómez J, Barnett GH. A case series discussing the anesthetic management of pregnant patients with brain tumors [v1; ref status: indexed, http://f1000r.es/y7]F1000 Research 2013;2:92.

33. Ivana H, Patricia G. Cesarean section in spinal anesthesia on a patient with mesencephalic tumor and ventriculoperitoneal drainage—a case report. Korean J Anesthesiol 2012;63(3):263–5.

34. Shashikala K, Sheela CN, Manmeet C. Malfunction of ventriculoperitoneal shunt during pregnancy: A case report. Int J Pharm Biomed Res 2011;2(4): 266–8.

35. Bajwa SJ, Kwatra IS, Bajwa SK, Kaur M. Renal diseases during pregnancy: Critical and current perspectives. J Obstet Anaesth Crit Care 2013;3: 7–15.

36. Beena KP, Veena RS, Guruprasad B. Anesthesia for parturient with renal transplantation. J Anaesthesiol Clin Pharmacol 2012;28(4):524–7.

37. Michelle JS, Brian RM. Management of urolithiasis in pregnancy. Int J Womens Health 2013;5: 599–604.

38. Fernando K, Eduardo CR, Ita PH. Urolithiasis and Pregnancy. J Bras Nefrol 2014;36(3).

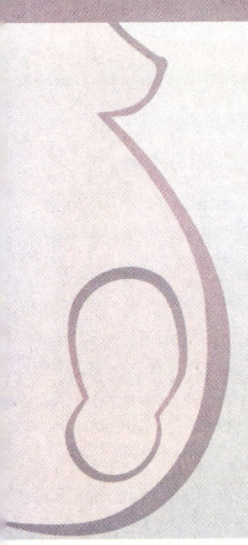

Trauma in Pregnancy

Indu Lata, Sandeep Sahu, Sanjay Agarwal

INTRODUCTION

When any trauma patients are transported to an emergency department, the doctors must be prepared to handle the physiologic complexity of their injuries due to trauma. This is particularly important in the case of the pregnant trauma patients who are special because of two life concerns and trauma management is further confounded by its physiological changes. Trauma in pregnancy is currently a leading cause of non-pregnancy-related maternal deaths and fetal demise.[1] The management of trauma in pregnancy requires a multidisciplinary team involving the anesthesiologist, obstetrician, emergency physician, intensivist and the trauma surgeon.

INCIDENCE

The incidence of trauma in pregnancy ranges from 6 to 8%.[2] Maternal death rates have been reported as high as 11% after trauma.[3] The overall rate of hospitalizations due to trauma-related injuries in pregnant women was 4.1 per 1,000 deliveries in the USA.[4] Trauma is the leading cause of death for all women of childbearing age. Motor vehicle accidents (MVA)/road traffic accidents (RTA) account

Table 17.1: Causes of trauma in pregnancy	
Motor vehicle accidents (MVA/RTA)	55%
Falls	22%
Assaults	22%
Burns	1%

for almost two thirds of all maternal trauma-related deaths, while falls and domestic violence comprise a large percentage of the rest.[5] The incidences of various causes of trauma in pregnancy are shown in Table 17.1.[6]

PHYSIOLOGICAL CHANGES IN PREGNANCY AND THEIR SIGNIFICANCE IN TRAUMA

The overall anatomical and physiological changes during various stages of pregnancy had been described in details elsewhere in this book. We are focusing here some important points for clinical management points of view. The clinician treating the pregnant trauma victims should consider the changes in anatomy and physiology of pregnancy (Table 17.2). During the first trimester of pregnancy, the bony pelvis protects the uterus and the fetus from direct injury. During the second trimester onwards, the uterus comes into the peritoneal cavity (Fig. 17.1). It protects

Table 17.2: Physiologic changes of pregnancy and their mimicking effect in trauma

Physiologic changes	Mimicking effect in trauma
Cardiovascular changes	
↑Blood volume	Mask signs of hypovolemia
↑Cardiac output may ↓blood pressure	Mimic myocardial ischemia or cardiac contusion
EKG changes ↓ cardiac filling pressures	Mimics severity of hemorrhagic shock
Aortocaval compression	
Pulmonary changes	
↓Functional residual capacity	Rapid onset of hypoxemia
↑Oxygen consumption	↓Buffering capacity and develops metabolic acidosis
↑Alveolar hyperventilation leads respiratory alkalosis	during periods of hypoperfusion and hypoxia
Gastrointestinal changes	
↓Gastric emptying	↑Incidence of reflux and aspiration
↓Gastroesophageal sphincter tone	↑Risk of upper abdominal penetrating injuries
Displacement of small intestine into the abdomen due to gravid uterus	
Renal changes	
↑Renal blood flow and GFR	Natriuresis
↓Blood urea and creatinine	Renal damage
Hematologic changes	
↓Hematocrit	Anemia, internal bleeding
↑White blood cells	Infection
↑Coagulation factors	Thromboembolic disease

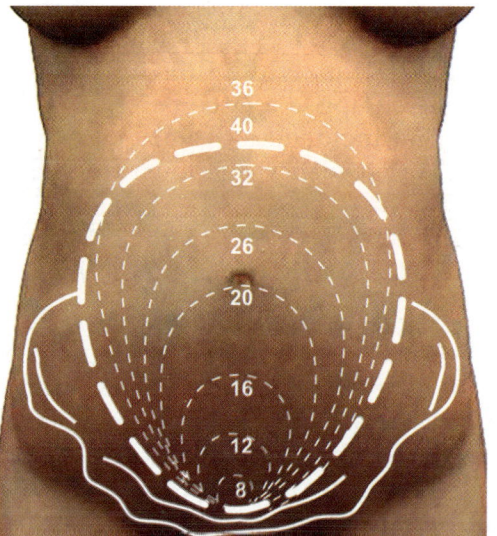

Fig. 17.1. Estimating gestational age by fundal height: Measure the vertical distance in the midline from the symphysis pubis to the top of the fundus in centimetres. This measurement correlates approximately with the gestational age *(Adapted from Queensland Clinical Guidelines: Trauma in Pregnancy)*

other maternal abdominal organs by displacing them (mesentery, stomach) and itself becomes more susceptible from direct traumatic injury.[7]

The cardiovascular changes during pregnancy may not accurately predict the status of the uteroplacental circulation. It may complicate the evaluation of intravascular volume, assessment of blood loss and management of hypovolemic shock. Physician treating the pregnant trauma patients should remember that uterine vasculature is maximally dilated in pregnancy with absence of the autoregulation. The uterine blood flow is solely dependent on maternal mean arterial blood pressure. The relative hemodilution and hypervolemic state due to pregnancy may be protective as fewer red blood cells (RBCs) are lost during blood loss. The hormonal effect of pregnancy leads to increased levels of coagulation factors that may improve hemostasis following trauma.

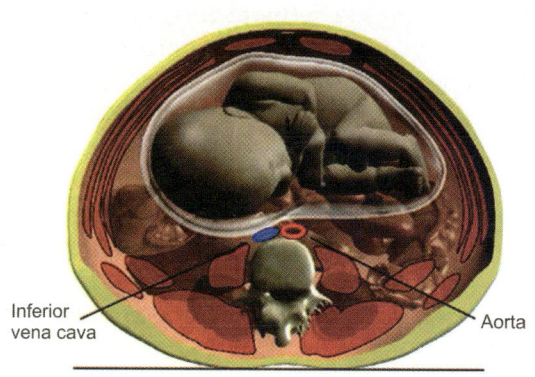
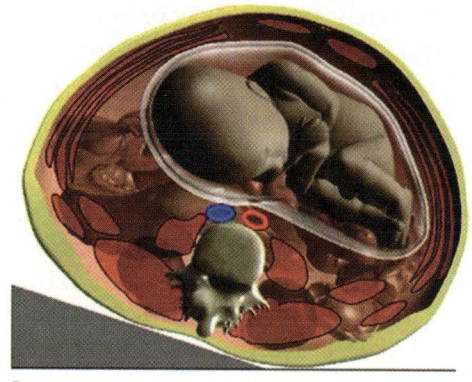

A   **B**

Inferior vena cava

Aorta

Figs 17.2A and B. *Aortocaval/supine hypotension syndrome:* (A) Inferior vena cava compression when positioned supine; (B) Left lateral tilt (right side up) 15–30° to relieve compression *(Adapted from* Queensland Clinical Guidelines: Trauma in Pregnancy*)*

But this hypercoagulable state may increase the risk for thromboembolic complications simultaneously and during periods of immobilization.[8]

Pregnancy increases the risk of difficult intubation due to various physiological and anatomical causes. Besides this, *the aortocaval syndrome/supine hypotension syndrome is also important considerations in pregnant patients while doing trauma and cardiac resuscitation* (Figs 17.2A and B).

MECHANISMS OF INJURY OF TRAUMA DURING PREGNANCY

Blunt Injury

The most common cause of blunt abdominal trauma in pregnancy is RTA/MVA followed by falls and violent accident. More challenging in MVAs is management of pelvic fracture, leading to massive hemorrhage, shock, and significant maternal and fetal death. The most common cause of fetal death is placental abruption, causing prematurity, exsanguination (bleed to death), and hypoxemia. During the placental abruption occurs, loss of placental surface 50% or greater had a high likelihood of fetal loss.[9,10]

Penetrating Injuries

Stab injuries and gunshot injuries are the frequent causes of penetrating injury. After 1st trimester, gravid uterus is the most likely organ to be injured in the 2nd and 3rd trimesters of pregnancy. The bowel is pushed upward by the enlarged uterus, so penetrating injury to the upper part of the abdomen is more likely associated with multiple gastrointestinal injuries.[11]If the bullet has penetrated, the uterus and the fetus is viable, cesarean delivery is indicated. Although maternal mortality is low but fetal mortality is high due to the injury to the uterus. The thick uterine musculature absorbs the energy from low-velocity penetrating injury.[12]

Burn Injuries

Burns are uncommon and unusual in pregnancy. Pregnancy should not affect the management of burns. Better maternal and fetal outcome depends on the severity and grade of burns and its associated complications. Third space fluid loss and intravascular volume depletion due to severe trauma can result in uteroplacental hypoperfusion, fetal hypoxia, and distress and thus can lead to premature labor and death. Management consists of supplemental oxygen,

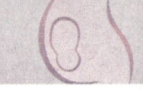

assessment of extent and severity of burn, and aggressive fluid management as per Parkland formula (4 mL/kg per% burn). Based on this formula, the 24-hour fluid requirement is calculated, with half of the fluid replacement is done within the first eight hours. Urine output monitoring provides a vital guide to assess the adequacy of volume resuscitation. Fetal mortality increases with increasing severity of burns with an almost 100% mortality rate with burns greater than 50%.[12]

Carbon monoxide (CO) poisoning should be considered early in managing pregnant burn patients with history of closed space burning. CO have high affinity for hemoglobin and rapidly crosses the placenta. Carboxy-hemoglobin level should be measured to label the severity (CO level greater than 25% normally (or >15% in pregnancy). The fetal hemoglobin has more affinity for CO than maternal hemoglobin. Because of this, the fetal carboxyhemoglobin levels are higher than maternal levels with slower fetal elimination. So even in mildly symptomatic mothers, the chances of anatomic malformations and death of the fetus are high. Hyperbaric oxygen therapy should be considered early in the care of the pregnant patients with CO poisoning.[12,13]

Electrical Injury

Electrical injury, though rare, but may cause injury in pregnancy. The clinical spectrum of electrical injury ranges from a transient unpleasant sensation felt by the mother and no effect on her fetus to fetal death. Severity of injury depends on several factors like the type of current, magnitude of the current, duration of contact and its path through the body. Every patient with history of electric injury should be admitted for observation. Patient's vitals, ECG and electrolyte monitoring for 24 hrs, as these patients are having higher chances of arrhythmias and myoglobinuria-induced acute renal failure.

TRAUMA-RELATED OBSTETRIC COMPLICATIONS AND THEIR MANAGEMENT

The possible maternal and fetal trauma-related injuries are summarized in Tables 17.3 and 17.4.[14,15]

Table 17.3: Maternal injuries associated with trauma

- Vaginal bleeding
- Maternal pelvic fractures
- Uterine rupture
- Placental abruption
- Premature rupture of membranes
- Premature labor/delivery
- Direct uterine/fetal injury from penetrating trauma more likely in the 2nd and 3rd trimesters
- Splenic rupture
- Retroperitoneal hemorrhage
- Hepatic injury
- Hematoma
- Bowel injury—uncommon due to protection from gravid uterus

Table 17.4: Direct and indirect fetal injuries from trauma

Direct injuries	Indirect injuries
• Fetal death	• Placental abruption
• Organ rupture	• Uterine rupture
• Feta fractures: Spinal/cranial and long bone fractures	• Fetomaternal hemorrhage
• Intracranial hemorrhage	• Preterm labor
• Umbilical cord rupture	• Rh isoimmunization
Direct injuries are primarily due to impact of trauma	Indirect injury is mostly because of fetal hypoxia and secondary to maternal hypotension

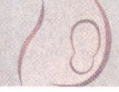
Placental Abruption

An acceleration-deceleration injury, such as an MVA or falls, may create shearing force that can cause placental detachment or abruption. Placental abruption occurs in up to 40% of severe blunt abdominal trauma and in the 3% of minor trauma with direct uterine force. The intrauterine cavity may accommodate one's entire blood volume. Tissue thromboplastin release from an abruption leads to plasminogen activator-mediated fibrinolysis, resulting in or exacerbating disseminated intravascular coagulation. Due to placental abruption, there is a compromise in fetal oxygen transfer, leading to signs of fetal distress and fetal death. Even non-severely injured pregnant women are at increased risk for placental abruption. Abruption may occur immediately after abdominal impact or be delayed even after several hours after the trauma.[16] The clinical manifestations, and complications of placental abruption, and their management have been described in Table 17.5.

Table 17.5: Placental abruption: Clinical manifestations, complications, and their management

Etiology	Hypertension Trauma Parity Tobacco use Premature rupture of membranes Prior abruption	
Clinical manifestation	**Symptoms** Abdominal pain Cramping or contraction Vaginal bleeding **Signs** Uterine tenderness Increased uterine activity Vaginal bleeding **Diagnosis** Continuous fetal monitoring Ultrasound: Retroplacental hematoma Kleihauer-Betke test	
Complications	**Maternal** Hemorrhagic shock Acute renal failure Coagulopathy Perinatal mortality and morbidity	**Fetal/neonatal** Fetal distress Fetal death Prematurity
Management	**Obstetric management** *Supportive management* • Close monitoring of FHR • Large bore intravenous access • Assess hematocrit • Assess coagulation • Blood for crossmatch • USG may help detect early • Left uterine displacement • Supplemental oxygen	*Definitive management* Continue pregnancy • Preterm fetus • Minimal abruption • No signs of fetal distress Induction of labor • No evidence of fetal distress • Favorable cervix Cesarean delivery • Maternal instability • Fetal distress

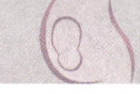

Uterine Rupture

Uterine rupture is a rare consequence of maternal trauma. Uterine rupture occurs in less than 1% of pregnant trauma victims but is associated with grave prognosis for the fetus and the mother. The increase in uterine vascularity and blood flow due to advance pregnancy makes more serious hemorrhage. Besides this, bleeding from other solid organ (liver and spleen) injuries also aggravates the severity of shock. The extent of such damage cannot be predicted by clinical presentation and will not be apparent until exploratory surgery is performed. Prompt hemodynamic resuscitation with fluids and replacement of blood products diminishes the potential for bleeding complications from disseminated intravascular coagulopathy.[14,15] The clinical manifestations and complications of uterine rupture, and their management have been described in Table 17.6.

Pelvic Fractures

Pelvic fractures are a common accidental injury. Three main mechanisms of injury of pelvic fracture are MVA, falls, and pedestrian struck by a car. Pelvic fractures are the independent factor for adverse fetal outcome. These patients can present with concealed hemorrhage of around 2–3 liters of blood and thus always have hemodynamic instability. It may be associated with other injuries like femur fracture, placental abruption or rupture of membrane. Mechanism of injury and injury severity were related to mortality rates. Management includes aggressive resuscitation with blood product, pelvic binder and transfer to designated trauma center with experience in managing such injuries.

Direct Fetal Injury

Direct fetal injury is rare because of protection by the uterus and amniotic fluid. Blunt

Table 17.6: Uterine rupture: Clinical manifestations, complications, and their management		
Etiology	Trauma, multiparity H/o previous cesarean section	
Clinical manifestation	**Symptoms** History of trauma Abdominal pain (lower) Maternal discomfort **Signs** Uterine tenderness Absence of fetal movement Hemodynamic instability (vaginal or concealed bleed) Palpation of fetal part on abdominal examination.	
Complications	**Maternal** Hemorrhagic shock Acute renal failure Coagulopathy Perinatal morbidity and mortality	**Fetal** Fetal death
Management	Oxygenation Left lateral tilt Large bore intravenous cannula Inotropes and vasopressors Aggressive resuscitation with fluids and blood products Exploratory laparotomy as early as possible Hysterectomy, if necessary	

abdominal trauma to the abdomen or pelvis can result in direct fetal trauma. Direct fetal injury complicates less than 1% of pregnancies with blunt trauma. The risks to the fetus are greatest in late 2nd and 3rd trimestes. There is a greater risk for fetal skull fracture and brain injury with maternal pelvic fractures. A trauma to the uterus injures the myometrium and destabilizes decidual lysosomes, releasing arachidonic acid that causes uterine contractions, and perhaps inducing premature labor.[17]

Head and Neck Injury

The most common etiologies of head injury include MVA and falls. In pregnant trauma patients with head injury, the possible problems are: full stomach, possibly elevated intracranial pressure, fractured cervical spine with head injury, an possibility of difficult airway, an uncertain volume status of patient, altered consciousness(comatose or combative), an uncertain oxygenation (possibly decreased), and an uncertain obstetrical status (about pregnancy) in reproductive age group patients.[18]

Management of Pregnant Patients with Head Injury[18,19]

- Consider MILS (manual in-line stabilization) of the head and neck for neck instability.
- May fiberoptic intubation of the trachea to prevent difficult airway and neck instability.
- Titrated dose of analgesic and sedative drugs to prevent aspiration and hypotension.
- Intubation and mechanical ventilation for the airway control in severe head injury GCS <8 and control of the intracranial pressure.
- Prevent rise in intracranial pressure by osmotic diuretics, hyperventilation, hypothermia, etc.
- Aggressive maternal resuscitation and avoidance of teratogenic drugs.

The resuscitation should always be an initial priority than control of ICP after head injury in any trauma patient.

RESUSCITATION OF PREGNANT TRAUMA PATIENT

The resuscitation of severe trauma patient includes primary survey that includes initial resuscitation of pregnant trauma patients with thorough evaluation and stabilization. It does not differ from evaluation of non-pregnant patients. When the patient is stabilized secondary survey that is detailed head to toe examination is done as per Advanced Trauma Life Support guidelines.[20] Detailed ATLS guidelines for the maintenance of ABCDE of life of trauma patient are shown in Tables 17.7 and 17.8.[21] Two large-bore (14- or 16-G) intravenous lines should be placed, and crystalloid 1–2 litters in the form of normal saline or lactated Ringer's solution should be given to replace the estimated blood loss over the first hour of acute resuscitation. Resuscitation during acute hemorrhage shock the current recommendations are maintenance of blood composition by early transfusion of red blood cells, plasma, platelets, and limiting the crystalloid transfusion to avoid dilutional coagulopathy and hypothermia called damage control resuscitation. O-negative packed red cell scan be used, if emergent transfusion is needed because crossmatching takes times. Overall summary of management, investigation and follow-up of pregnant patient for better understanding and clinical use is given in algorithm form in Figures 17.3 and 17.4.[21]

Goal of Resuscitation

Goal is to maintain adequate uteroplacental perfusion and fetal oxygenation by avoiding hypoxia and hypotension. It is important to preventing the lethal triad of acidosis and hypothermia and coagulopathy to decrease morbidity and mortality.[22]

- The first priority is identification of life-threatening injuries to the woman.
- Thoroughly assess the woman as fetal survival is directly related to maternal wellbeing.

Table 17.7: Primary survey—additional considerations for trauma in pregnancy (*Adapted from Queensland Clinical Guidelines: Trauma in Pregnancy*)

Aspect	Clinical care

1. **Airway and C-spine control**	• *Increased risk of failed intubation consider*
	   • Earlier intubation than for non-pregnant patients
	   • Use of a short handle laryngoscope
	   • Cricoid pressure
	   • A smaller endotracheal tube (ETT) due to laryngeal edema
	• *Increased risk of aspiration*
	   • If intubated, consider insertion of an orogastric tube
	   • Consider nasogastric tube, if not intubated
	• Apply cervical spine collar

2. **Breathing and ventilation**	• Routinely administer supplemental high flow 100% oxygen • Ventilation volumes may need to be reduced because of elevated diaphragm • If safe to do so, raise the head of the bed to reduce weight of uterus on the diaphragm and facilitate breathing • If a chest tube is indicated, place tube 1–2 intercostal spaces above usual fifth intercostal space landmark due to raised diaphragm

3. **Circulation and hemorrhage control**	• Control obvious external hemorrhage
	• Position with left lateral tilt 15–30° (right side up)
	• Obtain large-bore intravenous (IV) access
	   • Avoid femoral lines due to compression by gravid uterus
	• Commence crystalloid IV
	   • Assess response—maintain an awareness of pregnancy-related physiological parameters
	   • Aim to avoid large volumes of crystalloids (greater than 2 L) which may lead to pulmonary edema due to the relatively low oncotic pressure in pregnancy.
	• Avoid vasopressors to restore maternal BP as they may compromise uteroplacental flow.
	• Maintain a high index of suspicion for bleeding and an awareness of the limitations of clinical signs.
	• Perform a thorough search for occult bleeding as maternal blood flow is maintained at expense of fetus.
	• Conduct focused abdominal sonography for trauma (FAST) to assess for intra-abdominal hemorrhage.
	• If hypovolemia is suspected, initiate fluid resuscitation to ensure adequate maternal and uteroplacental perfusion.
	• Consider massive transfusion protocol (MTP) activation, if non-responsive to crystalloids.
	• Rapid transfer to operating theatre as indicated.
	• See blood/product replacement and MTP activation protocols.
	• Evaluate fetal heart rate, but do not delay resuscitation for fetal assessments.

4. **Disability**	• Rapid neurological evaluation utilizing the Glasgow Coma Scale
5. **Exposure and environmental control**	To avoid potential missed injuries and prevent hypothermia

Table 17.8: Secondary survey—additional considerations for trauma during pregnancy (*Adapted from Queensland Clinical Guidelines: Trauma in Pregnancy*)

Aspect	Clinical care
1. Obstetric history	• Gestation in weeks/estimated date of delivery • Previous pregnancy complications • Prenatal care • History of vaginal bleeding

2. Physical examination	• Head to toe examination as for non-pregnant trauma patients.
	• Inspect abdomen for ecchymosis or asymmetry
	• In cases of motor vehicle accident, incorrect positioning of the seat belt across the gravid uterus may:
	  ♦ Cause marked bruising of the abdomen
	  ♦ Increase the risk of placental abruption
	  ♦ Increase the risk of uterine rupture
	• Assess uterine tone, contractions, rigidity, tenderness, palpable fetal parts
	  ♦ The gravid abdomen may be relatively insensate to peritoneal irritation

3. Estimation of gestational age	• Can be estimated by measuring fundal height
	  ♦ Measure the vertical distance in the midline from the symphysis pubis to the top of the fundus in centimeters. This measurement correlates approximately with the gestational age
	  ♦ Estimation of gestational age
	• Ultrasound scan (US) estimation
	  ♦ Biparietal diameter (BPD) of 60 mm generally corresponds to a gestation age of approximately 24 weeks
	• Mark the top of the fundus to evaluate the possibility of concealed abruption as noted by increasing fundal height.

4. Fetal heart rate (FHR) monitoring	• Normal FHR 110–160 bpm.
	• FHR can be assessed using standard stethoscope from about 20 weeks and Doppler from about 12 weeks.
	  ♦ Differentiate maternal and FHR as maternal tachycardia may cause confusion.
	• For gestations greater than 24 weeks (major trauma), initiate continuous cardiotocography (CTG) as soon as feasible.
	  ♦ Good sensitivity for immediate adverse outcome
	  ♦ Detects uterine irritability and abnormal fetal heart rate patterns
	• Abnormalities may be the only indication of injury or compromise to the fetus
	  ♦ Persistent fetal bradycardia more than 5 minutes, loss of baseline variability or recurrent complex variable or late decelerations indicates fetal compromise
	  ♦ Sinusoidal trace indicates fetal anemia

Contd...

Contd...

Aspeact	Clinical care
	• CTG application and interpretation requires clinicians trained in their use • Physiological control of FHR and resultant CTG trace interpretation differs in the preterm fetus compared to the term fetus, especially at gestations less than 28 weeks • CTG trace review should be performed by a clinician experienced and confident with CTG interpretation relevant to the gestation • Move staff and equipment to the woman's location rather than transporting a woman to an obstetric unit for monitoring
5. Vaginal examination	• If major trauma, perform a rectal examination to assess for spinal cord damage or local trauma • Perform sterile speculum vaginal examination as clinically indicated (preferably by an obstetric/maternity team member) • Evaluate for ruptured membranes, vaginal bleeding, cord prolapse, cervical effacement and dilation in labor, fetal presentation. • Vaginal bleeding may indicate preterm labor, abruption, pelvic fracture or uterine rupture. • Consider urinary catheter insertion.

• Recognize maternal anatomical and physiological changes due to pregnancy.
• Clear, coordinated and frequent communication between care providers is essential.
• Generally, do not withhold medications, tests, treatments and procedures required for the woman's stabilization because of pregnancy.
• Refer all major trauma cases to a trauma center:
  • If less than 20 weeks gestation, transfer to the nearest trauma center.
  • If greater than or equal to 20 weeks gestation, transfer to a trauma center with obstetric services.
• Provide pregnant women with minor injuries, medical treatment for their injuries and appropriate fetal assessment.

The optimal management of hemorrhagic shock consists of maintenance of systolic blood pressure at 80 to 100 mm Hg, pulse oximetry above 95%, hematocrit 25 to 36%, platelet >50,000/cumm, normal serum calcium and lactate, along with providing adequate analgesia.[23]

Common Pitfalls for the Resuscitation of Pregnant Trauma Patient[24]

• Suspect or recognize shock in the presence of normal vital signs.
• Suspect or recognize abdominal injury because of a benign examination.
• Treat shock aggressively with volume replacement (crystalloids/blood).
• Suspect and screen for intimate partner violence.
• Recognize and treat supine hypotensive syndrome.
• Conduct necessary radiology studies secondary to fear of injury to the fetus.

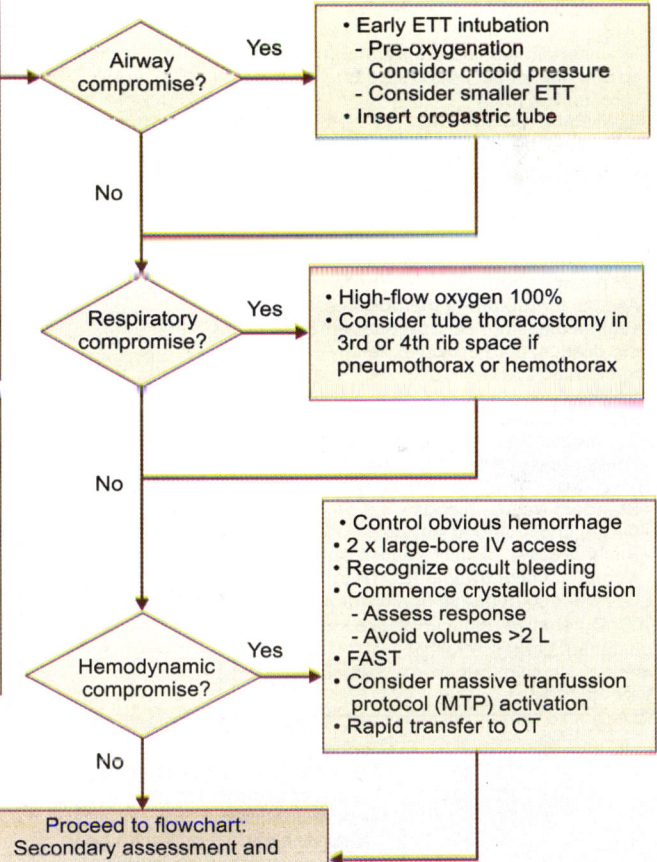

Principles of care for the pregnant trauma patient

- Follow ATLS guidelines
- First priority is to treat the woman
- Multidisciplinary team that includes an obstetrician is essential
  - Contact neonatal team early if birth imminent/likely
- Recognize anatomical and physiological changes of pregnancy
- Clear, coordinated and frequent communication essential
- Generally, medications, treatment and procedures as for non-pregnant patient
- Refer pregnant women with major trauma to a trauma center
  - <20 weeks gestation: To the nearest trauma center
  - ≥20 weeks gestation: To the a trauma center with obstetric services
- Thoroughly assess all pregnant women—even after minor trauma

Initial stabilization

- As indicated for all trauma patients
- Follow ATLS guidelines
- Initiate early obstetric consultation
- Contact QCC (1300 799 127) to expedite transport and identify receiving facility as required

Additionally for pregnancy
- Position (tilt or wedge):
  - Left lateral 15–30° (right side up) or
  - Manual displacement of uterus
  - Place wedge under spinal board if necessary
- Routinely administer oxygen therapy
- Large-bore IV access
- Volume resuscitation (crystalloid infusion)

Cardiac arrest

- Follow ATLS guidelines
- Defibrillate as for non-pregnant patient
- Advanced cardiac life support durgs as indicated for non-pregnant patients
- Perimorterm CS if:
  - ≥ 20 weeks gestation
  - No response to effective CPR after 4 minutes

Airway compromise?

Yes →
- Early ETT intubation
  - Pre-oxygenation
    Consider cricoid pressure
  - Consider smaller ETT
- Insert orogastric tube

No ↓

Respiratory compromise?

Yes →
- High-flow oxygen 100%
- Consider tube thoracostomy in 3rd or 4th rib space if pneumothorax or hemothorax

No ↓

Hemodynamic compromise?

Yes →
- Control obvious hemorrhage
- 2 x large-bore IV access
- Recognize occult bleeding
- Commence crystalloid infusion
  - Assess response
  - Avoid volumes >2 L
- FAST
- Consider massive tranfussion protocol (MTP) activation
- Rapid transfer to OT

No ↓

Proceed to flowchart:
Secondary assessment and management of pregnant trauma patient

Abbreviations
ATLS: Advanced trauma life support; CPR: Cardiopulmonary resuscitation; CS: Cesarean section; ETT: Endotracheal tube; FAST: Focused abdominal sonography for trauma; IV: Intravenous; OT: Operating theatre; QCC: Queensland Emergency Medical Coordination Centre; >: Greater than; ≥: Greater than or equal to; <: Less than

Fig. 17.3. Algorithm of initial assessment and management of the pregnant trauma patient *(Adapted from Queensland Clinical Guidelines: Trauma in Pregnancy)*

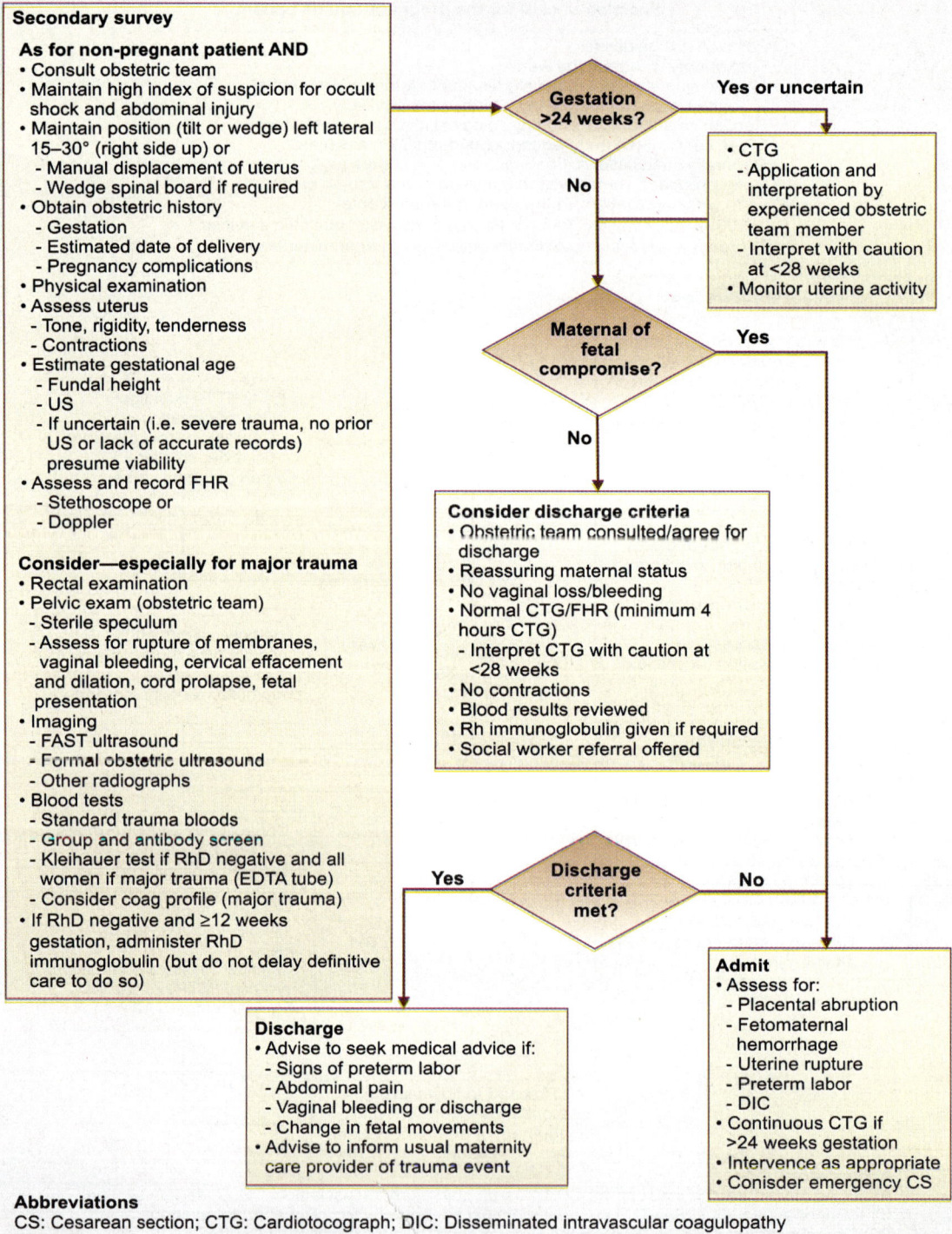

Secondary survey

As for non-pregnant patient AND
- Consult obstetric team
- Maintain high index of suspicion for occult shock and abdominal injury
- Maintain position (tilt or wedge) left lateral 15–30° (right side up) or
  - Manual displacement of uterus
  - Wedge spinal board if required
- Obtain obstetric history
  - Gestation
  - Estimated date of delivery
  - Pregnancy complications
- Physical examination
- Assess uterus
  - Tone, rigidity, tenderness
  - Contractions
- Estimate gestational age
  - Fundal height
  - US
  - If uncertain (i.e. severe trauma, no prior US or lack of accurate records) presume viability
- Assess and record FHR
  - Stethoscope or
  - Doppler

Consider—especially for major trauma
- Rectal examination
- Pelvic exam (obstetric team)
  - Sterile speculum
  - Assess for rupture of membranes, vaginal bleeding, cervical effacement and dilation, cord prolapse, fetal presentation
- Imaging
  - FAST ultrasound
  - Formal obstetric ultrasound
  - Other radiographs
- Blood tests
  - Standard trauma bloods
  - Group and antibody screen
  - Kleihauer test if RhD negative and all women if major trauma (EDTA tube)
  - Consider coag profile (major trauma)
- If RhD negative and ≥12 weeks gestation, administer RhD immunoglobulin (but do not delay definitive care to do so)

Gestation >24 weeks?

Yes or uncertain

No

- CTG
  - Application and interpretation by experienced obstetric team member
  - Interpret with caution at <28 weeks
- Monitor uterine activity

Maternal of fetal compromise?

Yes

No

Consider discharge criteria
- Obstetric team consulted/agree for discharge
- Reassuring maternal status
- No vaginal loss/bleeding
- Normal CTG/FHR (minimum 4 hours CTG)
  - Interpret CTG with caution at <28 weeks
- No contractions
- Blood results reviewed
- Rh immunoglobulin given if required
- Social worker referral offered

Discharge criteria met?

Yes

No

Discharge
- Advise to seek medical advice if:
  - Signs of preterm labor
  - Abdominal pain
  - Vaginal bleeding or discharge
  - Change in fetal movements
- Advise to inform usual maternity care provider of trauma event

Admit
- Assess for:
  - Placental abruption
  - Fetomaternal hemorrhage
  - Uterine rupture
  - Preterm labor
  - DIC
- Continuous CTG if >24 weeks gestation
- Intervene as appropriate
- Conisder emergency CS

Abbreviations
CS: Cesarean section; CTG: Cardiotocograph; DIC: Disseminated intravascular coagulopathy
FAST: Focused abdominal sonography for trauma; FHR: Fetal heart rate; US: Ultrasound scan
<: Less than; >: Greater than; ≥: Greater than or equal to

Fig. 17.4. Algorithm of secondary assessment and management of the pregnant trauma patient *(Adapted from Queensland Clinical Guidelines: Trauma in Pregnancy)*

- Observe and CTG monitor all women with minor trauma and a viable fetus (greater than 24 weeks gestation).
- Detect early pregnancy (by not ordering a urine pregnancy test).
- Test for RhD status and administer RhD immunoglobulin in RhD negative women.
- Initiate perimortem cesarean section within 4–6 minutes of no response to effective CPR.

A perimortem cesarean delivery should be performed by the present physician with the most surgical experience, preferably an obstetrician or surgeon, if available. If possible, a neonatologist should be available for resuscitation. Maternal resuscitation efforts—including definitive management of the airway, cardiopulmonary resuscitation (CPR), fluids, and advanced cardiac life support (ACLS) protocol-driven pharmaceutical therapy—should not be interrupted to allow more room for the surgical intervention team. Full CPR measures should continue during the delivery. The perimortem cesarean has been described in Figure 17.5.

Cardiopulmonary Resuscitation in Pregnant patients, ACLS Summary

Effective CPR is difficult in near-term pregnant woman because of a limited ability to perform chest compressions and displace the uterus.[25]

Summary of CPR in Pregnant Patients over 20 Weeks Gestation[26]

- Before starting compressions, turn the woman to lateral position 15–20° up.
- Defibrillation as in non-pregnancy (no significant shock is transferred to fetus). Remove fetal/uterine monitors prior to shock.
- Establish advanced airway early with C-spine stabilized.
- Breathing: Ventilation volumes may need to be reduced because of elevated diaphragm.
- Closed-chest compressions: 100 per minute using 30:2 ratio with ventilations.
- IV: avoid femoral or other lower extremity lines, as flow may be affected by vena caval compression.
- ACLS drugs as indicated in adult CPR.
- If no maternal response after 4 minutes of ACLS, immediate cesarean delivery should be performed in the emergency department by a qualified physician, with proper support and resources, who has determined the viability of the fetus.
- Thoracotomy and open cardiac massage may be considered at this time, if the patient or fetus is believed to be viable.
  - Age greater than or equal to 24 weeks: Attempt to save life of both mother and fetus.

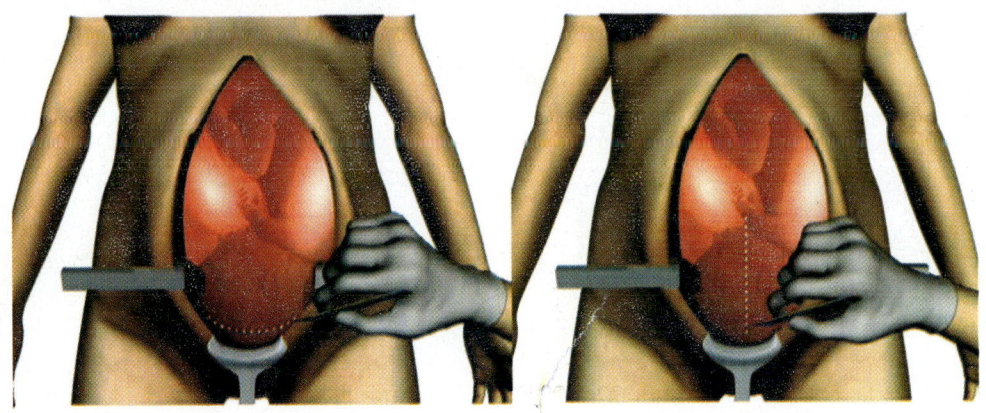

Fig. 17.5. **Perimortem cesarean section procedure:** Large vertical abdominal incision required. Uterine incision may be either vertical or horizontal (*adapted from* Queensland Clinical Guidelines: Trauma in Pregnancy)

- Age 20–23 weeks: Primary attempt to save life of mother by improving aortocaval blood flow and cardiac output. Fetal survival is unlikely.
- Age less than 24 weeks: Urgent cesarean unnecessary as aortocaval compromise unlikely.

Assessment of fetal heart tones should be done throughout, as allowed by circumstances.

PREGNANCY AND RESTRAINT USE

American College of Obstetrics and Gynecology recommends that restraint use during pregnancy reduces both maternal and fetal morbidity and mortality.[27]

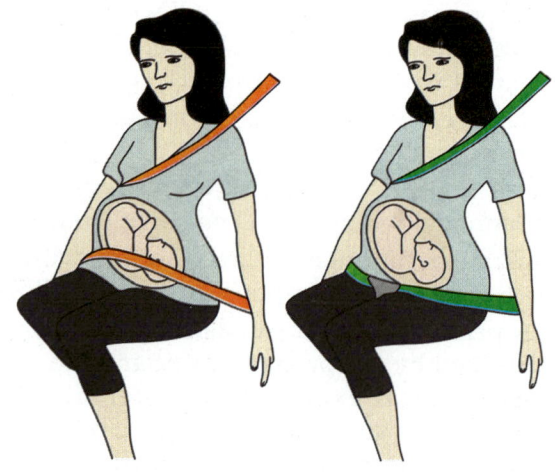

Fig. 17.6. Correct position of car seat belt in pregnant for prevention of seat belt-related injury

Seat Belt Restraints

Education on the proper use of restraints should be a standard component of all prenatal care programs. The use of three-point seat belt restraints or tummy shield (the device) during pregnancy is highly recommended (Fig. 17.6).[21] The National Highway Transportation Safety Administration of USA recommends that pregnant women wear their seat belts with the shoulder harness portion positioned over the collar bone between the woman's breasts, and the lap belt portion under the pregnant abdomen as low as possible on the hips and across the upper thighs and not above or over the abdomen (Fig. 17.7).[28,29]

ANESTHETIC CONSIDERATIONS FOR MANAGEMENT OF PREGNANT TRAUMA PATIENTS

Anesthesia management for trauma patient is challenging as most urgent cases comes during odd-hours in emergency, where lack of experienced anesthesia senior personnel and

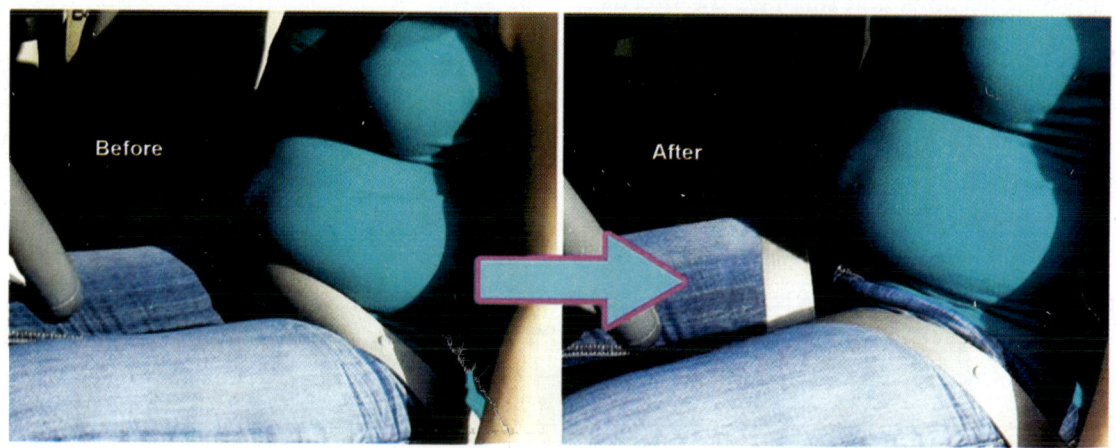

Before   After

Fig. 17.7. Use of triple point seat belt/tummy shield to protect pregnancy from impact of motor vehicle accident

technology may make simple operations more complex.[30] In trauma patient, detailed information regarding personal and medical history may be limited like of allergies, genetic abnormalities, and previous surgeries that may pose unexpected difficulties. Patients usually have multiple complex injuries which need to be prioritized during management like head injury with blunt abdominal trauma. Occult injuries, such as chest injuries, tension pneumothorax, pericardial tamponed and pelvic injuries, can manifest unexpectedly.[31]

Successful management of the pregnant patients with trauma requires a good understanding of pathophysiologic changes of pregnancy and sever trauma, with adequate preparation, team work, timely identification of the life-threatening conditions and their aggressive management for optimal maternal and fetal outcome.[32]

The difficulties in perioperative management of reproductive age female trauma victims are complexity of anatomic and physiologic changes of pregnancy, emergent nature of operations, difficult airway, full stomach and decrease 'safe apnea interval' and the margin of safety.[33,34] The general anesthesia with oral intubation with cuffed ETT should be done, with rapid sequence induction with cricoid pressure, lung de-nitrogenation with 100% oxygen is mandatory with taking care of any hypoxia and hypotension.[35] Intravenous induction agent etomidate is useful because of its cardiovascular stability. Ketamine may be a suitable alternative in hemodynamically compromised patients, but take care of its direct myocardial depressant effect that may lead to cardiovascular collapse. Succinylcholine is the muscle relaxant of choice for its fast onset and offset actions for rapid-sequence induction. Rocuronium with safer cardiovascular profile may be used in place of succinylcholine; to avoid its adverse effects.[36,37]

If coagulation is abnormal and same is not absolute contraindication for regional anesthesia, it can be used for anesthesia and analgesia with multimodal therapy for satisfactory pain relief in emergency during resuscitation and for postoperative period. Epidural analgesia provides potent analgesia and hastens recovery following most of the thoracoabdominal and orthopedic trauma in perioperative period.

One should use minimal mandatory monitoring in both emergency room and the operating theatres like electrocardiogram, blood pressure, oximetry, temperature and capnometry.[38] Invasive monitoring like arterial blood pressure, CVP and cardiac output and stoke volume variation can be considered in selective unstable cases with polytrauma. In addition, a tocotransducer to detect the onset of uterine contractions and cardiotocographic monitoring in viable fetus should be used to judge optimal resuscitation and identifying any adverse event.[39] A correlation between the maternal bicarbonate level and fetal outcome has been suggested. Therefore, it may be useful to monitor the maternal ABG for serum bicarbonate level.[40]

SUMMARY

The physiologic changes and hemodynamic instability due to trauma are two important considerations while managing trauma in pregnancy for optimal maternal and fetal outcome. There is need of a multidisciplinary team that is managing, evaluating and coordinating the care of the pregnant trauma patient. The most common mode of injuries is road traffic accidents, falls, intimate partner violence and the assault. About 90% of the injuries during pregnancy are minors, with around 60 to 70% of fetal losses after minor trauma due to various pitfalls. Management of the pregnant severe trauma patient requires a primary and secondary survey with emphasis on airway, breathing, circulation, and disability as per ATLS guidelines. It is important to consider mode of injury, severity of trauma, gestational age and fetal viability while managing the patient. Minor trauma can often be safely evaluated with simple diagnostic modalities. Pregnancy should not lead to under diagnosis or under treatment of trauma due to unfounded fears of fetal effects. The first 24 hours tocodynamometric monitoring and serial USG (for placental abruption), Kleihauer-Betke test to determine the degree of fetomaternal hemorrhage, regardless of Rh status is recommended.

To improve the effectiveness of cardio-pulmonary resuscitation after cardiac arrest, clinicians should perform left lateral uterine displacement by tilting the whole maternal body 25° to 30°. Unique aspects of advanced cardiac life support include early intubation, and performance of perimortem cesarean delivery should be done for viable fetus, if maternal cardiac arrest occur and CPR done within due time.

The anesthesiologist with the multidisci-plinary team can play an important role for resuscitation, triage, management and transfer of severely injured unstable pregnant trauma patient. Here two lives can be saved with aggressive resuscitation and monitoring of the mother that is priority over concerns for fetal wellbeing as per ATLS guidelines. The hypoxia and hypotension due to hemorrhage are to be prevented to have its deleterious secondary effects on fetus. Perimortem cesarean section can save viable fetus.

REFERENCES

1. Chang J, Berg C, Saltzman L, Herndon J. Homicide: a leading cause of injury deaths among pregnant and postpartum women in the United States, 1991–1999. Am J Public Health 2005;95: 471–7.

2. Pearlman MD, Tintinalli JE, Lorenz RP. A prospective controlled study of outcome after trauma during pregnancy. Am J Obstet Gynecol 1990;162:1502–7.

3. El Kady D, Gilbert WM, Anderson J, Danielsen B, Towner D, Smith LH. Trauma during pregnancy: an analysis of maternal and fetal outcomes in a large population. Am J Obstet Gynecol 2004; 190:1661–8.

4. Kuo C, Jamieson DJ, McPheeters ML, Meikle ML, Posner SF. Injury hospitalizations of pregnant women in the United States, 2002 [published erratum appears in Am J Obstet Gynecol 2007;196:614–5]. Am J Obstet Gynecol 2007; 196:161.e1–7.

5. Hyde LK, Cook LJ, Olson LM, Weiss HB, Dean JM. Effect of motor vehicle crashes on adverse fetal outcomes. Obstet Gynecol 2003;102:279–86.

6. Ikossi DG, Lazar AA, Morabito D, et al. Profile of mothers at risk: an analysis of injury and preg-nancy loss in 1195 trauma patients. Am Coll Surg 2005;200:49–56.

7. Mattox KL, Goetzl L. Trauma in pregnancy. Crit Care Med 2005;33:385–9.

8. Brooks DC, Oxford C. Chapter: the pregnant surgical patient. ACS Surg Princ Pract. 2007:1–21)

9. Maull KI. Maternal-fetal trauma. Semin Pediatr Surg 2001;10(1):32–4.

10. Rothenberger D, Quattlebaum FW, Perry JF Jr, Zabel J, Fischer RP. Blunt maternal trauma: a review of 103 cases. J Trauma 1978;18:173–9.

11. Ullmann Y, Blumenfeld Z, Hakim M, et al. Urgent delivery, the treatment of choice in term pregnant women with extended burn injury. Burns 1997; 23:157–9.

12. Rorison DG, McPherson SJ. Acute toxic inhalations. Emerg Med Clin North Am May 1992;10(2):409–35.

13. Gordon MC. "Chapter 3, Maternal Physiology" Gabbe SG, Niebyl JR, Simpson JL, et al. Gabbe: Obstetrics: Normal and Problem Pregnancies 6th ed. 2012.

14. Kuhlmann RS, Cruikshank DP. Maternal trauma during pregnancy. Clin Obstet Gynecol 1994; 37:274–93.

15. American College of Obstetricians and Gyneco-logists. Obstetric Aspects of Trauma Manage-ment. ACOG Educational Bulletin 251. Washington (DC): ACOG; 1998.

16. Pearlman MD. Trauma and pregnancy. In: Hankins GD, Clark SL, Cunningham FG, (Eds). Operative Obstetrics. Norwalk (CT): Appleton & Lange; 1999;pp. 651–6.

17. Schiff MA, Holt VL, Daling JR. Maternal and infant outcomes after injury during pregnancy in Washington State from 1989 to 1997. J Trauma 2002;53:939–45.

18. Pearlman MD, Tintinalli JE, Lorenz RP. Blunt trauma during pregnancy. N Engl J Med 1990; 323:1609–13.

19. Cusick SS, Tibbles CD. Trauma in pregnancy. Emerg Med Clin North Am 2007;25(3):861–72,xi.

20. American College of Surgeons Committee on Trauma. "Chapter 11, Trauma in Women" Advance Trauma Life Support (ATLS) for Doctors, 9th ed. 2012.

21. Queensland Clinical Guidelines: Trauma in Pregnancy. Maternity and Neonatal Clinical Guidelines. No. MN14.31-V1-R19.Feb 2014:1–31, available at *www.health.qld.gov.au/qcg*, assessed online on 1 July 2015.

22. Haywood L Brown. Trauma in Pregnancy. Obstet Gynecol 2009;114:147–60.

23. Muench MV, Canterino JC. Trauma in pregnancy. Obstet Gynecol Clin North Am 2007;34(3): p. 555–83, xiii.

24. Agran PF, Dunkle DE, Winn DG, Kent D. Fetal death in motor vehicle accidents. Ann Emerg Med 1987;16:1355.

25. American Heart Association: Cardiac arrest associated with pregnancy. Circulation: 112:IV-150IV–153,2005.

26. Vanden Hoek TL, Morrison LJ, Shuster M, et al. Part 12: cardiac arrest in special situations: 2010 American Heart Association guidelines for cardiopulmonary resuscitation and emergency cardiovascular care [published corrections appear in Circulation. 2011;123(6):e239, and Circulation 2011;124(15):e405]. Circulation. 2010;122(18 suppl 3):S829–S861.

27. Astarita DC, Feldman B. Seat belt placement resulting in uterine rupture. J Trauma 1997; 42:738–40.

28. American College of Obstetricians and Gyneco-logists. Car safety for you and your baby.http://www.acog.org/~/media/For%20Patients/faq018.pdf?dmc=1=20140703T2121569354. Accessed July 1, 2015.

29. National Highway Traffic Safety Administration. Buckle up in pregnancy.http://www.nhtsa.dot.gov/people/injury/airbags/Internet_Services_ Group/ISG-Restricted/Buckle-Up%20America/pregnancybrochure/BUA_PregnancyNHTSA change.pdf. Accessed July 1, 2015.

30. Hawkins JL, Goetzl L, Chestnut DH. "Chapter 16, Obstetric Anesthesia". Gabbe SG, Niebyl JR, Simpson JL, et al. Gabbe: Obstetrics: Normal and Problem Pregnancies, 5th ed.

31. Obstetric aspects of trauma management. ACOG Educational Bulletin No. 251. September, 1998.

32. Neil J Murphy, Jeffrey D Quinlan. Trauma in Pregnancy; Assessment management and Prevention. Am Fam Physician 2014;90(10): 717–24.

33. Mirza FG, Devine PC, Gaddipati S. Trauma in pregnancy: a systematic approach. Am J Perinatol 2010;27(7):579–86.

34. Mendez-Figueroa H, Dahlke JD, Vrees RA, Rouse DJ. Trauma in pregnancy: an updated systematic review. Am J Obstet Gynecol 2013;209(1):1–10.

35. Brown S, Mozurkewich E. Trauma during pregnancy. Obstet Gynecol Clin North Am 2013;40(1):47–57.

36. Cronholm PF, Fogarty CT, Ambuel B, Harrison SL. Intimate partner violence. Am Fam Physician 2011;83(10):1165–72.

37. Reddy SV, Shaik NA, Gunakala K. Trauma during pregnancy. J Obstet Anaesth Crit Care 2012;2. 3–9.

38. Deitch E, Saraswati D. Intensive care unit management of the trauma patient. Crit Care Med 2006;34:2294–2301.

39. AAP Committee on Fetus and Newborn and ACOG Committee on Obstetric Practice (Eds). Guidelines for Perinatal Care, 7th ed. Elk Grove, Ill.: American Academy of Pediatrics; 2012:131–2, 246–8.

40. American College of Obstetricians and Gynecologists. Intimate partner violence. ACOG Committee Opinion No. 518. Obstet Gynecol 2012;119(2 pt 1):412–7.

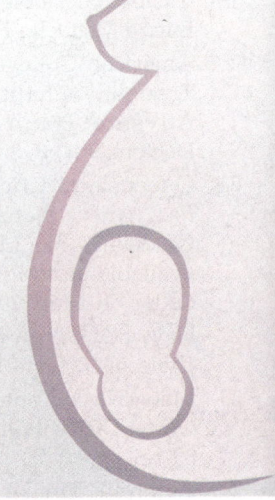

CHAPTER 18

Obstetric Anesthesia for Non-Obstetric Procedures

Sandeep Sahu, Chetna Shamshery, Indu Lata

INTRODUCTION

During the pregnancy, women are susceptible to any type of medical and surgical disorders. It is difficult to accurately quantify non-obstetrical disorders that complicate pregnancy. The overall antenatal hospitalization rate is 10.1 per 100 deliveries.[1] Approximately 1 in every 635 pregnant women will undergo a non-obstetrical surgical procedure.[2,3] As per American College of Obstetricians and Gynecologists, many of these non-obstetrical disorders are within the purview of the obstetricians and they can very well manage them.[4] But at the same time, non-obstetrician multidisciplinary specialists who also care for these pregnant women and their unborn fetuses should be well aware with pregnancy-induced physiological changes, special fetal considerations and pathological conditions during pregnancy.[5]

The Indian female fertility rate is over 2.7 during her lifetime, and approximately 0.75-2% of the pregnant females requiring surgery during the antenatal period, so the magnitude of pregnant ladies requiring anesthesia is huge. The situation is challenging especially because there are two lives at stake. But whether we perform surgery, anesthesia, trauma life support or resuscitation, the dictum is true, "Mother takes priority over her fetus".

SURGERY DURING PREGNANCY

The adverse effects of surgery during pregnancy usually not increased till the surgical procedures are uneventful. With the associated complications, however, risks will likely be increased. For example, perforative appendicitis with feculent peritonitis has significant maternal and perinatal morbidity and mortality rates. This may occur even if the surgical and anesthetic techniques are without any complications. Conversely, procedure-related complications may also adversely affect outcomes. Still, compared with non-pregnant women undergoing similar procedures, pregnant women do not appear to have excessive complications.[6]

Effect of Surgery and Anesthesia on Pregnancy Outcome

The most extensive data regarding anesthetic and surgical risks to pregnancy are from the Swedish Birth Registry as described by Mazze and Källén.[7] The effects on pregnancy outcomes of 5405 non-obstetrical surgical procedures performed in 720,000 pregnant women from 1973 to 1981 were analyzed. General anesthesia was used for approximately half of these procedures with nitrous oxide supplemented by other inhalational or intravenous medications. These procedures were performed in 41% of women in the first trimester, 35% in the second, and 24% in the third trimester (Table 18.1).

Perinatal Outcomes

Excessive perinatal morbidity associated with non-obstetrical surgery is attributable in many cases to the disease itself. There were no adverse effects of surgery and anesthesia. According to the Swedish Birth Registry that have most robost data about it, results were not significantly differ from that of non-exposed control.[7] Except with significantly increased rate of low birth weight, preterm birth, and neonatal death in pregnant woman who had undergone surgery, that may have synergistic effect. There are also no strong evidences that anesthetics may harm the fetus.[8]

DIAGNOSTIC IMAGING DURING PREGNANCY

The diagnostic imaging is very important to diagnose, manage and follow-up of different medical and surgical disorders in pregnancy.[9]

Ionizing Radiation

This is biggest concern regarding ionizing radiation to the developing fetus. The impor-tant factors reading the dose of radiation and the gestational age are described in Table 18.2.[10,11]

The first 2 weeks of conception are crucial; any significant radiation may result in a miscarriage. There is "all or none" phenomenon. If the fetus is viable after this early exposure, no adverse effects are expected. Post-conception 2–8 weeks, because of period of organogenesis, are sensitive to teratogenicity.[11] The fetal central nervous system is the most sensitive to radiation damage during 8–15 weeks.[12]

While evaluating a pregnant patient, she should counseled that the radiation exposure of a diagnostic test does not confer a significant risk or fetal harm.[13,14] In addition, the use of low-exposure techniques and abdominal lead shielding can also reduce the exposure and preventable methods. When suitable ultrasound or magnetic resonance imaging (MRI) should be used, that are quite safe.[15]

Non-Ionizing Radiation

Ultrasound: There have been no confirmed adverse effects of diagnostic ultrasound procedures. The safety and versatility of ultrasonography has made it the first-line diagnostic tool during pregnancy.

Magnetic resonance imaging: MRI had no reported harmful effects to the mother or fetus.

As per the American College of Obstetricians and Gynecologists (ACOG), "a single exposure with X-ray of less than 5 rads during pregnancy does not result in harmful effects."

Table 18.1: Results of birth outcomes in pregnant women undergoing non-obstetrical surgery (Adopted form Swedish Birth Registry)[6]		
Birth outcome	Rate (%)	p value
Major malformation	1.9	Not significant
Stillbirth	7/1000	Not significant
Neonatal death (within the 7 days)	10.5/1000	Significant
Preterm <37 weeks	7.5	Significant
Birth weight <1.5 kg	1.2	Significant
Birth weight <2.5 kg	6.6	Significant

Table 18.2: Effects on the fetus about radiation exposure (*Adapted from Williams Textbook of Obstetrics*)[8,9]

Gestational age (weeks)	Possible adverse effects	Radiation minimal dose (cGy)
3–4 (first 2 weeks post-conception)	Embryonal demise ("all or none")	5–20
4–8	Death, intrauterine growth retardation, congenital anomalies	20–50
8–15	Intrauterine growth retardation, micro-cephaly, mental retardation	6–50
16–25	Mental retardation	25–150

One should see urgency and utility of diagnostic modalities during pregnancy.[16]

PRE-ANESTHETIC CHECK UPS OF PREGNANT WOMAN

For better maternal and fetal outcomes, it is important to understand the maternal physiological changes during pregnancy, indication, urgency and timing of the surgery and complex interaction between all of them. A detailed history and physical examination as per trimester-wise pregnancy should be done. It is important to examine each system especially cardiovascular to rule out any pathological cardiac illness, respiratory system to rule out obstructive/restrictive lung disease, renal disorder and GI system. Routine blood investigations to assess severity of anemia, platelet and coagulation function, liver and kidney function are essential for guiding the selection of anesthesia techniques and required modification for patient safety. The ECG and ABG may be done according to indication, status of patient and type of surgery. Airway assessment should be done routinely to know anticipated difficult airway, and should be managed as per ASA/difficult airway guidelines. The Mallampati grade may increase to four from one in about 35% of the cases with term pregnancy.[17]

Obstetric consultation should be asked to continue tocolytics to maintain pregnancy while the active manipulations during surgery. The decision for the fetal monitoring depends upon the viability of the fetus. For the fetal heart monitoring, Doppler ultrasound can be used from 10 to 24 weeks of pregnancy, and then by the tocodynamometer.

Every pregnant patient should always be considered full stomach. The incidence of gastric regurgitation and aspiration is increased in more than 16 weeks pregnancy due to relaxed lower esophageal sphincter (LES). But the gastric emptying time may remain unaffected.[18-19] The resting LES pressure is almost similar to pre-pregnancy and early pregnancy period. But the physiological, pharmacological, and hormonal responses are blunted during the pregnnacy.[20] Hence aspiration prophylaxis as premedication with ranitidine a night before and early morning to increases pH of the gastric contents or 0.3M sodium citrate 30 mL before elective or emergency surgeries should be given as per institute protocols. The prophylaxis for venous thromboembolism depends individually as per risk stratification and institute protocols. It is always important to optimize and improve the co-morbid conditions in mother for better outcome.[21] Advance planning for choosing techniques and type of anesthesia should be done. The team that include obstetricians, pediatricians and radiologists should be present in the operation suite. In any adverse event, emergency delivery or Doppler USG for fetal heart rate monitoring should be planned. One should take informed consent for intra-operative maternal mishaps and events like of

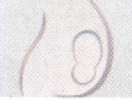

fetal intrauterine growth retardation, death or preterm labor.

MONITORING

The routine monitors, like ECG, NIBP, HR, ECG, pulse oximeter, temperature, urinary catheter, and EtCO$_2$, are a must. Specialized monitoring as neuromuscular monitor, Doppler USG, cardiotocography or stethoscope may be used to monitor fetus. Based on these monitoring, fetal distress can be diagnosed early to improve the oxygenation and ventilation and hemodynamic and perfusion status of mother or decision to early delivery.

Interpretation of CTG: Cardiotocography (CTG) correlates fetal heart rate with uterine contractions. Based on the interpretation and cause, intraoperative management can be altered (Table 18.3).[22]

INTRAOPERATIVE MANAGEMENT

1. **Maternal considerations:** Aim is to avoid maternal hypoxia, hypercarbia or hypocarbia, hypotension and decreased uteroplacental circulation. One should try to maintain preoperative maternal physiology.

2. **Aortocaval compression syndrome:** It usually occurs after 20th week of gestation. Right up tilt by 15–30° using a wedge of 4–6 inches of height is an important prerequisite to avoid it. This manure could augment around 30% return of the blood volume as preload and avoid maternal and fetal hypotension.

3. **Autoimmunization:** Rh isoimmunization is also a consideration different from the general population which is always implemented in a female who is Rh –ve with an Rh +ve fetus. It involves any surgery

Table 18.3: Interpretation of CTG [Adapted from Royal College of Obstetricians and Gynaecologists. Guidelines (8.2001)][22]

Parameter	Cause	Interpretation	Management
120–160		Normal FHR	
Baseline FHR less than 120	• Hypoxia • Prolonged cord compression/prolapsed • Epidural and spinal anesthesia • Maternal seizures • Rapid fetal descent	• 100–120: mild bradycardia • <80 FHR, severe bradycardia	• Increase FiO$_2$ • Increase BP • Treat maternal seizures and immediate C-section.
Baseline FHR more than 160	• Fetal hypoxia • Hypotension • Fever • Hyperthyroidism • Fetal or maternal anemia	• Tachycardia	• Increase FiO$_2$ • Increase BP • Antipyretics • Transfuse blood • IV propylthiouracil
5–25 beat to beat variation		• Normal variability	
<5 bpm variability	• Fetal acidosis • Fetus sleeping • Drugs—opiates, benzodiazepine, methyldopa, magnesium sulfate	• Reduced variability	• Increase FiO$_2$ • Increase BP • If due to drugs: ignore

Contd...

Contd...

Fetal heart rate	Causes	Interpretation	Management
	• Prematurity • Congenital heart abnormalities		
>15 bpm sudden increase in HR with uterine contractions		• Normal • At least 2 accelerations are desired/15 min	
>15 bpm decrease HR	When uterine contraction begins and recovers when uterine contraction stops. Cause: Increased fetal ICP	• Early deceleration	Physiological
	Rapid fall in baseline rate with a variable recovery phase Cause: Umbilical cord compression	• Variable deceleration	Fetus is adapting
	• Begins at the peak of uterine contraction and recover after the contraction ends Cause: Fetal hypotension • Fetal hypoxia • Fetal acidosis • Uterine hyperstimulation • Immediate blood sampling	• Late deceleration	• Increase FiO_2 • Increase BP • Stop uterine manipulation
		• Prolonged deceleration >2 min	Immediate C-section
Smooth, regular, wave-like pattern with frequency: 2–5/min Stable baseline HR	• Severe fetal hypoxia • Severe fetal anemia • Fetal/maternal hemorrhage	• Sinusoidal pattern	Immediate C-section

except those that are located distant from the torso site and would never involve fetomaternal blood contact (e.g. surgeries involving the extremities).

4. **Tocolysis:** Prophylactic tocolysis is not supported by evidence to have any beneficial effect, although it forms a part of the management in case of risk of preterm labor in the intraoperative and immediate postoperative period.

5. **Progesterone:** Obstetric consultation should be taken to decide if progesterone is to be given based on the timing of surgery.[23]

6. **Antenatal steroids:** Obstetric consultation should also be sought for steroid administration, if fetus has crossed the period of viability, as there are chances of preterm delivery or emergency cesarean section.

Apart from the above general considerations, the special cases have been discussed later in the chapter.

Fetal Considerations/Teratogenesis

Pathophysiology of fetal distress, a vicious cycle, has been discussed in Figure 18.1.

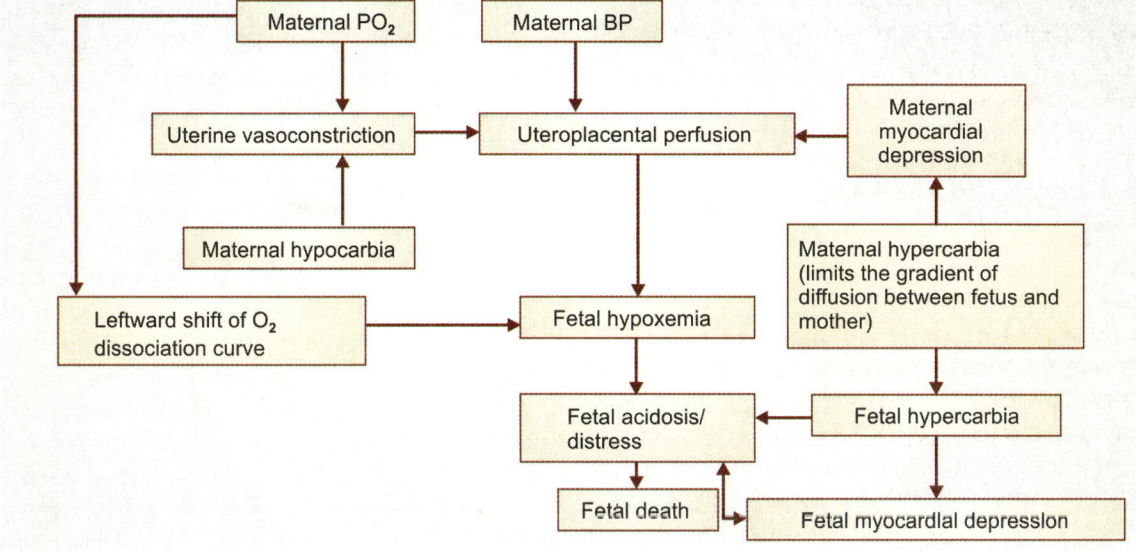

Fig. 18.1. Pathophysiology of fetal distress

The most important factor affecting the growing fetus is the time since conception. In the initial 3 to 14 days, either the zygote adheres to the uterine wall or behaves as ectopic pregnancy, so it is an all or none phenomenon. The most important time is 15th day to 60th day which is the period of organogenesis.[24] Hence, it can most aggressively affect the fetus. It is always better to avoid any anesthetic or drug exposure during this period until unavoidable. Incidence of abortion varies between 5.8 and 10.5% during the 1st trimester. Following these 60 days, the incidence of intrauterine growth retardation concerns and in the 3rd trimester the incidence of preterm delivery is raised.[25] Although anesthetic drugs have been found to affect cell division and signalling at cellular level in animal studies yet none has been found to have a teratogenic effect on the human fetus with single dose or the amount in which they are clinically used.[26–27] The significant risk for congenital malformations is less when surgery done in the first trimester. Doppler USG helps to monitor the fetal heart rate and flow from 10–24 weeks. During this period, usually two scans are done: preoperatively and post-

operatively, because evidence shows that after 28 weeks the fetus is viable, it is then that continuous fetal monitoring using cardiotocography should be used to show fetal heart rate variability.

Drugs should be used in minimal amounts without compromising the anesthesia, so that the fetus is safe. The main goals for fetal wellbeing are avoiding hypoxia, hypercarbia, hypocapnia and hypotension in mother, all of which can directly or indirectly affect uteroplacental perfusion as it is not autoregulated. Maternal hyperoxia does not affect the fetus because the PaO_2 levels fall by 90% by the time it reaches the fetus.

Regarding the Timing of Surgery

The timing and type of surgery has direct impact on the maternal and fetal outcomes, this has been described in Table 18.4, as per American Heart Association guidelines. Appendicitis is the most frequently performed urgent surgery followed by cholecystitis and trauma during pregnancy. Laparoscopic surgeries should be preferred in comparison to open surgeries. The elective surgeries should be deferred till 6 weeks postpartum or

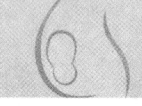

Table 18.4: Type and time of surgery (*Adopted from ACC, AHA, Circulation*)[28]

Type of surgery	Performed after diagnosis
Emergency surgery	<6 hrs
Urgent surgery	6–24 hrs
Time sensitive procedures	<1–6 weeks
Elective surgery	Up to 1 year

at least up to the 2nd trimester. The surgeries of urgent nature, done during the 1st trimester of pregnancy involving the torso of the mother, have the worst prognosis. There is lack of a significant increased risk for malformations among pregnancies exposed to non-obstetrical surgery and anesthesia. However, unless must, it is preferable to defer surgical intervention until the second trimester. Here theoretical risk for teratogenicity, spontaneous miscarriage, is almost decreased. Special considerations related to cardiac, trauma, laparoscopy and neurosurgeries are described later in the chapter.

TYPES OF ANESTHESIA

Equivocal results have been documented with regional and general anesthesia. The advantages and disadvantages of both the techniques have been described in Table 18.5. But whenever possible the regional anesthesia should be the preferred mode of anesthesia so

as to avoid any undue exposure of the fetus to medications. In cases of central neuraxial anesthesia, the drug dose with spinal or epidural route should be decreased because of two reasons:
1. The epidural space is decreased leading to a higher neuraxial cephalad spread of the drug.
2. Pregnant female has hypoalbuminemia due to which drug that is bound decreases, thus increasing the free fraction. This is the cause for local anesthetic toxicity.

Local anesthetic toxicity can also be precipitated by inadvertent intravascular access during central neuraxial procedure, as the vessels are engorged. Lignocaine with adrenaline should be avoided in epidural for pregnant females with hypertension, pregnancy-induced hypertension.[29]

To counteract hypotension, phenylepherine and ephedrine both have been found effective to counteract hypotension, in fact phenylephrine preserves the umbilical pH greater than ephedrine.[30,31] The comparison of the three vasopressors has been described in Table 18.6.[32,33]

ANESTHETIC DRUGS CROSSING PLACENTA

The choice of anesthetics based on their property to cross the placenta has been described in Table 18.7.

Table 18.5: Comparison of advantages and disadvantages of regional vs general anesthesia

	Regional anesthesia	General anesthesia
Advantages	Does not expose the fetus to intravenous drugs	With maternal coagulation abnormalities, it is the preferred mode of anesthesia.
	Causes uterine relaxation thus aids in tocolysis	Vital parameters are in better control
	Generally does not influence the fetal heart rate directly	
	No airway manipulation	Preferred with cardiac comorbidities.
	Analgesia is provided	
	Cannot be used in patients with coagulopathy	
Disadvantages	Due to increased sympathetic activity, central neuraxial block may causes hypotension to greater extent	All anesthetic drugs have been found to cross placenta. Drugs decrease basal and variability in FHR, thus interfering with CTG.

Table 18.6: Comparison of phenylephrine, ephedrine and mephentermine

	Phenylephrine	Ephedrine	Mephentermine
MOA	α1 agonist	Indirectly stimulates NE and affects α and β receptors, but without directly affecting uterine vasculature	Stimulates β receptors to release NE.
Vial	10 mg/mL	50 mg/mL	30 mg/mL
Administration as bolus	Dilute 10 mg in 100 mL 0.9% NaCl. Bolus of 100 µg can be given to counteract hypotension.	10–50 mg bolus dose.	Dilute 30 mg in 5 mL 0.9% NaCl. Bolus of 6 mg could be given to counteract hypotension.
Infusion	0.4 to 9.1 µg/kg/min	5 mg/min	
Side effects	Reflex bradycardia, severe peripheral and visceral vasoconstriction	Mainly due to hypertension: nausea, vomiting, restlessness, tremors, palpitations, urinary retention.	Tachycardia, nausea, vomiting, anxiety, palpitations, headache.

The placental transfer of anesthetic drugs is mainly by simple diffusion based on the Fick's principle of diffusion, i.e.

$$Q/t = \frac{K * A (C_m - C_f)}{D}$$

(K: constant, $C_m - C_f$: concentration difference between mother and fetus, Q/t: diffusion speed, A: membrane area, D: thickness of membrane)

Placental transfer also gets affected by:
- pKA
- Protein binding (increased binding decreases the placental transfer of drugs)

- Maternal and fetal pH: Acidosis would cause increased drug transfer.

POINT-WISE APPROACH FOR GENERAL ANESTHESIA

1. After counseling and reconciling, connecting the monitors, anxiolysis could be achieved using 0.02–0.03 mg/kg midazolam.
2. **Preoxygenation:** Head-up position (as FRC is reduced), 100% O_2 for denitrogenation, for 3 minutes (as incidence of hypoxia is increased by 3 times due to decreased FRC

Table 18.7: Anesthetic drugs crossing placenta

Drugs	Placental crossing
Induction agent	Readily crosses placenta
Inhalationals	Diffuse through placenta
Opioids [34,35]	Remifentanyl > fentanyl > alfentanyl > sufentanyl
	50% of maternal remifentanyl concentration could be seen in fetus.
	Morphine also readily crosses placenta.
Local anesthetics[37]	Lidocaine > bupivacaine (maternal fetal ratio for lidocaine: 0.5 and bupivacaine: 0.2. Thus giving greater difference of toxicity and free drug level for bupivacaine)
Muscle relaxants[36]	Do not cross placenta (due to high molecular weight, quaternary structure and ionization)
Anticholinergics	Glycopyrrolate: does not cross (as it is a quaternary compound)
	Atropine: crosses

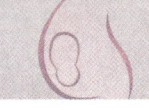

and increased O_2 consumption). The end tidal O_2 fraction should be >0.9.

3. **Drugs for induction** (difficult airway cart should always be prepared beforehand):
   - Opioids: Fentanyl 1–2 µg/kg (fentanyl causes minimal respiratory depression in fetus and morphine causes the most respiratory depression).
   - Thiopentone/propofol/ketamine/etomidate/benzodiazepines: None has been found to cause fetal teratogenicity.[38] In hemodynamically compromised patients, thiopentone/propofol should be avoided or use in low titrated doses. Also hypotension precipitates faster due to decreased SVR in pregnancy. Whereas, if patient is hemodynamically stable, ketamine should be avoided as it increases the abdominal pressure and uterine contractility, which are undesired as the patient is full stomach and uterine relaxation is required.
   - Medications should be given in low normal dose because of increased free fraction available due to hypoalbuminemia.
   - Muscle relaxant: Succinylcholine 1–2 mg/kg (increased response due to 30% decreased cholinesterase is compensated by increased volume of distribution.)

4. **Intubation**: Rapid sequence intubation (RSI) is to be performed in view of full stomach. Intubation is done by one size small endotracheal tube than anticipated, due to expected airway edema.

5. **Maintenance of anesthesia:** It is done using intermediate-acting muscle relaxant (atracurium/vecuronium), fentanyl and inhalational (sevoflurane is most preferred) agent.[39] MAC of inhalational anesthetics is reduced by 30%. Adequate depth and analgesia should be maintained to avoid sympathetic over activity. N_2O should be avoided; instead air should be used especially in the 1st trimester. Although N_2O effects on animals have been influenced

by timing, dose and duration (>16 hrs) of use, but it has not been found to affect human fetus.[40]

6. **Reversal:** It is done using neostigmine and glycopyrrolate. In the post-operation period, thromboprophylaxis is to be started along with early mobilization, physiotherapy and leg stockings. Aggressive monitoring should be done up to one week or not less than 48 hrs postoperative period.

SPECIAL PREGNANCY CONDITIONS

Pregnant Female with Valvular Lesion Non-Obstetric Surgery

Stenotic lesions are more bothersome for pregnancy especially in the 2nd and 3rd trimesters, because the mother has a low SVR, and tachycardia both of which oppose the hemodynamic required to manage stenotic valvular disease. On the other hand, they fulfil our management for the regurgitant lesions. Comparative management goals of both the lesions have been described in Table 18.8. A case of mitral/aortic regurgitation can be performed under central neuraxial anesthesia. For mild to moderate aortic/mitral stenotic cases, epidural anesthesia with graded top-ups can be tried, but for severe stenotic lesions general anesthesia is to be administered.

Pregnant Female with a Prosthetic Heart Valve Posted for Non-Obstetric Surgery

These patients are likely to be on anticoagulants and antiplatelet. In the 1st trimester, warfarin is to be avoided as it causes teratogenic effects, e.g. nasal hypoplasia, stippled epiphyses, limb deformities, and respiratory distress in the fetus also known as "fetal warfarin syndrome". Heparin is prescribed because it does not cross the placenta. In the 2nd trimester, heparin is replaced by warfarin, and again the changeover takes place in the 3rd trimester as now warfarin causes mental retardation, microcephaly, optic atrophy, and blindness in the fetus.[41] Moreover, warfarin

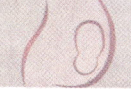

Table 18.8: Anesthetic goals for the stenotic and regurgitant lesions for non-cardiac surgery

	Stenotic lesion	Regurgitant lesion
Anesthesia preferred	General	Regional
HR	Low normal (<70)	High normal (>90)
BP	Avoid hypotension	Hypotension is tolerated well
SVR	Kept high	Kept low
Preload	Kept low	Kept high
Fluids	Low replacement	Judicious
Drugs to be used	Diuretics, vasopressors (phenyle-phrine/NA)	Ionodilators/vasodilators (NTG/dobuta-mine/milrinone)
Complication expected	AF, pulmonary edema	

also precipitates the incidence of bleeding at term. While taking up a case it is important to stop warfarin for 5 days and replace it by heparin either low molecular weight (LMWH) or unfractionated (UFH). Before taking up a case, last dose of LMWH should be withheld for 24 hours and UFH should be withheld 4–6 hours prior to surgery.[42] The coagulation status should be checked by measuring PT, INR after 3 days of stopping warfarin and if INR >1.5 then oral vitamin K, 1–2 mg is to be administered for 2–3 days. The aPTT should be done for unfractionated heparin. The activated clotting time (ACT) is a good bedside point of care. Normal ACT value is between 80 and 140 sec depending upon the manufacturer.[43] Platelet counts could also be investigated in case UFH has been used, because of the incidence of heparin-induced thrombocytopenia. If this comes to be normal, then regional anesthesia could be used without fear of an anticipated hematoma.

Pregnant Female for Cardiac Surgical Procedure

Any female with cardiac disease should be initially managed medically which is less dangerous than interventional procedures which are in turn less dangerous than open cardiac surgeries. The indication of any cardiac surgery depends upon the pathology and is not affected by the fact that the female is pregnant according to ACC, AHA guidelines.[28] Echocardiography should be performed, if there is a deterioration/change/appearance of new symptoms related to cardiac pathology, or else has to be performed once a year.[44] To perform the percutaneous interventional procedure, the main concern is fetal exposure to X-rays. Radiation of <50 is targeted for pregnant woman. Abdominal shield or lead apron covering the fetal area should be ensured and direct exposure of X-rays to abdomen should be curtailed.

Points to be remembered when taking up a case for open cardiac surgery:
1. Mean arterial pressure >70 mm Hg
2. Pump flow >2.5 L/min/m²
3. Adequate depth of anesthesia to be maintained to obtund the sympathetic response
4. Minimize the time on cardiac bypass
5. Temperature to be maintained >33°C
6. Use pulsatile flow
7. Hct >28%
8. α-stat pH management preferred.
9. CTG/FHR monitoring must be done.

Interventional Pain Procedures

Pregnancy leads to change in pelvis anatomy and orientation by laxity of ligaments to give more space to the enlarging fetus and uterus. Sacroiliitis results due to asymmetry in laxity

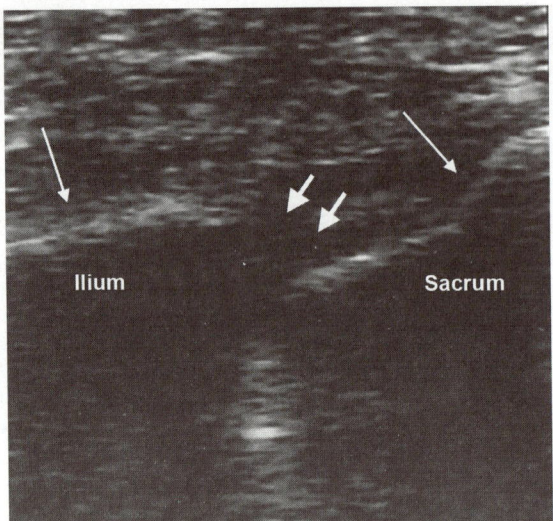

Fig. 18.2. USG-guided SI joint block

of SI joint during pregnancy.[45] Also pain of myofascial origin or certain uncommon etiologies result in crippling disability during pregnancy.[46] It might be difficult for her to walk or even turn sides in the bed. Initial management to these pain syndromes is medically dealt, but only paracetamol is prescribed (classified under Group B), as most of the other drugs of NSAIDs come under FDA drug classification (category: C/D). They may close the patent ductus arteriosus in third trimester after 32 weeks of gestation. Interventional procedures, if planned using fluoroscopy, have to follow similar norms of radiation prevention as have been described for cardiac interventional procedures. Moreover, nowadays, most of these pain problems could be managed using USG. Figure 18.2 shows ultrasound anatomy of sacroiliac joint, may be used for performing diagnostic and therapeutic pain relief blocks.

Laparoscopic Procedures during Pregnancy

Considering equivocal outcomes by laparotomy/laparoscopy, the later has become procedure of choice for abdominal surgeries during pregnancy.[47] Advantages of laparoscopy include small incision, less pain, less analgesic requirement, fast recovery, short hospital stay, decreased uterine manipulation.

Management Principles

- Gasless laparoscopy/targeted abdominal pressure <10 mm Hg
- Right up, left lateral position by 15°.
- Target PCO_2 to be maintained is between 30 and 35 mm Hg, despite which maternal and fetal hypercarbia is seen which emphasises large arterial and alveolar PCO_2 differences.[48]
- Open technique to enter into abdomen
- Maintain the respiratory alkalosis with PCO_2 <35 mmHg

LAPAROSCOPIC SURGERY DURING PREGNANCY

Laparoscopy has become the most common first-trimester procedure used for diagnosis and management of several surgical disorders.[6] In addition to management of ectopic pregnancy with laparoscopy, it is used preferentially during pregnancy for exploration and treatment of adnexal masses, for appendectomy, and for cholecystectomy. In 2011, the Guidelines Committee of the Society of American Gastrointestinal and Endoscopic Surgeons (SAGES) updated its recommendations concerning laparoscopy use in pregnant women are listed in Table 18.9.[49] Information regarding surgical approach selection in pregnant women comes from the American College of Surgeons database.[7] There are no randomized trials comparing laparoscopic with open surgery, however, most reviews report equally satisfactory outcomes.[50–52] At first, 26 to 28 weeks became the upper gestational-age limit recommended, but as experience has continued to accrue, many now describe laparoscopic surgery performed in the third trimester.[53] There are also reports of laparoscopic splenectomy, adrenalectomy, and nephrectomy done in pregnant women.[54–56]

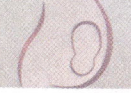

Table 18.9: Guidelines for the performance of laparoscopic surgery in pregnancy (Sages)[49,50]

Indications	Same as for non-pregnant women
	Adnexal mass
	Excision investigation of acute abdominal processes
	Appendectomy, cholecystectomy, nephrectomy, adrenalectomy, splenectomy
Timing	All trimesters
	Technique
Position	Left lateral recumbent
Entry	Open technique, careful Veress needle, or optical trocar; fundal height may alter insertion site selection
Trocars	Direct visualization for placement; fundal height may alter insertion site selection
CO_2 insufflation pressures	10–15 mm Hg
Monitoring	Capnography intraoperatively, FHR assessment pre- and postoperatively
	Perioperative pneumatic compression devices and early postoperative ambulation

CO_2=carbon dioxide; FHR=fetal heart rate.

Relevant Points for Laparoscopy in Pregnancy from Sages[49]

1. Diagnostic laparoscopy is safe and effective when used selectively in acute abdominal processes in pregnancy.
2. Laparoscopic treatment of acute abdominal processes has the same indications in pregnant and non-pregnant patients.
3. Laparoscopy can be safely performed during any trimester of pregnancy.
4. $EtCO_2$ monitoring by capnography should be used.
5. Pneumatic compression devices and early postoperative ambulation are recommended prophylaxis for deep venous thrombosis.
6. Laparoscopic cholecystectomy is the treatment of choice in the pregnant patient with gallbladder disease regardless of trimester.
7. Laparoscopic appendectomy may be performed safely in pregnant patients with suspicion of appendicitis.
8. Laparoscopic adrenalectomy, nephrectomy, and splenectomy are safe procedures in pregnant patients when indicated, and standard precautions are taken.
9. Laparoscopy observation is safe and effective in symptomatic adnexal cystic masses. When ultrasound is not worrisome for malignancy and tumor markers are normal, initial observation is warranted for most adnexal cystic lesions smaller than 6 cm.
10. Laparoscopy is recommended for both diagnosis and treatment of adnexal torsion unless clinical severity warrants laparotomy.
11. Fetal heart monitoring should occur before and after operation in the setting of urgent abdominal surgery during pregnancy.
12. Obstetrical consultation can be obtained before and after operation and tocolytics should not be used routinely (only when signs of preterm labor are present.

Perinatal Outcomes

The perinatal outcome about surgery during pregnancy discussed in details above, here it is in relation to laparoscopy. Because precise

Table 18.10: Physiological effects of CO_2 insufflation

System	Effects	Mechanisms	Possible maternal fetal effects
Respiratory	PCO_2 increases, pH decreases	CO_2 absorption	Hypercarbia, acidosis
Cardiovascular	Increased—heart rate, systemic vascular resistance, pulmonary, central venous, and mean arterial pressures	Hypercarbia and increased intra-abdominal pressure	Uteroplacental hypoperfusion—possible fetal hypoxia, acidosis, and hypoperfusion
	Decreased—cardiac output	Decreased venous return	As above
Blood flow	Decreased splanchnic flow with hypoperfusion of liver, kidneys, and gastrointestinal organs	Increased intra-abdominal pressure	As above
	Decreased venous return from lower extremities	Increased intra-abdominal pressure	As above
	Increased cerebral blood flow	Hypercarbia possibly from shunting due to splanchnic tamponade	Increased CSF pressure

CO_2=carbon dioxide; CSF=cerebrospinal fluid; PCO_2=partial pressure of CO_2

effects of laparoscopy in the human fetus are unknown, animal studies are informative. Pregnancy outcomes in women are limited to observations. As per updated Swedish Birth Registry database to analyse a 20-year period and more than 2 million deliveries.[7] There were no differences, however, when outcomes of women undergoing laparoscopy versus laparotomy were compared.[55]

Hemodynamic Effects

Abdominal insufflation for laparoscopy causes hemodynamic changes that are similar in pregnant and non-pregnant women, and these are summarized in Table 18.10. Effects intensified when insufflation pressure >20 mm Hg in baboons.[56]

Technique

Aortocaval compression is avoided and taken care by a left-lateral tilt. Positioning of the lower extremities in boot-type stirrups maintains access to the vagina for fetal sonographic assessment or manual uterine displacement. Vaginally placed instruments that enter the cervix or uterus for uterine manipulation should not be used during pregnancy. Most reports describe the use of general anesthesia after tracheal intubation with monitoring of end-tidal carbon dioxide $EtCO_2$.[57,58] Beyond the first trimester, technical modifications of standard pelvic laparoscopic entry are required to avoid uterine puncture or laceration. Many recommend open entry techniques to avoid perforations of the uterus, pelvic vessels, and adnexa.[3,59]

Complications

Risks inherent to any abdominal endoscopy are possibly increased slightly during pregnancy. The obvious unique complication is perforation of the pregnant uterus with either a trocar or Veress needle.[60]

SUMMARY

- Mother management should take priority over the fetus.

- Obstetric consultation should be sought before taking up a case.

- Evidence-based studies suggest equivocal outcomes for general and regional

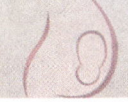

anesthesia. But regional anesthesia should be preferred whenever possible.

- Multidisciplinary approach to all pregnant cases should be undertaken, including pediatrician, surgeon, obstetrician and anesthesiologist.
- The anesthetic management varies with the type, timing, and urgency and comorbid conditions of the female. Aim is to maintain presurgical maternal physiology.
- Aortocaval compression release can contribute up to 30% of the circulating blood volume.

REFERENCES

1. Gazmararian JA, Petersen R, Jamieson DJ, et al. Hospitalizations during pregnancy among managed care enrollees. Obstet Gynecol 2002;100: 94–100.

2. Corneille MG, Gallup TM, Bening T, et al. The use of laparoscopic surgery in pregnancy: evaluation of safety and efficacy. Am J Surg 2010;200:363.

3. Kizer NT, Powell MA. Surgery in the pregnant patient. Clin Obstet Gynecol 2011;54(1):633–11.

4. Nonobstetric surgery during pregnancy. Committee Opinion No. 474. American College of Obstetricians and Gynecologists. Obstet Gynecol 2011;117:420–1.

5. Gary Cunningham F, et al. Williams Textbook of Obstetrics, 24th ed. McGraw-Hill Education. 2014, p. 926–9.

6. Silvestri MT, Pettker CM, Brousseau EC, et al. Morbidity of appendectomy and cholecystectomy in pregnant and nonpregnant women. Obstet Gynecol 2011;118(6):1261–5.

7. Mazze RI, Kallen B. Reproductive outcome after Anesthesia and operation during pregnancy: a registry study of 5405 cases. Am J Obstet Gynecol 1989;161:1178–85.

8. Kuczkowski KM. Laparoscopic procedures during pregnancy and the risks of anesthesia: what does an obstetrician need to know? Arch Gynecol Obstet 2007;275:53–66.

9. Brent RL. Saving lives and changing family histories: appropriate counseling of pregnant women and men and women of reproductive age, concerning the risk of diagnostic radiation exposures during and before pregnancy. Am J Obstet Gynecol 2009;200(1):4–24.

10. Patel SJ, Reede DL, Katz DS, Subramaniam R, Amorosa JK. Imaging the pregnant patient for nonobstetric conditions: algorithms and radiation dose consider-ations. Radio Graphics 2007;27: 1705–22.

11. Lee CI, Haims AH, Monico EP, et al. Diagnostic CT scans: assessment of patient, physician, and radiologist awareness of radiation dose and possible risks. Radiology 2004;231:393–8.

12. ACOG Committee Opinion. No. 299, September 2004 (replaces No. 158, September 1995). Guidelines for diagnostic imaging during pregnancy. Obstet Gynecol 2004;104:647–51.

13. Goldstone K, Yates SJ. Radiation issues governing radiation protection and patient doses in diagnostic imaging. In Adam A: Grainger & Allison's Diagnostic Radiology, 5th ed. New York: Churchill Livingstone, 2008.

14. McCollough CH, Schueler BA, Atwell TD, et al. Radiation exposure and pregnancy: when should we be concerned? Radio Graphics 2007;27.909–18.

15. Nijkeuter M, Geleijns J, De Roos A, et al. Diagnosing pulmonary embolism in pregnancy: rationalizing fetal radiation exposure in radiological procedures. J Thromb Haemost 2004; 2:1857–8.

16. Winer-Muram HT, Boone JM, Brown HL, et al. Pulmonary embo-lism in pregnant patients: fetal radiation dose with helical CT. Radiology 2002;224(2):487–92.

17. Wyner J, Cohen SE. Gastric volume in early pregnancy: effect of metoclopramide. Anesthesiology 1982;57:209–12.

18. Wong CA, McCarthy RJ, Fitzgerald PC, aikoff K, Avram MJ. Gastric emptying of water in obese pregnant women at term. Anesth Analg 2007;105: 751–5.

19. Wong CA, Loffredi M, Ganchiff JN, Zhao J, Wang Z, Avram MJ. Gastric emptying of water in term pregnancy. Anesthesiology 2002;96:1395–1400.

20. Fisher RS, Roberts GS, Grabowski CJ, Cohen S. Altered lower esophageal sphincter function during early pregnancy. Gastroenterology. 1978;74(6):1233–7.

21. Cohen-Kerem R, Railton C, Oren D, Lishner M, Koren G. Pregnancy outcome following non-obstetric surgical intervention. Am J Surg 2005; 190:467–73.

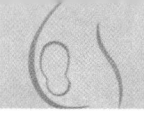

22. The use and interpretation of cardiotocography in intrapartum fetal surveillance. Royal College of Obstetricians and Gynaecologists. Evidence-based Clinical Guideline Number 8. 2001 available at www.ctgutbildning.se/Course/referenser/referenser/RCOG%202001.online assessed on 22 september 2015.

23. Visser BC, Glasgow RE, Mulvihill KK, Mulvihill SJ. Safety and timing of HYPERLINK "http://www.ncbi.nlm.nih.gov/pubmed11721118"non obstetricHYPERLINK "http://www.ncbi.nlm.nih.gov/pubmed/11721118" abdominal surgery in pregnancy. Dig HYPERLINK "http://www.ncbi.nlm.nih.gov/pubmed/11721118"SurgHYPERLINK "http://www.ncbi.nlm.nih.gov/pubmed/11721118" 2001;18:409–17.

24. Shnider SM, Webster GM. Maternal and fetal hazards of surgery during pregnancy. Am J Obstet Gynecol 1965;92:891–900.

25. Kuczkowski KM. The safety of anaesthetics in pregnant women. Exp Opin Drug Saf 2006;5:251–64.

26. Langmoen IA, Larsen M, Berg-Johnsen J. Volatile anaesthetics: cellular mechanisms of action. Eur J Anaesthesiol 1995;12:51–8.

26. Sturrock JE, Nunn JF. Mitosis in mammalian cells during exposure to anesthetics. Anesthesiology 1975;43:21–33.

27. Koren G, Pastuszak A, Ito S. Drugs in pregnancy. N HYPERLINK "http://www.ncbi.nlm.nih.gov/pubmed/9545362"EnglHYPERLINK "http://www.ncbi.nlm.nih.gov/pubmed/9545362" J Med 1998;338:1128–37.

28. ACC/AHA Guideline on Perioperative Cardiovascular Evaluation and Management of Patients Undergoing Noncardiac Surgery. A Report of the American College of Cardiology/American Heart Association Task Force on Practice Guidelines. December 2014. Assessed online on 17/09/2015 at circ.ahajournals.org/content/early/.../CIR.0000000000000106.full.pdf

29. Takahashi Y, Nakano M, Sano K, Kanri T. The effects of epinephrine in local anesthetics on plasma catecholamine and hemodynamic responses. Odontology 2005;93:72–9.

30. NganKee WD, Khaw KS. Vasopressors in obstetrics: what should we be using? Curr Opin Anaesthesiol 2006;19:238–43.

31. Lin FQ, Qiu MT, Ding XX, Fu SK, Li Q. Ephedrine versus phenylephrine for the management of hypotension during spinal anesthesia for caesarean section: an updated meta-analysis. CNS Neurosci Ther 2012;18(7):591–7.

32. Christopher B. Overgaard, Vladimír D•avík. Contemporary Reviews in Cardiovascular Medicine. Inotropes and Vasopressors. Circulation. 2008;118:1047–56.

33. Kang YG, Abouleish E, Caritis S. Prophylactic intravenous ephedrine infusion during spinal anesthesia for cesarean section. Anesth Analg 1982;61(10):839–42.

34. Hewitt M, Madden JC, Rowe PH, Cronin MT. Structure-based modelling in reproductive toxicology: (Q)SARs for the placental barrier. SAR QSAR Environ Res 2007;18:57–76.

35. Kopecky EA, Simone C, Knie B, Koren G. Transfer of morphine across the human placenta and its interaction with naloxone. Life Sci 1999;65: 2359–71.

36. Abouleish E, Abboud T, Lechevalier T, et al. Rocuronium (Org 9426) for cesarean section. Br J Anaesth 1994;73.336–41.

37. Tucker GT. Pharmacokinetics of local anesthetics. Br J Anaesth 1986;58:717–31.

38. Shepard TH. Catalog of Teratogenic Agents, 7th ed. Baltimore, Md, The Johns Hopkins University Press, 1992.

39. Heinonen OP, Slone D, Shapiro S. Birth Defects and Drugs in Pregnancy, Littleton, Mass, Publishing Sciences Group, 1977.

40. Reitman E, Flood P. Anaesthetic considerations for non-obstetric surgery during pregnancy. British Journal of Anaesthesia 2011;107(S1):72–78.

41. Allaert SE, Carlier SP, Weyne LP, Vertommen DJ, Dutré PE, Desmet MB. First trimester anesthesia exposure and fetal outcome. A review. Acta Anaesthesiol Belg 2007;58(2):119–23.

42. Holzgreve W, Carey JC, Hall BD. Warfarin-induced fetal abnormalities. Lancet 1976;2:914–5.

43. Regional Anesthesia in the Patient Receiving Antithrombotic or Thrombolytic Therapy: American Society of Regional Anesthesia and Pain Medicine Evidence-Based Guidelines (Third Edition). Regional Anesthesia & Pain Medicine: 2010;359(1):64–101.

44. Byars TD, Ling GV, Ferris NA, Keeton KS. Activated coagulation time of whole blood in normal dogs. Am J Vet Res 1976;37(11):1359–61.

45. Léonie Damen, H. Muzaffer Buyruk, Füsun Güler-Uysal, Frederik K. Lotgerin, Chris J. Snijders and Hendrik J.The Prognostic Value of

Asymmetric Laxity of the Sacroiliac Joints in Pregnancy-Related Pelvic Pain. Spine 2002;27(24): 2820–4.

46. Anuj Jain, Anil Agarwal, Chetna Shamshery, Sanjay Dhiraaj. Fluoroscope-guided celiac plexus block in a pregnant patient: a case report. Journal of Clinical Anesthesia 2015;27(1):57–9.

47. Reedy MB, Källén B, Kuehl TJ. Laparoscopy during pregnancy: a study of five fetal outcome parameters with use of the Swedish Health Registry. Am J Obstet Gynecol 1997;177:673.

48. Hunter JG, Swanstrom L, Thornburg K. Carbon dioxide pneumoperitoneum induces fetal acidosis in a pregnant ewe model. Surg Endosc 1995;9:272.

49. Yumi H. Guidelines for diagnosis, treatment, and use of laparoscopy for surgical problems during pregnancy: this statement was reviewed and approved by the Board of Governors of the Society of American Gastrointestinal and Endoscopic Surgeons (SAGES), September 2007. It was prepared by the SAGES Guidelines Committee. It was prepared by the SAGES Guidelines Committee. Surg Endosc 2008;22(4):849–61.

50. Bunyavejchevin S, Phupong V. Laparoscopic surgery for presumed benign ovarian tumor during pregnancy. Cochrane Database Syst Rev 2013;1:CD005459.

51. Fatum M, Rojansky N. Laparoscopic surgery during pregnancy. Obstet Gynecol Surv 2001; 56(1):50–9.

52. Lachman E, Schienfeld A, Voss E, Gino G, Boldes R, Levine S, Borstien M, Stark M. Pregnancy and laparoscopic surgery. J Am Assoc Gynecol Laparosc 1999;6(3):347–51.

53. Donkervoort SC, Boerma D. Suspicion of acute appendicitis in the third trimester of pregnancy:

pros and cons of a laparoscopic procedure. JSLS 2011;15(3):379–83.

54. Aubrey-Bassler FK, Sowers N. 613 cases of splenic rupture without risk factors or previously diagnosed disease: A systematic review. BMC Emergency Medicine 2012;12:11.

55. Koo YJ, Kim HJ, Lim KT, Lee IH, Lee KH, Shim JU, Yoon SN, Kim JR, Kim TJ, Koo YJ, Kim HJ, Lim KT, et al. Laparotomy versus laparoscopy for the treatment of adnexal masses during pregnancy. Aust NZJ Obstet Gynaecol 2012;52(1): 34–8.

56. Miller MA, Mazzaglia PJ, Larson L, Ankner GM, Bourjeily GR, Curran P. Laparoscopic adrenalectomy for phaeochromocytoma in a twin gestation. J Obstet Gynaecol 2012;32(2):186–7.

57. O'Rourke N, Kodali BS. Laparoscopic surgery during pregnancy. Curr Opin Anaesthesiol 2006;19:254–9.

58. Hong JY. Adnexal mass surgery and anesthesia during pregnancy: a 10-year retrospective review. Int J Obstet Anesth 2006;15:212–6.

59. Ribic-Pucelj M, Kobal B, Peternelj-Marinsek S. Surgical treatment of adnexal masses in pregnancy: indications, surgical approach and pregnancy outcome. J Reprod Med 1999;44: 279–87.

60. Azevedo JL, Azevedo OC, Miyahira SA, Miguel GP, Becker OM Jr, Hypólito OH, Machado AC, Cardia W, Yamaguchi GA, Godinho L, Freire D, Almeida CE, Moreira CH, Freire DF. Injuries caused by Veress needle insertion for creation of pneumoperitoneum: a systematic literature review. Surg Endosc 2009;23(7):1428–32.

Medicolegal and Ethical Principles in Obstetric Anesthesia

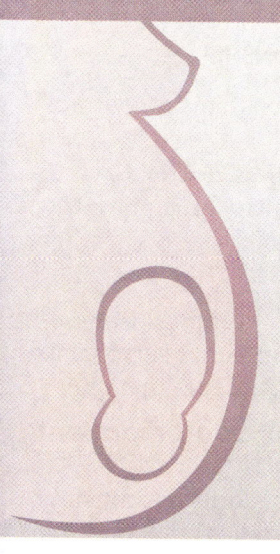

Medicolegal and Ethical Aspects, Negligence, Consent, Doctor—Patient Relationship in Obstetric Anesthesia

Sushila Baldwa, Mahesh Baldwa, Varsha Gupta, Namita Padvi

"The patient will never care how much you know, until they know how much you care."

ETHICAL ASPECTS: FOUR ETHICAL PRINCIPLES OF IMPORTANCE IN BRIEF

There are four basic ethical principles[1] underlying good medicoethical practice in western countries. These are *autonomy, justice, beneficence* and *non-maleficence*. They sound tongue twisters and also of little help in day-to-day practice yet we shall discuss the age old principles in brief to benefit our insight about ethics.

- The first principle is *autonomy*: The right of a fully informed patient party to choose out of the anesthesia offered to the obstetric patient.

- The second principle is called *justice*: The right to receive what is recommended by obstetric anesthesiologist.

- The third principle is *beneficence*: The obligation of obstetric anesthesiologist to do good in a given situation before, during and after the administration of anesthesia. This does *not* necessarily **imply to preserve life at all costs.** In situations, where outcome in a given situation is living a poor quality life, that it is considered less beneficial for the patient than death itself. In that case death is allowed. [Euthanasia is and was illegal and unethical, immoral in India and confirmed after latest Aruna Shanbhag Supreme Court Judgment][a]

- The fourth and final principle is *non-maleficence*: The obligation to avoid doing harm while giving anesthesia (Latin—*primum non-nocere*).

But we are not going to discuss these ethical principles in detail here since India has codified law on medical ethics-2002.[3] Nor are we going to discuss basic fundamental legal principles to prove malpractice and negligence which are described in detail in Supreme Court judgment of IMA versus VP Shantha[4] and several other Supreme Court judgments.[5] We briefly touched upon them to give you insight.

FOUR FUNDAMENTAL LEGAL PRINCIPLES TO PROVE MALPRACTICE AND MEDICAL NEGLIGENCE

1. **Duty:** The obstetric anesthesiologist's duty to the patient arises moment he/she undertakes to contemplate giving anesthesia to his

patient. If there is no fiduciary obstetric anesthesiologist–patient relationship, there is no malpractice risk. The relationship is usually created through performance of preanesthetic check up, but may be created without an actual face-to-face meeting between the obstetric anesthesiologist and patient party evolves in implied way through obstetric surgeon.

2. **Breach of duty:** Once the obstetric anesthesiologist/doctor–patient relationship has been established, then they shall conduct anesthesia within a reasonable standard of care equivalent of ordinary specialist with that qualification in same circumstances in same locality. Failure to meet the standard of care has been laid by Bolam's law.[6] While often difficult to define, a reasonable standard of care, which is says is average, not very high and not very low. Breach of such standard of duty constitutes negligence and is the central issue in most medical malpractice litigation.

3. **Proximity of causation/cause of action:** To be successful in a medical malpractice suit, the plaintiff/patient party must prove that substandard medical care was the proximate cause of injury to the particular patient.

4. **Actual injury/damage:** Further, to succeed, the plaintiff/patient party must establish that some type of physical or mental or psychological injury actually occurred. Having shown that a breach of duty caused an injury, one or more of three types of damages might be awarded in the form of monetary payments. These include general damages for pain and suffering; special damages for past, present and future medical expenses and for loss of income, wages, and profits. Punitive damages are generally not awarded by courts in negligence and malpractice suits. Punitive damages are usually granted for gross negligence caused by intentional harm, conscious indifference, or fraud in criminal suits.

DOCTOR–PATIENT RELATIONSHIP

Doctor–patient relationship is a pure 'contract' in law.

So both patients as well as doctor have to agree for this relationship and that too voluntarily.

When it starts?

It arises the moment anesthesiologist agrees to provide his or her professional services to the patient and the patient accepts this offer.

What is the domain of doctor–patient relationship?

Obstetric anesthesiologist is only responsible to patients whom he undertakes to manage by written/implied, tacit or presumed consent. Hence a consent document becomes vital piece of evidence in crystallizing doctor–patient relationship, e.g. helping other anesthesiologist in emergency.

Who are out of the domain of doctor–patient relationship?

Legally, doctor is not responsible towards all patients in general or/at large, but is responsible towards specific patients developing/establishing doctor–patient relationship.

Rights emanating from doctor–patient relationship.

A doctor has a right to choose his/her patient. (Regulation 2.4-ETHICS, 2002) A doctor retains the right to choose his or her patients. Ultimately, treatment today is a pure contract between two consenting adults and cannot be forced on a doctor. A doctor is, therefore, well within his right to refuse treatment to a patient at the outset, but cannot abandon patient having undertaken to give anesthesia.

Duty of particular standard of care emanating from doctor–patient relationship.

Hence next question is to whom a obstetric anesthesiologist has duty of care? The next logical question is who amongst the patients are entitled to this standard of care, all, or only some? The answer is that a doctor is under a legal obligation to provide the 'standard of care' only to those patients to whom the doctor owes the 'duty of care'. Doctor does not have duty to care towards anyone and everyone whom the doctor meets or speaks, even if that particular conversation is regarding medical science related to unidentified patient. The legal obligation of duty of care starts when legal dctor–patient relationship is established.

To summarize, the standard of care can be stated in simpler terms.

- A doctor must act as other doctors of the same specialty would have acted in same or similar situation.
- The fact that others would have acted differently or the majority does not subscribe to a particular course is simply irrelevant. In fact the courts have gone to the extent of accepting that doctors may even have their personal prefcrcnccs.
- An injury, death, complication or unfavorable result of treatment will not necessarily mean that the doctor has deviated from the standard of care.

Two more cautions:

i. Nowadays, the latest judicial trend in Indian courts is higher standard of care expected from a specialist is higher. A specialist is expected to give a higher standard of care than a non-specialist.

ii. Greater degree of care is expected for legally incompetent patients, i.e. newborn children, lunatics, etc. Greater the disability, greater is the degree of care expected by law from doctors. Greater degree of care is expected for incompetent patients.

What is that conduct obstetric anesthesiologist which signals doctor–patient relationship as established and when it gets terminated?

Duty of care arises in physical/telephonic/web consultations and emergencies. Duty of care may arise:

- By a physical consultation
- By a telephonic conversation or web consultation or

- By legal compulsion—in case of emergencies.

Once the duty of care has arisen, it continues till the happening of any of the following contingencies:

- The patient is relieved of the ailment/anesthesia.
- The patient is discharged or transferred.
- The patient voluntarily seeks discharge from the care of the doctor. The doctor terminates his treatment on valid grounds after giving proper notice.
- The patient is dead.
- In case of emergency patients, the emergency ceases to exist.

Some perfectly legal and valid reasons for termination are as follows:

- Failure of patient to pay
- Refusal by the patient to allow implementation of the anesthesia plan
- Refusal by the patient to follow instructions
- Doctor's change of practice
- Doctor's abandonment of practice

MEDICOLEGAL ASPECTS OF CONSENT AND RISK EXPLANATION

Informed consent: Consent should be patient-specific, procedure-specific, with full disclosure about disease, its investigations and treatment without hiding anything, without misrepresentation, coercion, fraud, undue influence in writing and signed by authorized signatory which is witnessed by two adult people is good enough.

Information: Information to be given to patient party as per MCI Regulation Chapter 2.3 which says about disclosure by obstetric anesthesiologist—he should neither exaggerate nor minimize the gravity of the patient condition. He must ensure himself that the patient, his relatives or his responsible friends have such knowledge of patient's condition as well serve the best interest of the patient and the family.

It is usual for an obstetric anesthetist to explain to relatives of patient and obtain their ascent procedure of anesthesia, plan of anesthesia, co-existing conditions influencing general medical status of patient as per ASA state and also obtain ascent for further treatment in case patient deteriorates.

Reality about informed consent in India: It needs to be ensured that privacy will be maintained. In the context of developing countries, obtaining informed consent has been considered many times as difficult/impractical/not meeting the purpose on various grounds such as incompetence to comprehend the meaning or relevance of the consent and culturally being dependent on the decision of the head of the family, e.g. husband in case of obstetric patient. However, there is no alternative to obtaining individual's informed consent.

Who can consent: Any person who has completed 18 years of age as per Indian Majority Act-1975 is considered an adult. An adolescent is less that 18 years old so legal adult status for him is a far-fetched legal dream but at the same time parents and adult relatives cannot arrogate[7] with adolescent rights.

Proxy Consent (Substitute Consent)

Minors/Incompetent/Emergency Patients—Proxy Consent

a. Consent and age:
  i. Minor/emancipated child patient between 12 and 18 years—take consent of the patient as well as the parents'/guardian.
  ii. Adult patient above 18 years—take consent of the patient only.

b. Proxy consent 'giver' for incompetent/emergency patients:
  i. The lineal descendant or ascendant blood relative, or natural biological parents
  ii. The person/s or crowd who may have bought such a patient (e.g. in accident or emergency cases), or

  iii. Medical superintendent or such other responsible person in institutions/hospitals.

c. Taking proxy consent:
  i. Record specifically the name, address and telephone number of the person from whom proxy consent has been obtained in the consent.
  ii. Record specifically the reason for obtaining proxy consent in the consent.
  iii. Further future directions/consent during the treatment may be sought from such a person.

d. Consent of any one of the parent for adolescent obstetric patient is valid and binding even though there may be difference between both the parents.

Situations where consent may not be obtained: Like in medical emergencies. The wellbeing of the patient is of paramount importance hence medical treatment precedes legal considerations.

a. Do not wait for consent in emergencies. Proceed with oral consent or even without consent.

b. Take proxy consent, only if possible and without much effort.

c. Record specifically in the patient's medical records and/or the consent form the emergency as well as the reason/s for not obtaining consent or for obtaining proxy consent. This exercise can be done once the emergency is over.

Duty of care during emergency requires no consent: A 'duty of care' on each and every doctor to attend emergency patients irrespective of specialty or whether he/she is your patient or not. This does not apply to routine and cold patients. The Supreme Court in the case of Parmanand Katara v/s Union of India[8] wherein it was stated, "Every doctor whether at a government hospital or otherwise has the professional obligation to extend his services with due expertise for protecting life,

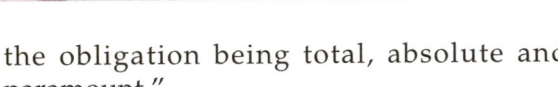

the obligation being total, absolute and paramount."

When consent is not valid: Consent given under fear, fraud or misrepresentation of facts, or by a person who is ignorant of the implications of the consent, or who is under 12 years of age is invalid (Sec. 90 IPC[9]).

What is implied consent?

Consent that is inferred from the conduct or action of the concerned persons.

What is tacit consent?

Consent can be silently or passively by omission/passage of time/ignored/waiver.

What is presumed consent?

Consent is presumed on the basis of knowledge, intelligence and values and beliefs of the patient.

Implied Consent (Presumed/Tacit Consent) for Obstetric Anesthesiologists

This is by far the most common variety of consent obstetric anesthesiologists in India do not obtain separate consent in practice and usually depend upon consent obtained by surgeons/hospital. The fact that a patient comes to you though indirectly for administering anesthesia you cannot depend on implied consent obtained by surgeons/hospital when a legal trouble arises.

Consent form should at least contain:

a. Printed consent form in English can have printed translated version in the local language appended.

b. Consent form can also be filled in the local language or the language understood by the patient.

c. Printed consent forms must have enough space to fill complete additional information.

d. Take the patient party's signature/initials on every page of the consent form.

e. Doctor-in-charge of the patient/principal surgeon/anesthetist should also sign the consent form in whose presence parents/relatives have given consent with date and time written below signatures.

f. Consent form can have suitable directions from the patient indicating names of relatives/attendants whose directions should be followed in case the patient is not in a position to give direction regarding what needs to be done be his/her doctor in case patient is incapacitated to communicate. Patients can fill column/ space provided for such direction with full name, address and telephone numbers of such relatives/friends and can also indicate the order of preference amongst them.

Risk explanation/information:

a. Explain the potential risks of anesthesia to the patient, especially the commonly occurring one and enumerate such risks in the consent.

b. Risks having probability of 10% or more must be specifically spelt out to the patient and duly recorded in the consent.

c. Answer any specific question raised by the patients about risks and record the same in the consent. Risk involving loss of vision, hearing, mental function, loss of function of limbs and organs must be specified even though the risk may be rare.

Take 'high-risk consent'/postoperative ventilatory support consent:

i. PPH, excessive bleeding needing internal iliac ligation during LSCS.

ii. CPD, transverse lie, LSCS for premature baby sonographically baby weighing more than 4 kg.

iii. LSCS for cord prolapsed, dry labor, antepartum passage of meconium.

iv. Post-LSCS amniotic fluid or pulmonary embolism.

v. Consent for tracheostomy.

vi. Hemodynamically unstable patients/ metabolically unstable patients, patient with electrolyte imbalances, patient in surgical shock, bacteremia, toxemia, septicemia, DIC serious and complicated nature of surgery/latest/new—surgical procedures.

vii. Removing uterus during obstetric hysterectomy to control bleeding under anesthesia given by obstetric anethesiologist. Insist for sending uterus for histopathological examination after removing.

viii. High-risk patients specify and justify medically, scientifically in consent form.

ix. Proceeding with a surgery/procedure in spite of any abnormal parameter. Record both the abnormality as well as the reasons for proceeding for anesthesia.

x. Obstetric patient with heart disease, trauma or associated with syndrome pattern.

Because complications and error are common so do not hold out any guarantee/ warrantee: Do not hold out any guarantee/warrantee for no mishap. Never hold out for 100% mishap freedom. Tell patient that risks though exist are rare.

Always minimize patient-related mishaps to minimum by issuing written warnings and restrictions:[10] Give warnings and restrictions regarding nil by mouth in writing, time and type of food before anesthesia and post-anesthesia care.

Consent for Postmortem (PM)

1. Legally two types of death may need PM:
   a. PM after natural death, where cause of death is not known.
   b. PM for all unnatural death which includes table death, postoperative death.
2. If death is natural, then the dead body is property of relatives but if unnatural death; then dead body becomes property of state.
3. For PM in natural death, consent of nearest relatives (husband, father, mother, son, daughter, etc.) is required.

4. PM for unnatural death—the consent for PM is not required but information to local police is required.

SUMMARY

1. Informed consent is the legal embodiment of the concept of the right to make decisions regarding one's wellbeing.
2. Informed consent should be based on the 'professional standard' or peer 'accepted risks' approach, or the 'materiality risk' or 'prudent patient' approach.
3. If the risk involved can have severe consequences, like death or serious disability, it is material and should be disclosed independent of the frequency of the occurrence.
4. Severe risks (e.g. death, removal of uterus, internal iliac ligation) should always be disclosed, even when the probability of their occurrence is almost negligible.

REFERENCES

1. Gillon R. "Medical ethics: four principles plus attention to scope". British Medical Journal 1994;309:184.Doi:10.1136/bmj.309.6948.184.
2. Aruna Ramchandra Shanbaug vs Union of India & Ors. on 7 March, 2011, Bench: Markandey Katju, Gyan Sudha Misra.
3. The Indian Medical Council (Professional conduct, Etiquette and Ethics) Regulations, 2002.
4. Indian Medical Association vs VP Shantha & Ors on 13 Nov., 1995: 1996 AIR 550, 1995 SCC (6) 651.
5. Jacob Mathew vs State of Punjab & Anr on 5 Aug., 2005, Bench: R Lahoti, G Mathur, PK Balasubramanyan, CASE NO.: Appeal (crl.) 144–5 of 2004, Martin F D'Souza vs Mohd. Ishfaq on 17 Feb., 2009, Bench: G Singhvi JJ, Katju JJ, Civil Appellate Jurisdiction, Civil Appeal No. 3541 of 2002, V Kishan Rao vs Nikhil Super Speciality Hospital on 8 March, 2010, Bench: GS Singhvi, Asok Kumar Ganguly. In the Supreme Court of India, Civil appellate jurisdiction, Civil appeal no.2641_of 2010.
6. Bolam vs Friern Hospital Management Committee (1957) 1 WLR 582.

7. Arrogate means not undermine and prevail over welfare of adolescent, law ensures under S.125 of Criminal procedure code, 1973 and S. 317 of Indian Penal code, 1860 along with S. 68 of Indian contract Act, 1872 that minors are looked after for their physical, mental, economic safety and generally and normally adults responsible are 1. Natural parents, 2. Legally appointed guardians by court of law 3. Court itself shall ensure safety under Guardians and wards act, 1890 their safety and security. If law enforcing authority or any person complaints welfare of adolescent legally breached then law court shall be put in motion. If doctor or any other social spirited person or police asks for permission for benefit of such adolescent court shall be prompt to grant it for adolescent's benefit.

8. Pt. Parmanand Katara vs Union of India & Ors on 28 August, 1989: 1989 AIR 2039, 1989 SCR (3) 997.

9. Aruna Ramchandra Shanbaug vs Union of India & Ors. on 7 March, 2011, Bench: Markandey Katju, Gyan Sudha Misra.

10. Padvi N, Padvi A, Gupta V, Baldwa M. Textbook of Paediatric Anaesthesia, CBS Publishers & Distributors Pvt Ltd, Delhi, Ch.42:546–51, Ch.43:551–6;2015.

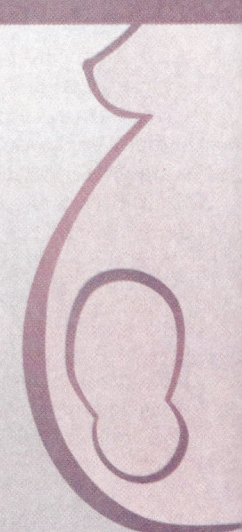

CHAPTER **20**

Record Keeping, Sudden Death, Table Death, Violence, Police Arrest, Vicarious Liability, Blood Transfusion and Indemnity in Obstetric Anesthesia

Varsha Gupta, Mahesh Baldwa, Sushila Baldwa, Namita Padvi

RECORD KEEPING IN OBSTETRIC ANESTHESIOLOGY

"Doctors and patients may forget but records will always remember."

Record Keeping as per Ethics 2002[1]

The issue of medical record keeping has been addressed in the Medical Council of India Regulations 2002 guidelines answering many questions regarding medical records. The important issues that have been addressed are as follows:

1. Maintain indoor records along with anesthesia records in a standard proforma for 3 years from commencement of treatment (Section 1.3.1 and Appendix 3). For anesthesia records, no particular format is prescribed. Customarily anesthesia records should contain pre-anesthetic check up, anesthesia details during surgery with monitoring of vital parameters, anesthesia reversal notes, and post-anesthesia recovery room notes.

2. Request for medical records by patient or authorized attendant should be acknowledged and documents issued within 72 hours (Section 1.3.2).

3. Maintain a register of certificates with the full details of medical certificates issued with at least one identification mark of the patient and his signature (Section 1.3.3).

4. Efforts should be made to computerize medical records for quick retrieval (Section 1.3.4).

Medical records as evidence: Medical records are accepted usually as irrefutable piece of evidence as per Section 3 of the Indian Evidence Act[2] in a court of law established in India.

How long to maintain records?

1. Ideally records of adult patients are maintained for 3 years and for newborn children, for 21 years. (3+18 years), or till newborn child grows up to become adult to be able to sue. For mentally retarded newborn children, one needs to keep records forever till the person is practicing.[3]

2. From income tax point of view, for six years from the end of the relevant assessment year.[4]

3. As per code of medical ethics April 2002, for three years

278

4. As per section 24 A of Consumer Protection Act,[5] for two years
5. As per Limitation Act,[6] for three years

How to destroy records?

1. By giving public notice in one in English and other in vernacular newspaper, with a time limit of usually one month from date of publication in which any one wants the relevant case paper can come and take a copy of record needed.
2. After one month, destroy record for everyone, except:
   a. Where litigation is going on.
   b. Pre-litigation process of notice exchange is going on.
   c. Mentally ill or retarded patients.
   d. Where you expect that there could be future trouble.

One can maintain records in electronic formats,[7] but avoid electronic format of record keeping in following situations:

1. They are:
   a. Frequent monitoring of vital parameters and investigations are required
   b. Moribund patient
   c. Patients who develop complications of disease, drug, surgery, anesthesia or procedure
   d. Patients who suddenly take a serious turn involving lot of expenditure
   e. Patients who are transferred or referred to other hospitals/doctors
   f. Accident/suicide/attempted homicide/poisoning/burns/fracture/tetanus and cases involving violence, aggravating obstetric disease or causing injury
2. Consent needs to be on hard copy.
3. Transfer to other hospital needs hard copy.
4. Referral to doctor/investigations need hard copy.
5. Police cases need hard copy.

Tampering/manipulation and alteration and keeping records blank are not permitted by law: The National Commission in another case held that the hospital was guilty of negligence on the ground that the name of the anesthetist was not mentioned in the operation notes though anesthesia was administered by two anesthetists. There were two progress cards about the same patient on two separate papers that were produced in court.[8]

SUDDEN OPERATION TABLE DEATH DURING ANESTHESIA RESORTING TO VIOLENCE/EXTORTION/DEFAMATION BY PATIENT PARTY

Odious Situation

It is rather impossible to find a medical professional, who would say that they never faced a medicolegal situation called 'Sudden unexpected death' and world at large, gazing in their face as if they were responsible for death. This type of scenario where treating team of doctors are made to feel guilty about sudden unexpected death by relatives is not uncommon.[9]

A spectrum of medicolegal reactions from patient party affecting medical professional may be as below and probable legal solution:

Violence by Patient Party

Sometimes in the event of sudden unexpected death of mother or newborn child occurring in front of lot of accompanying relatives then at slightest provocation they may take law in their own hands and bash doctors and other staff members along with destroying medical equipment and hospital property. In this case, file FIR in nearest police station under antiviolence law of respective state like one in Maharashtra by the name of Medicare Service Persons & Medicare Service Institution (Prevention of Violence, Damage or Loss to Property) Act, 2010. The antiviolence law says anyone who attacks a doctor will be punished with a fine of ₹ 50,000 and imprisonment up to 3 years. Therefore, any attack against doctors is considered as a non-bailable offence. Similar acts are passed by your states. Insist for arresting hooligans.

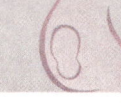

Arrest of Doctor

Some other times, no sooner than expected instead relatives asking you explanations about sudden unexpected death, you have policemen coming for medicolegal questioning to anesthetist/doctor your staff as to what happened to deceased mother or newborn child as they have received a medicolegal complaint from relatives and worst doctor may be arrested by police on the basis of FIR.[10] Two legal solutions come handy to arrested doctor:

1. Keep a copy handy to show the police Jacob Mathew judgment[11] of Supreme Court which say without affirmative opinion of expert opining about alleged negligence, police cannot arrest the doctor (last page of judgment).
2. Doctor can obtain regular bail Sec. 437(1) of CrPC or for imminent arrest once can apply for anticipatory bail under Sec. 438 of CrPC.[12]

Extortion by People

So often in the event of sudden unexpected death, you may receive a politician's telephone to resolve the issue amicably or some social worker actually walking in your office to pay for sudden unexpected death or a local goon threatening you to cough up money immediately for sudden unexpected death without asking your explanation. The legal solution is to file a police case and move the court for being subjected to extortion under Sec. 383/384 of IPC.[13]

Defamation

So often in the event of sudden unexpected death, you may find media and press people gathering around you and your staff members to speak details of sudden unexpected death, which are flashed in defamatory way on TV or newspapers leaving you disgusted. The legal solution is to file a police case and move the court for being subjected to defamation under Sec. 499/500 of IPC.[14]

Pleader/Advocate Notice

In the event of medicolegal sudden unexpected death, you should feel lucky and blessed if police does not walk to make inquiry about sudden unexpected death but so often your comfort is disturbed weeks later or sometimes months later by a lawyer's notice probing in sudden unexpected death and asking for case papers related to medical treatment of deceased along with astronomical compensation. The legal solution is to reply the notice through your lawyer.[15]

As per the media projection,[16] one out of ten doctors is dragged in unnecessary prosecutions for medical negligence. Court summons for sudden unexpected death and complaints narrating absurd allegations and asking astronomical sum of money as compensation is going to be on rise in coming days.

It is surprisingly true that in spite of wearing good, empathetic, sympathetic attitude and observing courteousness in communications, allegations of negligence in sudden unexpected death may put medical professional in a medicolegal maze of alleged medical negligence and leave them disgusted. Medical professionals feel they are framed in alleged medical negligence even though there is no medicolegal issue in sudden unexpected death. A new breed of legal advisors in medicolegal issues of medical negligence on internet are on rise who lure relatives of sudden unexpected death and show them big money in prosecuting doctors which cannot be traded off by medical professional wearing good, empathetic, sympathetic attitude and observing courteousness in communications in event of sudden unexpected death.

General Solutions to Odious Situation

1. Membership of large professional organization like Indian Medical Association
2. Good relationship with medical fraternity
3. Insuring oneself for professional work with professional indemnity with reputed

general insurance companies every year without fail.

This subtopic is designed to reduce the trauma accompanied with alleged medical negligence in sudden unexpected death, where there is no medical negligence of doctor. Some knowledge of medicolegal aspects of sudden unexpected death may sharpen your:

a. Record keeping skills

b. Communication skills while dealing with relatives, police, and politician or for that matter a goon walking in your office.

> **Pearl**
>
> In the case, violence breaks after death of an obstetric patient, file FIR in nearest police station under antiviolence law of respective state like one in Maharashtra by the name of Medicare Service Persons & Medicare Service Institution (Prevention of Violence, Damage or Loss to Property) Act, 2010. There are similar acts in your own state also.

MEDICOLEGAL ASPECTS OF DIFFICULT SITUATIONS, DECLARATION OF DEATH AND COMMUNICATION WITH PATIENT PARTY

Most legal problems in health care systems arise from poor communication hence good communication can play a significant part in avoiding complaints and malpractice claims.

One Big Barrier to Good Communication: Arrogance and Paternalistic Attitude

Arrogance and paternalistic automatic antagonism towards patient party is deeply ingrained into doctors. Doctors presume that they know the best about their patient hence they always issue commands. Doctors expect patients to follow commands unquestioningly. Doctor should willingly change this situation by being more adaptive, interactive and communicating.

Delivering Bad News

- **Preparing to deliver bad news**/declaration of death

- **Percepting self-reflection:** Anesthesiologist will invariably have strong negative emotions when they have to give bad news. In near death situations, anesthesiologist should not spontaneously discuss their own emotional reaction with a preceptor; therefore, they should be introducing this topic. "This is a really hard case, and what is being done medically for patient, yet patient is not responding".

- **Create an appropriate setting:** Say mother or newborn child is serious and every bit of best is being continuously done.

- **Make sure you know basic information** about the patient's disease, current situation, prognosis, and treatment options before delivering bad news.

> **Pearl**
>
> **Situations Requiring Extra-caution**
>
> Medical professional should keep in mind certain high-risk surgical and anesthetic situations, which are common causes for allegation of medical negligence actions; situations that require extra cautions are anesthesia resulting in coma, PPH, amniotic fluid embolism, DIC, loss of sight, hearing, paralysis, cesarean hysterectomy, vegetative life and death.

MEDICOLEGAL ASPECTS OF VICARIOUS LIABILITY

Only delegation of work is allowed by law: Delegation of medical work to junior obstetric anesthesiologist, nurses (be those qualified or unqualified staff), employed or contracted, the medical professional owes vicarious liability to patient on the basis of sound legal principle that, one can delegate medical work not responsibility.

Delegation of responsibility not allowed by law: 'Vicarious' means arising out of a vicar or a deputy or an agent. Vicarious liability indicates liability arising out of an agent's, a deputy's, or a substitute's wrongful actions or omissions of their duties, and not out of the medical professional's own wrongs. In the course of their professional duties, obstetric anesthesiologists often have to requisition the services of nurses, technicians and para-medical staff. In hospitals, there are other categories employed to assist the medical professional in charge of the patients: house-men and registrars, technicians, ward boys and ayahs. The vicarious civil liability is to compensate the victim monetarily for loss/damage. This liability is applicable only for civil liabilities, not criminal actions.

There is no criminal vicarious liability: There is no principle of employer's liability in criminal law. There is no indirect or secondary or vicarious criminal liability.

MEDICOLEGAL ASPECTS OF EUTHANASIA, DNR, VEGETATIVE LIFE AND ACTIVE AND PASSIVE WITHDRAWAL OF LIFE SUPPORT SYSTEMS

Advance directives/do-not-resuscitate instructions by patients for neonatal resuscitation:

a. Take a high-risk consent from the patient party for continuing neonatal resuscitation in spite of failure to resuscitate after 10 minutes.

b. Record specifically in the consent the patient's advance directive/s, if parents want the neonatal resuscitation be discontinued at the end of 10 minutes.

c. Take signature of two independent witnesses on DNR document.

Removing active life support system and passively keeping alive obstetric patient by feeding tubes, etc.

a. Make sure patient is brain dead as per guidelines given in Human Organs Transplant Act (HOTA)-1994.

b. Take High Court order after taking consent from the patient's closest relative and caretaker that in the given circumstance it is no use continuing active/passive life support.

c. Take signature of two independent witnesses.

Information for parents and families about ventilator withdrawal of obstetric patient: The anesthesiologist's counseling of families is a critical aspect of care for the dying patient who is to be removed from a ventilator. Ideally the family will be involved in the decision to withdraw the ventilator. Before withdrawal, the following issues should be discussed.

Potential outcome of ventilator withdrawal: Assuming all other life-sustaining treatments have been stopped, including artificial hydration and nutrition, there are several potential outcomes: rapid death within minutes or death within hours to days and very rarely patient may survive also.

The procedure of ventilator withdrawal: Never make assumptions about what the family understands; describe the procedure in clear, simple terms and answer any questions. Families should be told before-hand the steps of withdrawal and whether or not it is planned/desired to remove the endotracheal tube. In addition, they should be counseled about the use of oxygen and medications for symptom control. Assure them that the patient's comfort is of primary concern. Explain that breathlessness may occur, but that it can be managed. Confirm that you will have medication available to manage any discomfort. Ensure they know that the patient will likely need to be kept asleep to control their symptoms.

If asked, explain that they can show love and support through touch, wiping of the patient's forehead, holding a hand and talking to her.

Support the decision: Even though a family is able to make a definite decision for ventilator withdrawal, such a decision is always emotionally charged. Families will constantly second-guess themselves, especially if the death appears to linger following ventilator withdrawal. Anesthesiologist's support, guidance and leadership are crucial, as the family will be looking to the anesthesiologist to ensure them that they are 'doing the right thing'. Furthermore, support needs to continue following death during the bereavement period.

MEDICOLEGAL ASPECTS OF BLOOD TRANSFUSION

a. Blood is an FDA approved product and needs to come from registered blood bank for transfusion.

b. Counsel that transfused blood is tested for HIV, HCV, Hep B yet no one can guarantee that these diseases will not be transmitted to recipient. The window period of diseases cannot be detected by tests done in blood banks.

c. Take separate and specific consent for blood, blood products transfusion, if transfusion is foreseeable and anticipated since bleeding might be excessive.

d. Take consent for blood transfusion for all surgeries/procedures along with consent for surgery/procedure.

e. Do not administer blood to Jehovah's witness.

MEDICOLEGAL ASPECTS OF OPERATING THEATRE MISHAPS NOT CAUSING DEATH

"Errors are an inevitable and unfortunate reality of medical practice."

Iatrogenic injuries caused by medical errors are moving from the realm of death conference of medical professionals to courtroom. In old times, a doctor was considered next to god and his authority and actions were rarely, if ever, questioned. But times have changed; doctors as well as patients are more aware of the inner nuances of the medicine hence should do everything possible to reduce errors and reduce the chances of harm to the patient

Single Most Common Cause of Medical Error

Overwork and tiredness of medical staff called on to perform extra duties. Sleep deprivation has also been cited as a contributing factor in medical errors. One study found that being awake for over 24 hours caused medical interns to double or triple the number of preventable medical errors, including those which resulted in injury or death.

Anesthesia-related Complications

i. Misdiagnosis of an illness/condition, failure to diagnose or delay of a diagnosis.

ii. Oxygen deprivation is one major cause.

iii. Not able to read labels of injectable medicines and depend blindly on color and size of vial/ampoule.

iv. Use of arterial line for administration of drugs instead of venous line.

v. Exchange of O_2 with N_2O gas pipes/flow meters.

MEDICAL INDEMNITY POLICY[17]

The purpose of medical professional indemnity is to protect the medical professional persons against legal liability to pay damages to patients who have sustained loss arising from their own professional negligence.

The medical indemnity policy offers indemnity guided by law of contract and strictly covers civil legal liability/loss due to medical negligence only. The premium paid on the policy is on yearly basis and doctor has to renew every year without fail to maintain retroactive date. Retroactive date is the date of taking such policy for the first time.

The rate of premium of obstetric anesthesiologist is ₹ 3 per thousand rupees per year plus service tax.

Note: Obstetric anesthesiologist is not covered for criminal/prison sentence awarded by courts but the cost of defense can be received.

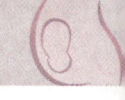

INVESTIGATION OF ALL MATERNAL MORTALITY OF CASES IRRESPECTIVE OF ANY ALLEGED NEGLIGENCE

Health is concurrent matter as per constitution of India. Each state in India has central and state acts. Most states investigate maternal mortality in detail. Anemia, PPH, and obstructed labor are leading causes of maternal mortality during parturition. Obstetric anesthesiologist is sucked in the situation and enquiry passively. Obstetric anesthesiologist may have to reply to various questions asked by police, local authority, district authorities and state authorities with respect to anesthesia part. Remember, plea of emergency comes handy to obstetric anesthesiologist to steer clear from various enquires.

SUMMARY

This chapter describes medical record keeping in obstetric anesthesiology. How to tackle legally sudden operation table death during anesthesia leading to violence, extortion, and defamation is described. This chapter also describes medicolegal aspects related to difficult obstetric situations, declaration of death and communication with patient party. There are notes made for medicolegal aspects of vicarious liability, euthanasia, DNR, vegetative life and active and passive withdrawal of life support systems, blood transfusion, operating theatre mishaps not causing death and medical indemnity.

REFERENCES

1. The Indian Medical Council (Professional conduct, Etiquette and Ethics) Regulations, 2002.
2. The Indian Evidence Act, 1872 as amended up to date.
3. Section 6 in The Limitation Act, 1963.
4. Form of daily case register, FORM NO. 3C [See rule 6F(3)] under s. 44AA of Income Tax Act 1961.
5. Consumer Protection Act, 1986 as amended up to date.
6. The Limitation Act, 1963 as amended up to date.
7. Information Technology Act 2000 as amended up to date and the Indian Evidence Act, 1872 as amended up to date.
8. Meenakshi Mission Hospital and Research Centre vs Samuraj and Anr., I (2005) CPJ (NC).
9. Jacob Mathew vs State of Punjab and Anr on 5 August, 2005 [Jacob Mathews case].
10. Supra at 15, Jacob Mathews case.
11. Supra at 15, Jacob Mathews case.
12. The Code of Criminal Procedure, 1973 (CrPC).
13. Indian Penal Code, 1860.
14. Indian Penal Code, 1860.
15. Advocates Act, 1961.
16. Outlook Magazine April 2002 issue.
17. Padvi N, Padvi A, Gupta V, Baldwa M. Textbook of Paediatric Anaesthesia, CBS Publishers & Distributors Pvt Ltd, Delhi. Ch.42:546–51, Ch.43:551–6,2015.

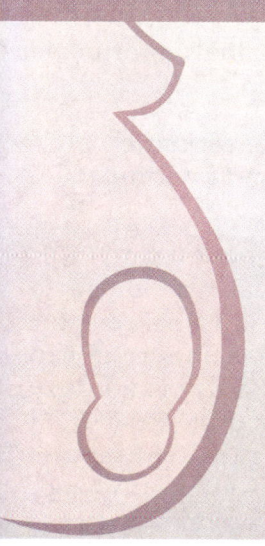

Do We Need Solutions for Grey Areas of Medicolegal Aspects Creating Controversies in Obstetric Anesthesia

Mahesh Baldwa, Namita Padvi, Varsha Gupta, Sushila Baldwa

High-risk branch of medicine involving two lives—hence high chances of litigations

Obstetric anesthesia subspecialty is a high-risk branch involving welfare of mother as well as newborn child. Obstetric anesthesiologists in US were once upon a time the most sued doctors. Although most anesthesiologists do everything in their power to prevent accidents, errors, mistakes do happen, further leading to litigation. With more awareness of the people about anesthesia, litigation is likely to increase in medicolegal issues.

We do not have authentic Indian statistics about anesthesia risk. Decades ago in USA, an estimated 6,000 Americans died or remained brain damaged because of avoidable errors during anesthesia. Since then outdated methods have been replaced with comprehensive safety guidelines, including a bar against leaving patients unattended during surgery, as well as using equipment that minimize human error. Indian healthcare system concurrently lives in previous century vis a vis in current century with respect to anesthesia infrastructure. Even today, some of the hospitals in some cities still do not have Boyles machine or any monitoring system. On the other side, five star hospitals in metro cities have state of art latest anesthesia infrastructure for both administering and monitoring. Such vast gap divides equally qualified anesthetists administering anesthesia with respect to infrastructure. Legal eagles are confused. They do not understand what standard to apply! When mishap occurs, everyone wants first world infrastructure even when the patient party consciously chose cheaper hospitals for delivery of their child. Post mishap, blame game starts with blame pointer pointing to obstetrician and hospital but usually ends up pinning pointing blame to anesthetist.

We in India should be doing what USA did way back in the 1970s; the death rate from anesthesia was about one of every 10,000 patients. Today in USA more than 25 million procedures are performed under anesthesia with reduced mortality. American anesthesiology association took measures to reduce errors, better training, and establishing safety procedures, identifying patterns of mistakes and improving the technology. In late 1990s, USA mortality due to anesthesia dropped to one in 200,000 patients due to above safety measures. Lawsuits resulting in payouts were nearly halved and malpractice insurance costs fell. By the year 2002, in USA, anesthesiologists had to pay lower premiums than they were paying in 1985 due to this fall in mortality. Even today in USA with all improvements in anesthesia-related adverse event rates, negligence can still occur, and the effects can have devastating results for both anesthetist and patient party. In USA, anesthesia practice aims at prevention of errors which includes developing electronic controls for anesthesia equipment and standardizing terminology on anesthesiology records. If, we in India do it, it will reduce litigation along with mortality as well as morbidity.

Doctor–patient relationship is nebulous since customarily anesthetist is called just in the nick of the time

Relationship between the surgeon and the anesthetist has been evolving over a long time. In the present system of anesthesia practice in India, customarily, anesthetist is called just in the nick of the time by obstetrician. This leaves no scope for interaction between the patient party and the obstetric anesthesiologist. Hence there is no rapport like doctor–patient relationship established between anesthetist and patient party. Legally doctor–patient relationship is presumed between anesthetist and patient by implication and conduct even though there was not much interaction between patient party and anesthetist. The public at large are even today are not aware of the risks involved in anesthesia because of absence of personal interaction between anesthetist and patient party. In India, obstetrician and hospital are still captain of ship and incharge and boss of anesthetist. The obstetricians are doing more and more major and demanding operations with bare minimum anesthesia equipment provided to anesthetist. Customarily anesthetists are paid paltry sum by obstetricians or hospitals. Anesthetist has to forego even that paltry sum also, if mishap occurs, worst the obstetricians and hospitals stop calling that unfortunate anesthetist after that mishap.

Joint/combined consent or separate consent for obstetrician and anesthetist

On several occasions, even consent for anesthesia is challenged by patient party. This happens because obstetrician also forgets to take proper separate or joint consent for anesthesia. The matter is raked up after mishap happens by patient party. But it is not very difficult to dissect duties of obstetrician from that of anesthetist. Legally consent is presumed. Implied consent is invoked. Though of course, legally written consent is always preferable but not taken.

Most feared mishap is pregnant women walking to operation theatre to return Back to ICU in serious condition or operation table death due to complications

The issue of anesthesiology malpractice or negligence has never been as newsworthy item to be discussed. In recent years due to speed of transmitting information about mishaps in anesthesia, it has gathered importance. Most feared mishap is women walks to operation theatre to return back to ICU in serious condition or table death. This usually does not happen due to negligence. It happens due to known complications but in this situation allegations of negligence are commonly hurled on anesthetist. Patient party's tendency is that table deaths even due to known documented complications of anesthesia are dubbed as alleged negligence. Under such circumstances, when something goes wrong, the patient party reacts in a hostile manner towards the anesthesiologist taking law in their own hand by behaving violently towards anesthetist and some other times they land up in a police station or court to seek redressal.[1] Every obstetric anesthetist should only be wishing away such bad situation to happen to them.

Can patient party seek redressal by complaining to multiple authorities?

Patient party can also file a case with police, courts, medical council, human rights panel, district health authorities, and politicians in addition to above host of other places simultaneously. The problem with multiple complaints with different authorities is that patient party becomes wiser and picks up holes with each explanation given by anesthetist at each forum. The newly found weakness in the defense of anesthetist is used against anesthetist in next forum/authority. This makes it difficult to plead innocence even though medically anesthetist is correct. Technical loopholes let the anesthetist down. Thus, anesthetist may be morally and ethically right but legally proved wrong at least technically. The most technical legal faults pointed out are about written consent and written medical records.

Most commonly patient party drags anesthetist to civil or criminal court or both. In a criminal case, the aggrieved party files a complaint or FIR against the anesthesiologist in a police station where investigation officer [IO] investigates the case. The government or state prosecutes the anesthesiologist in criminal court of judicial magistrate or session's court. This happens only when the offense is of a serious nature like death or disability. Appeals against orders of lower court can be filed in High Court or Supreme Court. The idea of judicial proceedings in criminal cases is to punish the anesthesiologist for the negligence. Complainant cannot get any compensation in criminal cases but anesthetist, if found guilty, may land in serving jail term. In a civil case, the aggrieved party itself approaches the court to seek compensation for the harm caused by bringing action against anesthesiologist. These cases can go to the common civil courts like District Civil Court or High Court or one of the consumer courts. In India initiation of litigation is perceived as starting of punishment by anesthesiologist. The time taken for mitigation

of litigation is long prolonged one. Legal battle even when won by anesthesiologist become sour with filing of appeal in higher court.

Should there be 'capping' of claims?

Several countries have capped medical compensation claims. In India, there is no capping on medical negligence claims. Landmark highest claim has been marked by awarding Dr Kunal Saha with more than 11 crores by honorable Supreme Court.[2] There are two aspects in this claim. The court ordered a compensation of ₹ 5.96 crore, with interest comes to more than ₹ 11 crore. In India initiation of litigation is perceived as starting of punishment by anesthesiologist. The time taken for mitigation of litigation is long prolonged one. Legal battle even when won by anesthesiologist become sour with filing of appeal in higher court.

Paying interest on court proceedings delay

First aspect is awarding above claim of compensation of ₹ 5.96 crore is aright if it was awarded within 90 days as per Consumer Protection Act. But second aspect of interest on ₹ 5.96 crore due to court proceedings delay is too harsh as per legal luminaries. Legal eagles felt medical professionals had no role in delaying court proceeding which went on for 15 years. In fact interestingly in this case Kunal Saha initially lost his fight as the West Bengal Medical Council and Calcutta High Court both dismissed his case against AMRI Hospitals. The national commission [NCDRC], however, found the hospital and its doctors guilty of medical negligence and fixed a compensation amount of ₹ 1.7 crore. Finally Supreme Court awarded ₹ 5.96 crore, which with interest crossed ₹ 11 crore. Leaders of Indian Medical Association (IMA) and famed cardiac surgeon Dr Devi Shetty have demanded that there should be a maximum limit ("cap") of compensation that any doctor or hospital may pay for causing death of a patient from medical negligence.

Indian health care system is as such over-burdened by application of "first world regulatory standards with third world infrastructure" making single MBBS doctor clinics redundant and extinct and soon small obstetric nursing homes shall perish since cost of implementing first world regulatory standards will make them shut shop vis a vis lurking fear of huge compensations without any cap on award as well as interest their-on.

The then US President Bush pushed for cap on medical malpractice awards to relieve doctors of frivolous lawsuits in USA. This made some states in USA to cap damages in medical negligence cases to a maximum of ₹ 1.5 crore (as converted in terms of Indian currency).

Should we make contractual capping of compensation claims?

Legal luminaries have, for the time being, suggested to incorporate in consent/contract forms to include limiting clause for compensation to a certain limit (say for example maximum ₹ 10 lakhs) as declared by patient himself, in case of litigation. These consent/contract documents showing limiting compensation clause of capping claim as part of pleadings when negligence or malpractice litigation is initiated before any authority of competent jurisdiction.

Apportionment of liability for what anesthetist is liable in case of mishap

It is well known that anesthetists have key role to play when a patient is critical and serious. Just because anesthetists resuscitate the patient, they are not liable for mishap. Often our legal fraternity and judiciary are extremely slow in appreciating these difficulties faced by anesthetist and adapting and dissecting to apportion the liability to obstetrician, hospital owner and anesthetist in cases of alleged medical negligence because most decrees are passed holding responsible everyone jointly and severally. It should be brought forward before judiciary while they award compensation for damage to patient they should be shown evidence apportioning the liability of

each and accordingly grant compensation rather than granting jointly and severally for obstetrician, hospital owner and anesthetist.

Allegations of medical negligence which are nothing more than well-explained, well-documented complications

First set of allegations which haunt anesthetists are not administering oxygen, not undertaking pre-anesthetic check up, overdose of anesthetic drugs, uses of expired drugs, use of poisonous and very potent drugs, postoperative spinal headache, post-spinal anesthesia meningitis, post spinal anesthesia pain and weakness/paralysis in lower limbs or radiculitis.

Worst of all situations are OT table death, high spinal or total spinal, sudden laryngospasm in unintubated patient, Mendelson's syndrome.

Last set of allegations are regarding postoperative recovery. They are related to inadequate reversal and premature extubation, cardiac or respiratory arrest in immediate postoperative period, malignant hyperthermia, etc.

Sometimes allegations made by patients against anesthetist are wild and disturbing without evidence of any proof like cutting of nerve, cutting of artery, etc. Allegations require evidence before it becomes proof of negligence.

How to save anesthetist from legal maxim of res ipsa loquitur?

If you do not explain mishap, then legal maxim of res ipsa loquitur is slapped. To save anesthetist from legal maxim of res ipsa loquitur (negligence speaks for itself and requires no proof), allegations require detailed proper explanation supported by medical literature and expert witness. Some allegations require explanations from obstetricians like why anesthetists were not called for prior to surgery, delay in calling anesthetist, surgeon giving spinal anesthesia himself and operating and later calling anesthetist when mishap occurred.

Not calling an anesthetist by obstetrician: In one case, complainant admitted his wife to the nursing home where patient could not deliver normally, a cesarean section was performed and male child was delivered. The parturient complained of severe pain, had two bouts of vomiting and subsequently died. It was alleged that the doctor neither tested her blood nor called an anesthetist. District Forum granted him compensation of ₹ 1,25,000/= with interest. But State Commission held that there was no deficiency in service, even then it held that the appellant was liable to ₹ 5000/= to the complainant with interest. On revision petition to NCDRC, it was observed that-once the State Commission found the doctor not deficient in service, there was no ground to award compensation. Therefore, the impugned order set aside in Dr M Radhakrishna Murthy vs Parakulam Elishama Babu (NCDRC) CTJ 2007, p.955.[3]

In a case, patient suffered cardiac arrest whilst under anesthesia. The court held that a fit heart does not stop under anesthesia without negligence. Res ipsa loquitur was applied. There was no need for the patient to show the cause of cardiac arrest as the doctor had offered no explanation to prove that the cardiac arrest was not due to his negligence. Saunders vs Leeds Western HA, (1993) 4 MedLR 355:(1994) CLY 2320.[4]

When will routine pre-anesthetic check-up (PAC) start for obstetric anesthesia?

There are no PAC OPDs though obstetric patient's entire antenatal period has several visits to obstetricians but prospective anesthetist only gets chance to know patient just prior to anesthetic intervention on emergency basis even for planned surgeries. PAC not only allows physical examination but also allows ordering separate set of pathological, biochemical, electrocardiography, imaging and other investigations. All these need to be recommended and documented to know the cardiorespiratory status of patient as per ASA

grades clearly, precisely and accurately in order to repudiate the future allegation of negligence. Even though pre-anesthetic check up (PAC) as routine preoperative protocol and discussion with the patient party about the choice of suitable anesthetic is not only necessary and mandatory in new medicolegal milieu but not done. Before surgery patients should be informed of the statistical possibility of death involved in anesthetic procedure, damage to brain and special senses. Legally, it is not only obligatory on the part of the anesthetist to explain the anesthetics administered but it is necessary to explain the anesthetic technique being administered to patients and their relatives.

Medical errors which are not known to patient party Should they be informed and documented or wrapped under carpet?

Sometimes anesthetists are worried about errors which are potentially harmless to look at. Anesthetist keep worrying about patient with cardiac and respiratory arrest who is revived and shifted to ICU, damage or displacement of loose teeth, crowns and bridgework, damage to the soft tissues of the lips, mouth, tongue, pharynx and larynx. Barring emergency intubation, the duty of the anesthetist is to inspect the patient's dentition preoperatively and to make note of loose teeth, crowns, bridgework, and missing teeth. The displacement of a tooth may be defensible, but failure to search for and retrieve the missing tooth will be indefensible. The careful use of laryngoscope and the use of plastic protector over the upper anterior teeth in anticipation of difficulty are advisable.

Patient party should be informed about revived cardiac and respiratory arrest displacement and dislodgement of loose teeth, dental crowns and bridgework during anesthesia, damage to the soft tissues of the lips, mouth, tongue, pharynx and larynx. It should also be documented. Patient party hardly knows that there is a possibility of postoperative headache after spinal anesthesia because there is no discussion with the patient party in pre-operative period. This should also be documented and informed.

Hidden box of errors—hide it or lay open

Due to prevailing and current customary practice of calling anesthetists just before operation, one cannot take neurologist's opinions regarding avoiding regional blocks in patients with neurological disease so as to avoid subsequent allegation of worsening of neurological disease due to regional anes-thesia. So often one needs to tell and document—breaking of new plastic intra-venous catheter in vein, breaking of epidural catheter while removing it, guide wire breakage, damaged cuff of endotracheal tube, while removing it. Who is responsible—manufacturing company or anesthetist? All are potentially worrisome. Should they be documented, should we complain to manu-facturing company or not is a million dollar question? Should patient party be told even though practically no harm is done to patient? Yes, it should be informed and documented. Not doing so and subsequent discovery by patient party will lead to litigation.

Obstetricians, nursing home owners and hospitals provide suboptimal anesthesia infrastructure

Traditionally, obstetricians are usually nurs-ing home or hospital owners. The provision of infrastructural facilities for administering anesthesia and monitoring facility for obstetric surgery is suboptimal. So, obstetricians even sometimes question need for Boyles machine or even oxygen when anesthetist gives spinal anesthesia for LSCS. The constant vigil and monitoring of vitals during anesthesia is prime duty of the anesthetist. Delegation of duty to inexperienced anesthetist or person is not permissible in law similarly working in poor infrastructure cannot be valid excuse in law courts. There are cases stating that it is anesthetist's duty to check that equipment are in good order. In Kalawati vs Himanchal Pradesh HC, 1988 ACJ 780,[5] where death of two patients in government hospital occurred due to exchange of gas pipes of nitrous oxide with oxygen were interchanged by ward boy during cleaning of OT, state government was held vicariously liable. Anesthetist must ensure cylinders are containing required gases and anesthetic machine is working prior to operation and to ensure that the equipment are functioning correctly throughout the period when the patient is under anesthesia. The gadgets and standard of monitoring is judged by the tenets of current, accepted professional practice.

Medicolegal Aspects of Mishaps Related to Intubation

Failure to detect failed/difficult airway leading to hypoxia constitutes negligence on the part of anesthetist. It is obligatory on the part of the anesthetist to verify the correct placement of the endotracheal tube. The anesthetist was held negligent by Andhra Pradesh High Court for removal of endotracheal tube without giving fresh breaths of oxygen and failure to resuscitate the patient with mask and bag or by mouth-to-mouth ventilation before inserting the tube for the second time, which led to cerebral anoxia and ultimately permanent brain damage of the patient—Dr P Narasimha Rao vs Gundavarapu Jaya Prakash AIR 1990 AP 207; 1990(1)ACJ 350:(1990)1. ACC468:(1989)3 Andh LT 564:(1989) 2APU (HC)491.[6] As per the minimum monitoring standard protocol, medically correct place-ment of endotracheal tube should be confirmed ideally by end-tidal carbon dioxide monitoring.

Medicolegal Aspects of Complications in Regional Anesthesia

It is obligatory on the part of the anesthetist to ensure that regional block carried out is safe, effective and useful. Spinal, epidural and

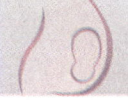

peripheral nerve blocks are used both for anesthesia and analgesia during surgery and for pain relief in labor. The possibility of headache due to spinal anesthesia cannot be ruled out, when large-bore needle is used. Administration of central neuroaxial and Peripheral nerve blocks should be done carefully in anticoagulated patients after proper documentation of coagulation parameters like PT, aPTT, INR, etc.

In a case of alleged death due to criminal negligence where deceased was admitted for delivery and for that purpose a cesarean section operation under spinal anesthesia was performed. Soon after the spinal anesthesia was administered, blood pressure began to fall and doctors did their best to save the deceased and the child but it was all in vain. A case was filed against the doctor who administered anesthesia contending that he was not an anesthetic expert and he did not give a test dose before giving spinal anesthesia. As postmortem was not conducted so anesthesia as cause of death could not be verified. Court enquired into "Whether death caused due to rash and negligent act of the doctor?" but it was held that anesthesia used was a common spinal anesthesia that is normally given to all the patients and court also said that non-giving of a test dose was not an indication of rashness or negligence; treatment given was proper, fair, competent and reasonable. Therefore, criminal proceedings were quashed under section 304-A of Indian Penal Code, 1860, read with section 482 Code of Criminal Procedure, 1973 in Dr Krishna Prasad vs State of Karnataka, 1989 ACJ 393 (Karn.-HC).[7]

Medicolegal Aspects of Awareness during Anesthesia

There are number of causes of awareness during anesthesia, e.g. inadequate doses of anesthetic drugs, entrapment of air into the gas mixture and abnormal resistance to anesthetic agents (drug abusers and alcoholics). It is difficult to defend the allegation of awareness

on the part of the anesthetist (a) where faulty equipment were not detected prior to operation, (b) where there was a failure to make constant vigil and proper monitoring during the period of anesthesia, (c) where there was a failure to keep adequate record of anesthetic procedure, and (d) where there was a failure to adhere to generally accepted clinical practice in the choice of anesthetic technique. Maximum chances of awareness are during anesthesia in hemodynamically unstable patients (trauma) and parturient. To avoid the allegation of awareness during anesthesia, the anesthetist is required to keep constant vigil on the following clinical signs: (a) a rise or fall in pulse or blood pressure which cannot be accounted for any other physiological/ pathological event. (b) The appearance of sweating and lacrimation, (c) the corneal reflex and reaction of the pupil to light

GA Given to Patient with 'Common Cold'

In several cases, obstetricians and anesthesiologists have been held negligent and liable for proceeding with non-emergency, elective surgery in which inhalation anesthesia was used when the patient had a cold. Since cold symptoms are usually obvious from casual observation of the patient, courts usually find that performance of the surgery was negligent. Quintal vs Laurel Grove Hospital, 397 P 2d 161, Cal 1964; Butler vs Lay ton, 164 NE 920, Mass 1929; Jackson vs Mountain Sanitarium, 67SE 2d57, NC 1951.[8]

Patient party is paying so the outcome should always be favorable irrespective of risks

There are two types of risks, ones which are theoretically possible to occur and others which are likely to be commonly encountered. A reasonable man may foresee the possibility of many risk factors, but life would be almost impossible, if he were to attempt to take precautions against every risk, which one can foresee. One takes precautions against risks which are reasonably likely to happen. Medicine is not a perfect science. It is combination of science and art. Worsening and cure depends upon several factors beyond the control of physician. Physician can give diligent care but healing or worsening depends on individual variation of body processes. Negligence is opposite of diligence. Negligence means failure to take reasonable care resulting in damage to patient. What is that reasonable care? Care not very high nor very low, but average care is what is required. As Lord Denning LJ has justifiably commented, "it is so easy to be wise after the event and to condemn as negligence that which was only misadventure". We ought to always be on our guard against it, especially in cases against hospitals and doctors.

Law requires particular standard of care

The legal standard of care should be reasonable not very high and not very low, but just an average. Are minority of practitioners committing legal wrong if they practice well recognized procedures instead of the latest ones, e.g. administering general anesthesia instead of neuraxial blocks for cesarean sections.

Legal fraternity should realize; unless the doctor does not conduct some patently illegal procedures. All other procedures practiced by majority or minority practitioners be considered legal. For example, administering anesthesia for cesarean sections in patients who are not fasting for six hours (patients have habit of not following doctors instructions relating to fasting). Legally, can such patients be taken up for operations after giving precautionary prokinetic medications with H_2 inhibitors. Sometimes obstetricians force anesthetists to waive off some investigations and preoperative precautions needed for giving safe anesthesia for planned surgeries. Surgeons want to take an unprepared patient on the pretext of emergency surgery. Unless these are documented, anesthetists will fail to prove in court of law.

Who will decide preoperative investigations—surgeon or anesthetist or both?

A reasonable anesthetist may foresee the possibility of many risk factors, but life would be almost impossible if one were to attempt to take precautions against every risk, which one can foresee. One should take precautions against risk which are reasonably likely to happen. Legal fraternity should understand and desist applying "first world regulatory standards for investigations, monitoring for third world people already under monetary constraint". This will only make health care costly and illusory in a long run. This is already promoting quacks thriving to conduct deliveries since qualified doctors are out of the reach of common people.

Reuse—resterilized 'single use'

Medicolegally, is it possible to reuse–resterilized 'single use' consumables like catheters, endotracheal tubes, spinal needles, epidural catheters to reduce cost for third world people already living under monetary constraint. One need not sterilize cheaper items like syringes. But costly items can be resterilized and reused. Authorities must come out with proper guidelines for third world economies for re-use, re-sterilization.

What is safe hemoglobin level prior to surgery?

Who will decide as to what is safe hemoglobin level prior to surgery with all risks of administering blood products with fear of window period diseases getting transmitted. Can legal fraternity dictate on case-to-case basis the safe hemoglobin level to operate or not to operate? Will protocols and standard operating procedures (SOP) work in patient who is stable and becomes serious suddenly? Again it should be reemphasized that reasonable anesthetist may foresee the possibility of many risk factors, but life would be almost impossible, if one were to attempt

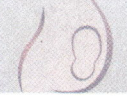

to take precautions against every risk, which one can foresee, while relieving pain. Hemoglobin of 10 is safe, below 6 is unsafe and in between falls in medicolegal grey area requiring anesthetist's explanation and risk taking appetite of anesthetist and co-morbidities patient is harbouring will tilt balance for administering anesthesia rather than legal fears.

Should risky patients be destined to suffer pain because of defensive medicine?

Risky patients be left to their destiny to suffer pain for sake of legal safety required for anesthesia under non-emergency situations. Anesthetists shall venture to do more investi-gations during PAC, monitor more rigorously during and after anesthesia with advanced gadgetry which has self-storing or printout options to be produced as evidence to prevent future litigations.

Taking decisions for end of life situations (EOS)

Who will take decisions for "End of life situa-tions" where neither patient party nor patient himself is capable of giving decision who will consent for medical and anesthetic procedures? Who will foot the bill? Is it alright to allow patient party to continue with costly life support systems till they mentally, monetarily are totally broke. How long legal fraternity will continue to equate EOS with euthanasia. When legal fraternity and legislators decriminalize EOS? How long physicians will survive this grey area around EOS and keep practicing slow imperceptible euthanasia or keep forcibly discharging patient DAMA or LAMA to allow to die at home.

Is use of ultrasound in obstetric anesthesia cross specialty practice?

Use of ultrasound for regional anesthesia and regional blocks is being taken over from use of *transcutaneous electrical nerve stimulation* [TENS]. There are no specialized MCI recognized PG fellowship/diploma available for practice of USG. In India, USG machine needs to be registered under PCPNDT Act. Anesthetist cannot use unless he/she has degree or diploma in radiology or six months training in use of USG.

Off Label Use of Drugs

a. Doses—higher or lower doses, sometimes extra top ups, sometimes given for longer duration than recommended situation similar to like inj Amikacin causing deafness in Martin F D'Souza vs Mohd. Ishfaq, Supreme Court of India, Civil Appeal No. 3541 of 2002, D/d 17.2.2009, (2009) 3 SCC 1.[9]

b. Using in combination with drugs with inter-action, where manufacturer contraindicated the use.

c. Used for children and pregnant women where manufacturer contraindicated the use.

d. Used in specifically contraindicated age group, conditions like avoiding using halothane in male child to avoid malignant fever.

Video or Audio Recording of Operating Rooms

Days have come when one will have to do video and audio recording in operation theaters, procedure rooms and labor rooms as evidence. This will require separate set of counseling and consent and assurance that such recordings will not be used unless required by judicial or quasi-judicial autho-rities. Privacy and confidentiality will be newer issues to be studied and applied in proper context in a quest to generate evidence to prevent future litigations.

SUMMARY

Everyday, newer advances challenge older established paradigms. The approved practices of today shall be replaced by newer, safer, better ones. The medical and legal fraternity is slow to absorb the same. This brings more grey areas of concerns requiring revised solutions in future.

REFERENCES

1. Padvi N, Padvi A, Gupta V, Baldwa M. Textbook of Paediatric Anaesthesia, CBS Publishers & Distributors Pvt Ltd, Delhi, Ch 42:546–51, Ch.43:551–6,2015.
2. Supreme Court civil appeal no. 2867 of 2012 Dr Balram Prasad vs. Dr Kunal Saha & Ors.
3. Dr M Radhakrishna Murthy vs Parakulam Elishama Babu (NCDRC) CTJ 2007, p.955.
4. Saunders vs Leeds Western HA (1993) 4 MedLR 355:(1994)CLY 2320.
5. Kalawati vs Himanchal Pradesh HC, 1988 ACJ 780.
6. Dr P Narasimha Rao vs Gundavarapu Jaya Prakash AIR 1990 AP 207;1990(1) ACJ 350:(1990) 1. ACC468:(1989) 3 AndhL T564: (1989) 2APU (HC) 491.
7. Dr Krishna Prasad vs State of Karnataka, 1989 ACJ 393 (Karn.-HC).
8. Quintal vs Laurel Grove Hospital, 397 p.2d 161, Cal 1964; Butler vs Lay ton, 164 NE 920, Mass 1929; Jackson vs Mountain Sanitarium, 67 SE 2d 57, NC 1951.
9. Martin F D'Souza vs Mohd. Ishfaq, Supreme Court of India, Civil Appeal No. 3541 of 2002, D/d 17.2.2009, (2009) 3 SCC 1.

Index